The Yellow Flag

Until the middle of the nineteenth
European nations mandated the dete
soldier, sailor, merchant, missionary,
Ottoman Empire and North Africa. M
large, ominous fortresses in Mediterran
examines Britain's engagement with thi
multiple angles. He explores how quaran
the state provision of public health and
European integration. Situated at the inters
matic, and medical history, *The Yellow Flag*
as an experience, its power as an administra
an example of a continental border built fr
bureaucrats.

ALEX CHASE-LEVENSON is Assistant Professo
of Pennsylvania.

Global Health

Series editor:

Sanjoy Bhatta

Global Heal
history of pu
which the i
described i
books in th
actors and
writing ab
global eco

The Yellow Flag

Quarantine and the British Mediterranean World, 1780–1860

Alex Chase-Levenson

University of Pennsylvania

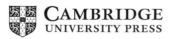

CAMBRIDGE
UNIVERSITY PRESS

CAMBRIDGE
UNIVERSITY PRESS

University Printing House, Cambridge CB2 8BS, United Kingdom

One Liberty Plaza, 20th Floor, New York, NY 10006, USA

477 Williamstown Road, Port Melbourne, VIC 3207, Australia

314–321, 3rd Floor, Plot 3, Splendor Forum, Jasola District Centre, New Delhi – 110025, India

79 Anson Road, #06–04/06, Singapore 079906

Cambridge University Press is part of the University of Cambridge.

It furthers the University's mission by disseminating knowledge in the pursuit of education, learning, and research at the highest international levels of excellence.

www.cambridge.org
Information on this title: www.cambridge.org/9781108485548
DOI: 10.1017/9781108751773

First published 2020

Printed in the United Kingdom by TJ International Ltd, Padstow Cornwall

A catalogue record for this publication is available from the British Library.

ISBN 978-1-108-48554-8 Hardback

For Karen and Michael Chase-Levenson

Contents

Figures

Acknowledgments

A work that has carried me through many years, different institutions, and multiple continents has also generated a significant number of debts, too many to mention here, but all felt deeply. Quarantine's records are widely distributed, and the jumble has only been possible to make sense of because of the resourceful archivists and scholars who have organized the system's remains. I am in debt to the staff members of Malta's National Library and National Archives; the UK National Archives; the British Library; the Wellcome Library and Archive; the French National Archives (both in Paris and Pierrefitte); the Departmental Archives of the Bouches-du-Rhône; the State Archives of Genoa, Livorno, Venice, and Naples; and the Haus-, Hof-, und Staatsarchiv in Vienna. Special thanks are due to Marlene Borg of Malta's National Archives for her assistance with files relating to the plague of 1813–14 and to Vicky Green of Southampton Central Library for her help in addressing an outbreak of "plagueomania" in Hampshire in the 1840s. For exceptionally stimulating tours of lazarettos, heartiest thanks are due to Walter Gatt, Edward Said, Giorgia Fazzini, and David Barnes. Much needed research support has come from the History Departments of the University of Pennsylvania and Princeton, Princeton's Institute for Inter-Regional Studies, Harvard's Center for European Studies, and the IHR-Mellon fund.

This project began as a doctoral dissertation completed at Princeton University under the direction of Linda Colley. I am grateful for her generous advice and for the example she has provided, in her own work, of transnational scholarship that remains attuned to ordinary people and individual stories. For their sage advice as this project was first conceived, thanks to David Barnes, Phil Nord, Molly Greene, David Cannadine, David Bell, Katja Guenther, and Jeremy Adelman. For their support of this idea in its very earliest stages, and for stimulating conversations since then, thanks to Anna Henchman and Maya Jasanoff.

There have been many moments while working on this project that I have found myself praying for an archival find that would enable a particular point to stand out more clearly. For pointing me toward such satisfying discoveries, leading me to new ideas, and other assistance at crucial junctures, I am indebted to more scholars than I can remember, but thanks in particular to Nükhet Varlık, Mark Harrison, Alison Bashford, Astrid Swenson, Peter Mandler, Tim Alborn, Catherine Kelly, and Arnab Dey.

I am grateful to my colleagues who have helped make the University of Pennsylvania a congenial scholarly home. Among others, I would like to thank especially Warren Breckman, Sophie Rosenfeld, Peter Holquist, Cheikh Babou, Ben Nathans, Firoozeh Kashani-Sabet, Antonio Feros, Dan Richter, Heidi Voskuhl, Etienne Benson, Yvie Fabella, Amy Offner, Ada Kuskowski, Melissa Teixeira, Oscar Aguirre-Mandujano, and Octavia Carr. And thanks to Beth Wenger, in her capacity as History Department chair, for allowing me to take the leave necessary to bring this work to a conclusion. Over the many years I have worked on this project, conversations and general intellectual camaraderie with Adrian Young, Frederic Clark, Heidi Hausse, Rebecca Johnson, Margarita Fajardo, Iwa Nawrocki, Padraic Scanlan, Katlyn Carter, and Jon Connolly have been invaluable. Special thanks are due to Iain Watts for reading multiple chapter drafts.

For invaluable help guiding many of these chapters, I am deeply grateful to the members of Rutgers-Camden's Lees Seminar, Columbia's British Studies Workshop, Princeton's Modern Europe Seminar, Penn's History of Science Workshop, the Quarantine Studies Network, and the Global and Contemporary History Colloquia at the Freie Universität in Berlin. Particular thanks are due to the members of the Delaware Valley British Studies Seminar (and most especially Seth Koven, Tom Smith, and Lynn and Andy Lees) for their engagement with multiple chapters of this work. For exceptionally thoughtful comments and kind invitations, thanks to Daniel Brandau, Claudia Moatti, Carl Wennerlind, Emily Marker, Eileen Ryan, Alan Mikhail, Ellen Nye, and Francesca Trivellato.

At Cambridge University Press, I thank Lucy Rhymer for her consistent support of this project and both anonymous readers, whose trenchant advice has helped me to improve it. I also wish to thank Emily Sharp and Lisa Carter for their patience and assistance throughout the process of publication. Thanks also to Tanya Buckingham and the University of Wisconsin Cartography Lab for preparing the maps.

Certain arguments and quotations present in this work appeared in a chapter entitled "Early Nineteenth-Century Quarantine as a European System" in *Quarantine: Local and Global Histories*, edited by Alison Bashford and published in 2016 by Palgrave Macmillan.

Some debts are closer to home. For cheerfully and lovingly welcoming me into their family, thank you to Allison, Mark, and Rebecca Leja. For her enthusiasm, solidarity, and sense of fun, I thank my sister Sarah. And for making the nineteenth century an endless source of intellectual excitement, for providing thoughtful critiques of this work, and for giving me boundless love, perpetual thanks go to my parents, Karen and Michael Chase-Levenson. I dedicate this book to them.

Finally, though she did not assist in any way with the typing of this manuscript, my wife, Meg Leja, *did* sharpen every idea and help clarify every point. I cannot overstate the extent to which this work has been improved by her superb historical sensibility, how much in my life has been made better because of her clear mind and generous heart, or how much delight I derive from our shared interest in bubonic plague.

Note on the Text and Translations

In order to preserve common usage among the text and quotations from archival sources and travel narratives considered here, I have adopted the nineteenth-century English terms for major cities in the Ottoman Empire: Constantinople for Istanbul, Smyrna for Izmir, Salonica for Thessaloniki, etc.

All translations, unless otherwise noted, are my own.

Introduction

> Thirty years ago, Marseilles lay burning in the sun, one day . . . Everything in
> Marseilles, and about Marseilles, had stared at the fervid sky, and been stared
> at in return, until a staring habit had become universal there . . . There was no
> wind to make a ripple on the foul water within the harbour, or on the beautiful
> sea without. The line of demarcation between the two colours, black and blue,
> showed the point which the pure sea would not pass; but it lay as quiet as the
> abominable pool, with which it never mixed. Boats without awnings were too
> hot to touch; ships blistered at their moorings.
>
> Charles Dickens, *Little Dorrit*

More than two hundred years ago, in 1801, Marseille lay burning in the sun. Its
harbor was full of the eerie spectacle of ships sitting silently, onto which no one
boarded and from which no one disembarked. The most crowded spot in the
city was not one of its public markets, squares, or churches, but a massive
complex that sat on its northern edge, abutting the sea: the Lazaretto of Arenc.
This fortress, at the time, served as France's most important quarantine station.
It was legally mandated as the reception point for almost all ships and passengers entering the nation from the Middle East and North Africa,[1] and employees there prided themselves on their efficiency and rigor in managing the threat
of bubonic plague. Marseille's last experience of that disease, roughly eighty
years before this moment, had instilled in its merchants, its citizens, and above
all its Board of Health a sense of a mission – saving not only France but all of
Europe from ever experiencing the most deadly contagion again.

In 1801, the *Conservateurs de Santé* (as Marseille's health board
members were called during the Revolutionary Era), were put in charge
of the most ambitious exercise in sanitary defense up to that point: the
reception and detention of the remnants of Napoleon's *Armée d'Orient* as
its soldiers returned, defeated, from France's brief invasion of Egypt, the
greatest blunder for France at this stage of the Revolutionary and
Napoleonic Wars. Throughout the quarantine of these returning troops
(managed in stages, over the course of more than a year), some 30,000
soldiers were subjected to quarantine in Marseille's vast lazaretto

---

[1] Some military ships underwent quarantine at the nearby port of Toulon.

1

(quarantine fortress).[2] Given that, on average, the Lazaretto of Arenc received between 300 and 1,000 passengers in quarantine each year throughout the first half of the nineteenth century, this was a mammoth undertaking. Knowing that many of these soldiers would never have entered a lazaretto before, the *Conservateurs* prepared a pamphlet to help explain this extraordinary place: "Those places of reserve known as lazarettos" they began, "[are] where the redoubtable plague is annihilated, places subject to the harshest police regulations; terrible places, marked by enclosures and limits, which the gravest punishments, including that of death, have rendered inviolable."[3]

Managing the return of the French prisoners of war was a prolonged process, which lasted into 1802. Nevertheless, at times, more than 10,000 people were detained in the lazaretto together. A letter from the Marseille Board of Health to the responsible *Citoyen Ministre* in December 1801, for example, noted that within the next week, some 9,108 soldiers would be released.[4] Such staggering numbers demanded novel systems of administration. The French government developed a system of food vouchers granted to each soldier in detention. Meanwhile, lazaretto officials, desperate to stay on top of the arrivals in their harbor, coordinated closely with representatives of the hated British, as many thousands of French soldiers were returned in British *parlementaires* (prisoner-of-war ships). Britain and France were inveterate enemies at the time (in the midst of a war that would last, with one brief pause, for more than twenty years). That said, each saw the value of an efficient quarantine for returning soldiers, and each was willing to negotiate in order to maintain discipline and sanitary security.

Because of the vast numbers of people involved, the uneasy relations between wartime enemies, and the copious bureaucracy required, the afterlife of Napoleon's Egyptian Campaign stands out in the history of quarantine as an extraordinary event. It also set a precedent; only thirty years later, Marseille's sanitary bureaucrats had to contend with another army of more than 33,000 men as they received veterans returning from the French invasion of Algeria. Both episodes involved extreme expense and the deprivation of manpower at critical moments for France's armies. Yet, on both occasions, quarantine was considered absolutely necessary.

---

[2] The word *fortress* is appropriate not simply because some lazarettos were repurposed military fortifications but because even structures built originally as lazarettos retained a fortress-like architecture as a means of emphasizing their isolation from the cities in which they sat. See Quim Bonastra, "Recintos sanitarios y espacios de control. Un estudio morfológico de la arquitectura cuarentenaria," *Dynamis* 30 (2010): 20.

[3] "Proclamation des Conservateurs de la Santé Publique . . .," Archives Nationales, Pierrefitte-sur-Seine, henceforth, AN (Pierrefitte) F/8/1/Dossier V.

[4] *Conservateurs de Santé* to the Interior Minister, 21 Frimaire, An X (December 11, 1801), AN (Pierrefitte) F /8/1 Dossier V.

The quarantine of the *Armée d'Orient* highlights the extent to which the Revolutionary and Napoleonic Wars marked a watershed moment in the history of the expansion of the modern state. It also signaled a general expansion of all aspects of the quarantine system through the first half of the nineteenth century. Between 1800 and 1850, Mediterranean quarantine generated more correspondence, detained more ships, passengers, and trade goods, and involved greater diplomatic coordination than at any other point in history. In a period of global war and during the subsequent birth of a global economy, quarantine took on new reach.

In the early eighteenth century, quarantines were applied unsystematically and ports operated without significant concern about foreign practices. In the late nineteenth century, after our period, quarantines were applied more selectively (and more unequally). They primarily became a tool of imperial powers regulating the movement of colonial populations (as with cholera quarantines in the Red Sea) or a common practice required by immigration authorities (in countries such as Australia). By contrast, in the period covered by this book, quarantine operated as a universal check on sailors, travelers, workers, and trade goods moving across the Mediterranean *even in the absence of epidemic disease*. The presence of intermittent plague in the Middle East and North Africa provided the primary justification for quarantine at this time, but the vast majority of ships detained proceeded from uninfected cities (in the language of quarantine, they arrived with "clean" bills of health). The practice occurred across Southern Europe with standards formed in common. Boards of health in the Italian states, British Malta, France, Spain, and the Habsburg Empire corresponded regularly. Together, over time, and without external impetus they fashioned quarantine into a system in which deviation from minimum standards would result in retaliatory quarantines. Disinfection was mutually guaranteed.

In quite a different context, Ursula Q. Henriques has observed that the era of industrialization represented "the increase in scale of almost everything."[5] Far removed from the industrial cities of Britain, Mediterranean quarantine exemplifies such scalar expansion thanks to an uptick in trade, an increase in travel, and a greater threat from invader diseases around 1800. Whether or not we want to see "modernity" as something that began with the French Revolution, the quarantine system that cohered during the Revolutionary and Napoleonic Wars was clearly responsive to broad developments in European history during the first half of the nineteenth century. Critics of quarantine liked to cast the system as an atavistic remnant of a premodern world, but historians should not be seduced by their arguments. Quarantine was far from a holdover in the modern Mediterranean, and its persistence well into the age of steam indicates an

---

[5] Ursula Q. Henriques, *Before the Welfare State* (London: Longman, 1979), 2.

ongoing belief in its merits. The late eighteenth century saw both a recommitment to quarantine and an expansion of its reach.

From the Habsburg Empire, to France's successive post-Revolutionary regimes, to the medical and political establishment in Britain, governments broadly accepted that quarantine was a crucial line of defense against devastating epidemics. Spain's government helped fund a massive new lazaretto at Port Mahon in Menorca; Britain's government, meanwhile, saw a commitment of about £100,000 turn to dust as a planned lazaretto at Chetney Hill in Kent languished in bureaucratic stasis.[6] In an era when governments across Western Europe differed in size and in style, quarantine was accepted as a worthy expenditure of large sums of state money by many states, and its necessity was a shared article of administrative faith. The very existence of quarantine as a multipolar system is a startling fact in an era considered to be the golden age of the nation-state.

Certainly, inside the cavernous walls of Marseille's Lazaretto of Arenc, few doubted that the quarantine of Napoleon's returning soldiers was necessary. Outside, too, quarantine was considered essential. Why was this the case? What did the distinctive procedures of quarantine signify? And what precedents did they set or upend? The answers to these questions are the heart of this book. What follows, then, is not a broader history of quarantine as a tool, nor is it a comprehensive history of disease control in and around the Mediterranean or Middle East. This book is concerned with the history of Mediterranean quarantine *as a system*, and the way that system shaped the history of Britain, the major Mediterranean power of the era.

These dual commitments are deeply interpenetrated. If Mediterranean history (as opposed to history *in* the Mediterranean)[7] becomes harder to see in an age when nationalism, imperialism, and disparities of power were growing more important, it becomes increasingly necessary to examine planes on which the Middle Sea was drawn together. Britain was the ascendant Mediterranean power of the nineteenth century, and its diplomatic, economic, and imperial interests spanned sites across the Mediterranean Basin. British interest and investment in the Middle Sea skyrocketed during precisely the same timeline that quarantine expanded and achieved cohesion. By approaching the history of Mediterranean quarantine from the perspective of a country often seen to be on the margins of Europe, we gain a greater sense of its systematic quality. Finally, following the precedents of Mediterranean

---

[6] On the Chetney Hill lazaretto project, see P. Frogatt, "The Lazaret on Chetney Hill," *Medical History* 8 (1964): 44–62, and John Booker, *Maritime Quarantine: The British Experience, c. 1650–1900* (Aldershot, UK: Ashgate, 2007), chapters 9 and 10.

[7] I am drawing on the distinction between history *in* the Mediterranean and the history *of* the Mediterranean suggested in Peregrine Horden and Nicolas Purcell, *The Corrupting Sea* (Oxford: Blackwell, 2000), 9.

quarantine throughout the British world reveals that system's global influence.

The only author of a monograph to focus on British quarantine policy suggests that Britons found the system "impossibly difficult" and that a practice developed among Mediterranean autocracies could hardly "sit comfortably in a nation proud of democratic and parliamentary traditions."[8] In fact, the vast majority of Britons accommodated themselves to quarantine just as others did, and critics of the system were by no means limited to "free-born Englishmen." No one liked to find her or himself destined for a lazaretto. Spanish, Italian, Austrian, Egyptian, Moroccan, Greek, French and Turkish travelers railed against the system as often as the British did. Certainly, many Britons *did* see quarantine as an imposition of Continental bureaucrats. On the international stage, especially from the 1830s on, Britain was a frequent opponent of the practice, but I also demonstrate that British diplomats were willing to participate in what many called "the European Sanitary System," content to bend its rules in their direction. British consuls, ambassadors, and colonial administrators conducted quarantine diplomacy capably.

Just as a British perspective aids our study of Mediterranean quarantine, an analysis of that system gives meaning and shape to the nineteenth-century British Mediterranean – a Mediterranean of the imagination as well as one keyed to the realities of the map, a Mediterranean whose patterns and modalities influenced developments in Britain itself. Britain's growing web of investments in the Mediterranean stood midway between its diminished Empire in North America and its expanding zone of power in South Asia. Like the central squares on a chessboard, British strategists thought Mediterranean dominance might translate to broader victories elsewhere in the world. One of the reasons, then, that Mediterranean quarantine shaped British debates about contagion and served as such a strong precedent in British imperial practice was how extensively the Mediterranean region captivated a particularly diverse set of British thinkers.

***

Two hundred years before Napoleon's Egyptian Campaign, the quarantine undertaken in Marseille would have been unthinkable. Though lazarettos existed in some European ports, no one would have assumed that, without exception, each returning ship from the fleets engaging the Ottomans at Lepanto in 1571 should be quarantined on its return. And large-scale quarantine would be equally unthinkable a century after the detention of Napoleon's troops. In the

---

[8] John Booker, *Maritime Quarantine*, xvii. Booker's history is based almost entirely on the administrative records of quarantine (in particular, Privy Council records). While the work is an extraordinary resource as a chronicle of official acts and regulatory changes, it does little to connect quarantine to broader historical trajectories.

late nineteenth century, the nature of the practice was dramatically refocused on people that Europeans found suspicious rather than on places; a robust system of sanitary controls in the Red Sea area detained thousands of Muslim pilgrims to Mecca, especially after the cholera panic of the mid-1860s. Yet, few people called for the quarantine of Lawrence of Arabia, or other allied soldiers who fought the Ottomans in the Middle East during World War I.

In the late eighteenth and nineteenth centuries, however, contagion appeared to align to a rigid cartography that justified the quarantine of hundreds of thousands. Some regarded it as anachronistic, but they were quarantined anyway. From Trieste on the Adriatic to Semlin on the River Save, from Ancona on Italy's eastern coast to Genoa on its northwestern, from Malta to Marseille, and to floating hulks off the British coast, Western Europe marked itself off from the ostensibly plague-ridden "East" by a tangible *cordon sanitaire*. With no exceptions, even for armies like Napoleon's, this system required every trader, tourist, missionary, soldier, and crew-member traveling to Western Europe from the Ottoman Empire and North Africa to submit to a detention of several weeks, to the indignity of fumigation, to the forced opening of every piece of luggage, and to the smoking of every piece of mail. Transported livestock were quarantined too, and each bale, box, or barrel of trade goods was opened and fumigated, often for a period lasting longer than the detention of persons.

The future Emperor Napoleon and the crew members accompanying him on his secret return from the Egyptian Campaign constitute a rare exception to this system of universal detention. In the story memorialized after the event, the Corsican general was practically dragged to the shore by enthusiastic crowds professing themselves willing to suffer the consequences of ignoring quarantine by chanting "we prefer the plague to the Austrians" (in reference to Bonaparte's victories in 1797) (Figure 0.1).[9] Yet even this apparent patriotic exception to the quarantine laws elicited significant disquiet. Marseille's health authorities demanded that the Directory (France's national government from 1795 to 1799) impose disciplinary action on the wayward sanitary authorities of Ajaccio and Fréjus who apparently licensed this abrogation of the sanitary laws: "This event could provoke alarm throughout the Midi, in France, and across Europe. Our commerce will be considered suspected."[10] The Directory responded by expressing profound regret and by promising the event would never be repeated.[11] That even this one exception to the laws of quarantine for

[9] Louis Antoine Fauvelet de Bourrienne, *Memoirs of Napoleon Bonaparte* (Glasgow: Blackie and Son, 1830), 1: 223.
[10] *Intendants de Santé* of Marseille to the Interior Minister, 25th Vendémiaire, An VIII (October 17, 1799), AN (Pierrefitte) F/8/1 Dossier IV.
[11] Undated Memorandum from the Interior Minister, AN (Pierrefitte) F/8/1 Dossier IV. For more on this episode, see Daniel Panzac, "Un inquiétant retour d'Égypte: Bonaparte, la peste et les quarantaines," *Cahiers de la Méditerranée* 57 (1998): 271–80.

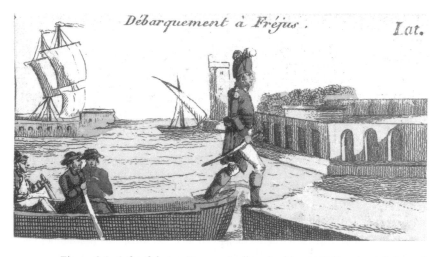

Figure 0.1 A fateful step. Bonaparte disembarking at Fréjus, in violation of the quarantine laws, as depicted in a contemporaneous 1799 drawing. Courtesy of the Bibliothèque Nationale de France.

Bonaparte himself should generate such controversy is a testimonial to the principle that, to remain valid, the laws of quarantine could admit no exceptions whatsoever.

Europeans, and others around the world, deployed quarantines against medical threats long before our period and long after. Though this book focuses on the universal quarantine against ships from the Middle East and North Africa, in the period under consideration the Americas were often under quarantine, too, due to the threat of yellow fever. Even among European nations themselves, quarantines were set up in times of cholera or other suspicious diseases. In contrast to these quarantines, the division of the plague-free West and the ostensibly plague-ridden East was unshakable. It did not vary based on the health of the Middle East at any given moment. In legislation, medical literature, and popular culture, the Ottoman Empire and the rest of North Africa were a special sanitary category justifying extra protection. And the quarantines that assumption justified, until they began to be dismantled in the 1840s, functioned as a permanent system coordinated from disparate poles of authority. Without the direction of either a particular national government or a supranational organization, Mediterranean quarantine functioned regardless of the vicissitudes of epidemic disease and was universal in its application.

"Universal quarantine," then, is the subject matter of this book. Universal, in the sense that boards of health across Western Europe's Mediterranean coast *never* exempted ships from the Middle East, *never* ceased to operate at certain times of year, and *never* relaxed the threat to apply retaliatory quarantines if foreign boards reduced the severity of their standards below an implicit common minimum standard. Furthermore, within this system, quarantine applied *universally* to all passengers, crew members, and trade goods on a particular ship based on its point of origin (regardless of ethnicity, race, religion, gender, or class, though the character of quarantine certainly did vary according to those categories, as we will see). This state of affairs lasted (roughly) from the late eighteenth century through the 1840s. In sum, universal quarantine applied within a unique geographical region and within a defined period of time. This book defends the specificity of both within the broader historiography of quarantine practice.

Quarantine: History and Tradition

Quarantine in Europe emerged not as a demarcation of the border between sickness and health but in the midst of epidemic disease. Though temporary periods of isolation and ad hoc quarantines were common during the Black Death of the fourteenth century, it was during the long recovery from this period of epidemic devastation that, in 1423, the Venetians built what may have been the first permanent lazaretto. So old is quarantine in Venice, that the "Lazzaretto Nuovo," built as a second station, is called "new" even though it was built in 1468. In Dalmatia, a lazaretto in Ragusa (Dubrovnik) was first built around the same time, or slightly earlier.[12] It is clear that early quarantine was an Adriatic affair – based on the idea that the sea could exist as a barrier against disease *and* a conduit for it. Both Venice and Ragusa had banned ships from foreign cities during a time of plague in the late fourteenth century, and the construction of permanent lazarettos was a logical next step.[13]

Other Italian city-states quickly took their cue from this Adriatic innovation. Naples and Genoa constructed lazarettos in 1464 and 1467, respectively. Even inland cities constructed quarantine structures to retard the approach of people and goods along major roads and waterways. Such a structure was built in Milan in 1448; the Florentine government decided to follow suit in 1464. Dedicated "plague hospitals" were first instituted on the Venetian mainland at Brescia and Padua in the 1430s; such institutions spread across Italy and into France throughout the mid-fifteenth century.[14] It is clear, then, that a growing

---

[12] For a recent articulation of the view that Ragusa/Dubrovnik was the site of the first European quarantine (and an overview of early quarantine procedures in that city-state), see Zlata Blažina Tomić and Vesna Blažina, *Expelling the Plague* (Montreal: McGill-Queen's University Press, 2015).

[13] See Jane Cranshaw, "The Renaissance Invention of Quarantine," in *The Fifteenth Century XII: Society in an Age of Plague*, ed. Linda Clark and Carole Rawcliffe (Rochester, NY: Boydell Press, 2013), 164.

[14] Ibid., 162–63.

consensus considered plague to be a "special" disease in need of a distinct prophylactic program. Jane Cranshaw notes the similarity between this new conception of the plague and long-standing ideas about the isolation of lepers, or even "unclean" professional activities such as leather tanning, which were often relegated to zones outside the city gates.[15] Lazarettos were one part of a rudimentary public health infrastructure, part of a logic of early modern healthcare based on the segregation of clean and unclean. Now permanent institutions, which operated regularly through the sixteenth century, they were not oriented against one particular geographic focus.

In other ways, though, these early modern developments anticipated elements of universal quarantine in the period under study here. In 1652, in the midst of a plague epidemic, the Republic of Genoa and Grand Duchy of Tuscany signed a treaty to coordinate quarantine procedures in their ports – a formal agreement that epidemic control necessitated cross-border coordination over sanitary regulation. Carlo Cipolla argues that though it lasted only four years, this agreement formed the most significant formal international agreement regarding prophylactic medicine before the International Sanitary Conference of 1851.[16]

In the course of the seventeenth century, bubonic plague epidemics diminished in frequency. By the century's end, many Western European cities experienced their final outbreaks of the plague. Britain was free of the disease after the famous Great Plague of 1665–66, and the last major outbreak on the Western European mainland was borne by the city of Marseille and other towns in Provence between 1720 and 1723. More cities built permanent lazaretto structures during this period as an association began to emerge between immunity from the plague and expanded quarantine infrastructure. Indeed, the Marseille plague epidemic was linked to that city's Board of Health failing to prevent the spread of the disease from the ship *Grand Saint Antoine* (recently arrived from Anatolia and Cyprus).[17] While Marseille had suffered from fourteen outbreaks of plague between 1505 and 1650, the 1650 plague was the last until 1720. This seventy-year interval coincided with an expansion of

---

[15] Ibid., 167.

[16] Carlo M. Cipolla, *Fighting the Plague in Seventeenth-Century Italy* (Madison: University of Wisconsin Press, 1981), 49–50. Indeed, Cipolla claims the 1652 conference actually achieved more than the 1851 Conference. This is misleading. While the 1652 agreement is a sign that many health authorities recognized the benefits of coordination, over the course of the eighteenth century, a much more durable understanding emerged of quarantine practice as a "general law" that applied to all Western Europe. And, as we will see in Chapter 9, the 1851 Conference was far from the "fiasco" Cipolla described.

[17] The Marseille plague of 1720 fostered an enduring belief that plague always spread to Western Europe from the "East." On this point, see Daniel Panzac, *Quarantaines et Lazarets: Europe et la Peste D'Orient* (Aix-en-Provence: Édisud, 1986), 38–45. Also Junko Takeda, *Between Crown and Commerce: Marseille and the Early Modern Mediterranean* (Baltimore, MD: Johns Hopkins University Press, 2011), chapter 4.

quarantine infrastructure, and the fact that the plague was nevertheless imported in 1720 was broadly construed as proof that only insufficiently strong quarantine could allow it into France.[18] After the plague, Marseille's health authorities saw prophylactic rigor as the most productive kind of atonement for previous laxity, and the plague was enshrined as a central point of reference in the "civic consciousness" of the city.[19] After a 1744 plague epidemic in Sicily, Western Europe remained free of the disease,[20] while just across the sea and just over the Austrian military frontier, the Ottoman Empire still suffered from routine epidemics.[21] Quarantine, it appeared, was working.

Most Mediterranean port cities had acquired permanent (if small) quarantine facilities by the late seventeenth century, while the early and mid-eighteenth century saw a construction boom, including the major lazarettos of Malta and Marseille. In the wake of the Marseille plague, the former grew from 8,000 to 30,000 square meters, while Marseille's lazaretto was surrounded by additional outer walls and built out to cover some eighteen hectares.[22] Pressure to increase government expenditure on quarantine in this period was constant; a French official complained in the 1780s of the many demands for funds from Marseille's Board of Health: "The degradation of one wall would alone establish communication [with the outside world]," he noted. "Such a fear makes one superstitious and abandon oneself blindly to those in charge of this business." Given the concession of moral authority to the boards of health, the official concluded that pursuing economy for quarantine budget line items was "extremely difficult."[23]

Although the structures that would define the nineteenth-century quarantine system came into being in the wake of the Marseille plague, quarantine was not yet the systematic institution it would become by the end of the century. As late

---

[18] See Pierre de Ségur-Dupeyron, *Rapport adressé a S. Exc. le Ministre de Commerce* (Paris: Imprimerie Royale, 1834), 21.

[19] Daniel Gordon, "Confrontations with the Plague in Eighteenth-Century France," in *Dreadful Visitations: Confronting Natural Catastrophe in the Age of Enlightenment*, ed. Alessa Johns (New York: Routledge, 1999), 16–17. Gordon suggests many Marseillaise exhibited a "morbid pride" about their city's experience with the plague.

[20] Free of the disease, with the small exception of the plague of Noja (1815), addressed in Chapter 1.

[21] For an argument that Ottoman plague epidemics were a continuation of the Second Plague Pandemic, which had been responsible for the Black Death, see Michael W. Dols, "The Second Plague Pandemic and Its Recurrences in the Middle East, 1347–1894," *Journal of the Economic and Social History of the Orient* 22 (1979): 162–89. While historians and bioarcheologists have not definitively settled on this classification, it is clear that Mediterranean plagues in the eighteenth and nineteenth centuries were distinct from the third plague pandemic, which emerged in China in the 1850s and spread worldwide from 1894.

[22] Panzac, *Quarantaines et Lazarets*, 37. On late eighteenth-century additions to Marseille's lazaretto, see extract of royal and ministerial ordinances from September 1778: Archives Nationales de France, C.A.R.A.N., hereafter, AN (Paris) AE/B/III/14, f. 166.

[23] Sénac de Meilhan, memorial to the Minister of the Marine Department (undated, but c. 1781), AN (Paris) MAR/D/2/42.

as 1729, for example, Britain's Levant Company felt it could petition the British government to exempt ships coming from Venice, Greece, and Anatolia from all quarantine procedures.[24] Only about fifty years later, such a petition would be unthinkable. This change accompanied a shift in travel narratives between roughly 1720 and 1780, in which the Ottoman Empire lost its favorable association with health and became identified as the most dangerous source of epidemic contagion. By the nineteenth century, its sanitary condition and political state were often seen (by Eurocentric observers) to be equally degraded.

It is clear that both shifts accompanied the transformation of Europe's political geography from an unsettled map in which the Ottomans might once again menace the West to an essentially stable division. Between the Treaty of Passarowitz in 1718 and the Congress of Vienna in 1815, although the frontiers of European nations and empires shifted radically, the boundary between the Christian "West" and the Islamic "East" remained largely constant.[25] Not coincidentally, by the mid-eighteenth century, European governments funded large, permanent lazarettos at Semlin, the Rothenthurm Pass, Messina, Trieste, Venice, Genoa, Ancona, Livorno, and Naples, in addition to the construction already mentioned in Malta and Marseille. Other substantial quarantine sites built or expanded at this time include those at Palermo, Ragusa, and Nice. Smaller quarantine facilities, tasked with keeping watch for shipwrecks and smugglers and usually under the control of a larger, nearby board of health also began to emerge throughout the eighteenth century on the French and Italian coasts (Figure 0.2).

Like so much about the practice, the word "quarantine" initially comes from Italy. After forty (*quaranta*) days, persons and goods suspected of plague were traditionally considered free of potential contagion (most quarantines were shorter by the nineteenth century, but the word did not change). Throughout the eighteenth century, Italy remained the heartland of the system – of the twenty-nine boards of health to which the Venetians sent out circular correspondence in the last third of the century, twenty-five were in what is now Italy.[26] In the early nineteenth century, thanks to a large new lazaretto in Menorca (Port Mahon) and expansions to lazarettos in Malta and Marseille, quarantine's geography changed. The shift coincided with the gradual rise of British and Austrian trade in the Mediterranean and the comparative decline of French and Italian mercantile dominance. As the practice became more

---

[24] Petition of the Levant Company, December 26, 1729, UK National Archives, Kew, London (hereafter, TNA) PC 1/4/108.

[25] There is, of course, the exception of the Ottoman–Russian frontier. But quarantine along that frontier was never as regular as in the Mediterranean, and even so, changes to it meant the hasty construction of new Russian lazarettos in the course of the eighteenth and nineteenth centuries.

[26] See Archivio di Stato di Venezia, Venice (hereafter, ASVe) Provv. Sanità 793.

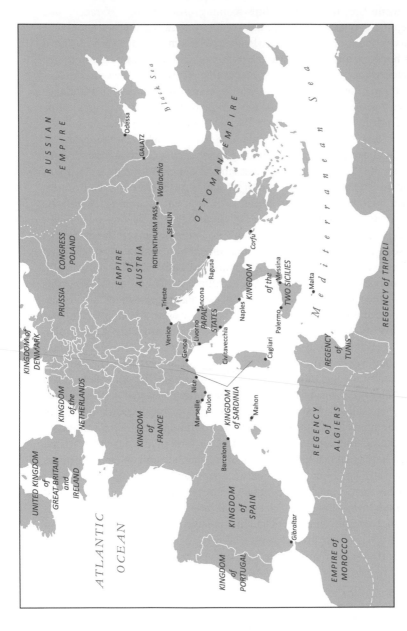

Figure 0.2 Map of major lazarettos and quarantine ports, c. 1820. British-run quarantine facilities in Corfu and Gibraltar were excluded from free pratique in most Continental ports for the majority of the period considered here and are noted in italics. "Terrestrial" lazarettos, along the land borders that the Habsburg and Russian Empires shared with the Ottoman Empire, are given in all caps. Map designed by the University of Wisconsin–Madison Cartography Lab.

transnational and subject to multiple authorities, it took on more coherence as an integral institution of European shipping.

As the epidemiological and political boundary between the West and the Middle East continued to harden (from a Western perspective), Italian-influenced *maritime* quarantine was only one way of imposing a barrier against the Ottoman Empire. After the 1718 Treaty of Passarowitz, the opening of the Austrian Empire's long land border with the Ottoman Empire (for trade and travel) provoked the organization of the extensive *"pestfront"* in 1728. This consisted of a military division, assembled via a *corvée* imposed on border provinces and tasked with guarding the entire frontier, which was mobilized whenever plague was found in the closest European provinces of the Ottoman Empire.[27] In 1740, the Habsburg government constructed a major lazaretto at Semlin, and smaller quarantine accommodations for travelers followed at the Rothenthurm Pass in present-day Romania. Terrestrial quarantine establishments often mandated shorter periods of detention if there was no plague present, given that travelers moving under the open air were thought to be less likely to retain pestilential matter than individuals confined to the close quarters of a ship. Nevertheless, the apparatus behind the terrestrial *cordon sanitaire* was at least as extensive as the maritime barrier. In addition to the lazarettos, smaller *rastels* (tiny quarantine establishments where goods or letters could be fumigated and passed through the frontier, though no individuals could cross) were built all along the Ottoman-Habsburg border, each with a small staff.

The entire network of institutions – major lazarettos in port cities, major land quarantine stations on the Ottoman-Habsburg frontier, smaller boards of health keeping a watchful eye on the coast, and Prussian and Austrian military quarantines that could be summoned up in a time of need – grew during the eighteenth century. As quarantine legislation was refined among the European powers, it became traditional to consign *all* ships coming from points eastern and southern to mandatory detention. It would take the epidemic and political pressures of the Napoleonic Era to produce the systematization and durability that quarantine experienced in the first half of the nineteenth century. That later period is the subject of this book. As we have come to its brink, it remains now to establish the basic elements of what constituted protection against the plague by 1780.

Across many areas of quarantine practice, administrators operated with a shared vocabulary. Every ship was required to possess a bill (or patent) of

---

[27] On this human *cordon sanitaire*, see Jovan Pesalj, "Some Observations on the Habsburg–Ottoman Border and Mobility Control Policies," in *Transgressing Boundaries*, ed. Marija Wakounig and Markus Beham (Zurich: GmbH & Co., 2013), 245–56, and Gunther Rothenburg, "The Austrian Sanitary Cordon and the Control of the Bubonic Plague, 1710–1871," *Journal of the History of Medicine* 28, no. 1 (1973): 15–23.

health, signed by a European consul stationed in the port of departure.[28] Bills were always classified in one of three or four categories: foul, touched/suspected, or clean.[29] In Britain itself, all ships proceeding from anywhere in the Mediterranean were potentially subject to quarantine, especially if their cargo contained trade goods considered most likely to harbor contagion ("enumerated goods"). In the rest of Europe, ships from other European ports were only quarantined in the case of disease outbreaks, while ships from the Levant and North Africa were always detained.[30] The length of detention depended both on the state of health in a ship's port of departure and on the supposed susceptibility of its cargo to infection. Though some ports were known to be harsher than others, there was an unspoken minimum standard of severity that was consistently negotiated by exchange and experiment among boards of health. If one port's board did not adhere to this threshold, ships from that port would be quarantined abroad.

Once in quarantine, goods (and often passengers) were subjected to a *spoglio*, or expurgation procedure, usually with a mix of smoking, airing, and dipping in vinegar, chlorine, or a substance euphemistically referred to as "perfume."[31] Indeed, trade goods (even more than people) were generally considered the most threatening sources of potential disease.[32] The most potentially infectious "enumerated goods" included cotton, wool, fur, hair, paper, flax, yarn, clothing, sponges, hemp, and other items, while more solid, harder, or finer items such as grains, salt, raisins, sand, alum, and ivory, were considered to be free from potential infection.[33] Lazaretto staff members developed specific fumigation techniques for each enumerated good; these were shared among lazarettos across Europe.

While bales of cotton were opened and aerated every day, once in the lazaretto, passengers were left more or less to their own devices. Contact

---

[28] It became standard for ships to carry a bill of health by the late seventeenth century, though throughout the 1700s, it was common for ships to purposely leave without one and so avoid certain ports' proscriptions against all foul bill ships. See Panzac, *Quarantaines et Lazarets*, 41.

[29] "Touched" and "suspected" bills were, in some cases, interchangeable and were both later inventions.

[30] See *Intendants de la Santé* of Marseille to Laurent Cunin-Gridaine, March 2, 1840, Archives départmentales des Bouches-du-Rhône, Marseille (henceforth, ADBR) 200 E 194.

[31] The Abbé Jean-Pierre Papon gave a recipe for "parfum" in 1800, which included sulfur, cardamom, black pepper, ginger, laudanum, and cumin. See Jean-Pierre Papon, *De la Peste, Ou, Époques Mémorables de ce Fléau et les Moyens de s'en Préserver* (Paris: Lavillette et Compagnie, 1800), 2:207.

[32] David Barnes, "Cargo, 'Infection,' and the Logic of Quarantine in the Nineteenth Century," *Bulletin of the History of Medicine* 88, no. 1 (2014): 75–101.

[33] John Howard, *An Account of the Principal of Europe* (Warrington: William Eyres, 1789), 17. Howard notes the ubiquity of this system of classification at various Mediterranean ports. Numerous examples also exist in the regulations of individual lazarettos. A British example can be found in an 1826 handbill: *Abstract of Quarantine Regulations* (London: George Eyre and Andrew Strahan, 1826). Wellcome Archive, London (hereafter, Wellcome).

with the outside world could come via letters (letters sent from the lazaretto were slit, smoked, and dipped in vinegar, as was all mail that passed through it) or at the *parlatorio* – usually a chamber divided by a narrow stream of water and/or iron grills separating individuals in quarantine from merchants, friends, and acquaintances "in free pratique" (i.e., not subject to quarantine).

The bulk of those who performed quarantine did so onboard ship (in most cases because they were sailors rather than paying passengers). Such individuals, more than anyone else, recognized quarantine's most famous sign: the yellow flag. This was the generally agreed signal, from the late eighteenth century on, that a ship was in isolation.[34] It was, as one ship's captain mournfully noted, "a public signal that we were tabooed."[35] Edwin Montague, a member of an American expedition to the Holy Land, performed quarantine on his return journey off the coast of Spain at the quarantine harbor of Port Mahon in 1848. To him, the flag itself was the most memorable aspect of sanitary detention: "The yellow flag, the abominable yellow flag, still marks our ship as 'plague smitten.' Every boat steers off from us, afraid of contamination."[36]

Encountering any person or thing supposed to have come into contact with the zone of infection clearly generated fear. Yet, it is important to remember that even this later phase of quarantine history occurred well before the emergence of germ theory. The understanding of what "contagion" meant, in the case of plague, clearly varied among doctors (was it a poison that spread through touch alone? an amorphous substance that could corrupt the air?). Some used the words "contagion" and "infection" interchangeably, others stressed differences.[37] Believers in quarantine (contagionists) defended an abstract idea of contagion, but the most persuasive arguments in favor of the system were based on the historical fact that the expansion of quarantine coincided with the retreat of the plague from Europe. The imprecision in imagining a discrete infectious agent provided fodder for quarantine's critics

---

[34] The origin of this symbol is unclear. It seems to have been required by Venetian authorities as early as the fifteenth century. In Britain, it was mandated by the Quarantine Act of 1788 (28th Geo. III, c. 34). According to John Booker, flying the yellow flag had been proposed several decades earlier only to be discarded. Given the increased number of ships in quarantine, the adoption of a universally recognized symbol was seen as more important by 1788. See Booker, *Maritime Quarantine*, 214.

[35] Capt. James Williamson, quoted in Lisa Rosner, "Policing Boundaries: Quarantine and Professional Identity in Mid Nineteenth-Century Britain," in *Mediterranean Quarantines, 1750–1914*, ed. John Chircop and Francisco Javier Martínez (Manchester, UK: Manchester University Press, 2018), 129.

[36] Edward P. Montague, *Narrative of the Late Expedition to the Dead Sea, from a Diary by One of the Party* (Philadelphia: Carey and Hart, 1849), 79.

[37] See Margaret Pelling, "The Meaning of Contagion: Reproduction, Medicine, and Metaphor," in *Contagion: Historical and Cultural Studies*, ed. Alison Bashford and Claire Hooker (London: Routledge, 2001), 15–38.

(anticontagionists), who believed atmosphere and environment, not contagion, caused the plague. The lack of clarity about what contagion was struck such critics as especially ridiculous when considered next to the extreme specificity of many quarantine rituals (the wiggling of cotton, the dipping of letters in vinegar, and the spectacle of the parlatorio).[38]

Still, defenders of the system emphasized that without understanding which procedure secured immunity from the plague, any reform was playing with fire. In this way, lack of certainty gave quarantine staying power. Because there had been no major outbreak of plague since the 1720 plague of Marseille, defenders of the system reasoned that something had to be working even while it was unclear what. In this way, one comes to appreciate the gravity and solemnity behind lazaretto practices, the careful gaze of the Guardians, and the endless series of fumigations. Augustus Bozzi Granville, a prominent London physician and staunch defender of the doctrine of contagion, was apoplectic when Parliament convened a Select Committee to examine that very doctrine in 1819: "Since the establishment of quarantine laws, no case of plague has occurred in England for the space of a hundred and fifty-four years! Are we tired of this species of security?"[39] Abolishing quarantine, one MP told Parliament, would be "a most frightful experiment."[40] Many accepted that it was better to be safe than sorry, and for most doubters, the economic arguments against unilateral reform (and the retaliatory quarantines that would follow) were enough.

For much of the period considered here, Britain was an outlier when it came to quarantine practice. I stress this, not for the reason assumed by some historians, that commercial pressures to reform the system were comparatively greater there.[41] In fact, I mean this in the sense that until an Order in Council of 1827, British quarantine laws were significantly *harsher* than Continental equivalents. Under the terms of the 1753 Quarantine Act, all ships from within the Strait of Gibraltar (i.e., from *any* Mediterranean port) were subject to quarantine, whether or not they carried enumerated goods. Throughout the late eighteenth and early nineteenth centuries, the Privy Council (hereafter, PC) applied this rule selectively, often reversing course over whether to allow certain ships (especially from Spain and Gibraltar) into British ports without quarantine. Ships with foul bills of health were not permitted to perform

---

[38] In 1843, for example, a shipping encyclopedia dismissively concluded that "the received distinction between susceptible and non-susceptible commodities is now held to be fanciful." See William Waterson, *A Cyclopædia of Commerce, Mercantile Law, Finance, and Commercial Geography* (Edinburgh: Oliver and Boyd, 1843), 566.

[39] Augustus Bozzi Granville, *A Letter to the Right Honorable F. Robinson, M.P.* (London: Richard and Arthur Taylor, 1819), 96.

[40] William Trant was the MP. Hansard, House of Commons Debate, May 19, 1825, Vol. 13, c. 792.

[41] See, for example, Anne Hardy, "Cholera, Quarantine, and the English Preventive System," *Medical History* 37 (1993): 251.

quarantine in Britain at all, being subjected to the "double quarantine" of enforced detention at a Mediterranean lazaretto, and then, in most cases, another quarantine off the coast of Britain. After lengthy debate, that rule changed in 1799 when ships with foul bills were granted the right to perform quarantine in Britain itself.[42] In the wake of the reformist Quarantine Act of 1825, the PC largely limited sanitary detention to ships from the Ottoman Empire and the rest of North Africa.[43] The unpredictability, inconvenience, and expense of the procedure in Britain meant that most Britons subject to quarantine usually performed it in a Mediterranean lazaretto; trade goods destined for the UK were the main targets of British quarantine acts.

Though quarantine as the formal response to ships with yellow fever and plague was only removed from British legislation in 1896, a series of PC orders limited the system to one-off usage in extraordinary circumstances from the late 1840s. Yet, even in this later era, Britain was hardly a Continental outlier given the eagerness of the governments of France (under the July Monarchy) and the Habsburg Empire to liberalize their own quarantine laws in the 1840s. While it is right to recognize that, at times, British officials were more impatient for reform than other Europeans, it is equally true that the broad trajectory of British quarantine policy was one of increasing symmetry with European powers – first by assimilating to common norms, then by pursuing reform internationally. At the first International Sanitary Conference in 1851 (discussed in Chapter 9), most European countries agreed in principle that quarantine should be limited to ships proceeding from ports actually infected with plague and yellow fever. Plague had begun to disappear from the Ottoman heartlands about a decade earlier, so, as the new consensus took hold, most ships in the Mediterranean managed to avoid quarantine from the early 1850s (though late nineteenth-century cholera quarantines directed against Muslim pilgrims both in the Mediterranean and around the Red Sea showed that Europeans remained concerned that the Mediterranean could be a conduit for disease to spread to Europe).

Freeing Quarantine from Quarantine

Quarantine is often thought of as a practice of isolation and exclusion. This book engages with that customary understanding; it investigates how the

---

[42] An Act to encourage the Trade into the Levant Seas (39th Geo. III c. 99).

[43] Though quarantine still applied to ships carrying "enumerated goods" from the Mediterranean that left from a port without a major lazaretto and lacked a certification that their enumerated cargoes were "not the produce of Turkey, or of Africa within the Straits, or of West Barbary." For a summation of this PC order, see Charles Greville to T. Whitmore, August 27, 1827. Quoted in *Quarantine: Return to an Order of the Honourable House of Commons* (London: House of Commons, 1831), 3–5.

prophylactic barrier deployed in Mediterranean ports shaped Western conceptions of "the sick man of Europe"[44] throughout the early nineteenth century
even as it reaffirmed an idea of health inside the barrier. That the most meaningful dividing line between West and East was a medical barrier made plague
into a metric by which Western Europeans judged the prospects of the Ottoman
regime – the extent of its problems, the chances for its "regeneration," and the
inevitability of its supposed "decline." Yet, I am equally interested in how
quarantine fostered transnational cooperation and coordination. Not only did it
undergird a sense of a protected interior but it also circumscribed the independent action of governments by its logic of mutually guaranteed protection.
Outside of international policing agreements or military alliances, quarantine
legislation was unique in that it depended on and assumed transnational
cooperation. In this way, quarantine gave a sense of sanitary congruity to
Western Europe.

Here, the history of quarantine is a history of networks and connections. The
archives of quarantine practice turn up not only people, goods, and things but
also rhythms of communication and a transnational process for responding to
threats current and implied. Just as an electrical system can be studied through
nodes and capacitors situated at individual points around circuits, so, too, can
the sites and records of quarantine capture the measure of Mediterranean
currents during a critical period of change. In many periodizations of the
Middle Sea, the Napoleonic Wars represent, simultaneously, a major dividing
line and an inscrutable black box from which emerged a modern dynamic, a sea
marked by the rhythms of globalization, colonialism, exploitative trade, and
increasing tension. As a history of the Mediterranean during this period of flux,
The Yellow Flag shows the development of a new regime but in a way that
highlights the surprising persistence (even reinvigoration) of premodern
precedents.

On the one hand, quarantine highlights regional divisions (sick vs. healthy,
"Europe" vs. "East"). On the other, its records reveal connective patterns by
drawing attention to the diverse individuals and goods moving back and forth.
Julia Clancy-Smith's evocative reading of a diverse base of sources from both
sides of the "Central Mediterranean Corridor" between Italy and Tunisia
demonstrates how workers from both the northern and southern coasts of the
Middle Sea formed a mobile, diverse group of "Mediterraneans."[45] Similarly,
the records of quarantine stations help us understand the patterns that drove
fishermen, sailors, merchants, diplomats, and leisure travelers to cross the
Middle Sea. Most cross-Mediterranean travelers experienced quarantine not

---

[44] This famous phrase, used by Western observers to refer to the Ottoman Empire, has been
    attributed to Tsar Nicholas I of Russia.
[45] Julia Clancy-Smith, *Mediterraneans: Europe and North Africa in an Age of Migration,
    c. 1800–1900* (Berkeley: University of California Press, 2010).

once, but regularly, and many came from the margins of national economies. The significant investment of time the lazaretto exacted helped to instantiate a sense, among elite and impoverished passengers and sailors alike, that to be a "traveler" was to be something identifiable – it was to understand a certain set of rituals of passage and disinfection, to be able to grapple with boredom during long months in a lazaretto, to incorporate a sense of contamination and expurgation into the experience of crossing the Mediterranean itself.

For these and other reasons, travel narratives are a powerful source for this book. After all, since any travel across the Mediterranean from Africa or the Levant to Europe involved detention at a lazaretto, such works often include thoughtful meditations on the experience of quarantine. The authors of such narratives mostly come from one elite stratum of the British Mediterranean world, yet as a historical source, travel narratives expand, rather than contract our apprehension of that world's contours. Many enjoyed a wide circulation back in Britain and served to fashion a mental landscape of the Middle East (and of quarantine) for those who never went abroad. Furthermore, travel narratives by relatively well-off Britons serve as a means of conveying glimpses of the lives of far more modest people as they negotiated the *cordon sanitaire*. They help put the *experience* of quarantine back at the center of its broader history.

Across a global backdrop, the history of quarantine has enjoyed a resurgence of interest among historians with considerably different perspectives. For Mark Harrison, debates surrounding quarantine serve as a barometer for measuring the competing fortunes of public health authorities and merchants.[46] For Alison Bashford, quarantine in the late nineteenth and early twentieth centuries has served as a fruitful way of understanding racial anxieties about the admission of refugees and immigrants,[47] a concern that also animates the work of Nayan Shah on San Francisco and Angel Island or Howard Markel's study of Jewish immigrants in late nineteenth-century New York.[48] David Barnes uses a *longue durée* history of a crucial American site of yellow fever quarantine to explore the evolution of ideas of infection among civic authorities in nineteenth-century Philadelphia.[49]

---

[46] Mark Harrison, *Contagion: How Commerce Has Spread Disease* (New Haven, CT: Yale University Press, 2012).

[47] See Alison Bashford, "At the Border: Contagion, Immigration, Nation," *Australian Historical Studies* 33, no. 120 (2002): 344–58. Also, Bashford, ed., *Medicine at the Border: Disease, Globalization and Security, 1850 to the Present* (New York: Palgrave Macmillan, 2006).

[48] Nayan Shah, *Contagious Divides: Epidemics and Race in San Francisco's Chinatown* (Berkeley: University of California Press, 2001); Howard Markel, *Quarantine! East European Jewish Immigrants and the New York City Epidemics of 1892* (Baltimore, MD: Johns Hopkins University Press, 1999).

[49] See D. S. Barnes, "'Until Cleansed and Purified': Landscapes of Health in the Interpermeable World," *Change over Time* 6, no. 2 (2016): 138–52. The regulation of yellow fever, more generally, has become a popular topic for historians of the Atlantic world. Two recent dissertations exemplify this. See Katherine Arner, "The Malady of Revolutions: Yellow Fever in the

The history of Mediterranean quarantine itself has increasingly interested historians from around the Mediterranean Basin. This rich historiography has focused on specific sites of quarantine practice and administrative histories that connect quarantine legislation to broader stories within national historiographies regarding territorial control, the articulation of borders, and imperialism.[50] Like much of this literature, *The Yellow Flag* seeks to restore a sense of specificity and distinction to quarantine practice in the Mediterranean. Yet, the tendency of such work to fall within distinct local or national historiographies of specific Mediterranean states tends to diminish the extent to which it conveys how quarantine operated as a universal system. Especially in France, Malta, and the Italian states, boards of health were oriented outward to foreign boards to a much greater extent than they were in sync with the priorities or ideologies of national ministers. Members of these boards viewed themselves as colleagues in a region-wide fight against epidemic contagion – the systematic quality of universal quarantine was the key to its staying power and its global influence.

Yet, one of the virtues of connecting the study of "universal quarantine" in the Mediterranean with a thorough engagement with one particular national historiography (Britain's) is that it highlights the importance of Mediterranean events and controversies to a history that has been almost exclusively recounted in a metropolitan context: sanitary reform in the 1830s and 1840s. The work of Anthony Wohl, Margaret Pelling, Graham Mooney, James Hanley, Christopher Hamlin, Tom Crook, and Matthew Newsom Kerr has carried the history of public health to the center of interpretations of moral and political understandings of British society.[51] By the end of the nineteenth century, Victorian Britain could boast a justly famous public health infrastructure; the existing

Atlantic World, 1793–1828," PhD diss., Johns Hopkins University, 2014, and Julia Mansfield, "The Disease of Commerce: Yellow Fever in the Atlantic World, 1793–1805," PhD diss., Stanford University, 2017. On links between yellow fever control in the Americas and the long history of quarantine against plague in the Mediterranean, see Arner, "Making Global Commerce into International Health Diplomacy: Consuls and Disease Control in the Age of Revolutions," *Journal of World History* 24, no. 4 (2013): 771–96.

[50] I refer, in particular, to the essays collected in Chircop and Martínez, eds., *Mediterranean Quarantines* (2018). Giuseppe Restifo, *I Porti della Peste: Epidemie Mediterranee fra Sette e Ottocento* (Messina: Mesogea, 2005), is a unique example of a monograph with a pan-Mediterranean frame, but in Restifo's narrative, epidemics tend to appear as irregular crises and quarantines as temporary, episodic responses.

[51] Margaret Pelling, *Cholera, Fever and English Medicine* (Oxford: Oxford University Press, 1978); A. S. Wohl, *Endangered Lives: Public Health in Victorian Britain* (Cambridge, MA: Harvard University Press, 1983); Christopher Hamlin, *Public Health and Social Justice in the Age of Chadwick* (Cambridge: Cambridge University Press, 1998); Graham Mooney, *Intrusive Interventions: Public Health, Domestic Space, and Infectious Disease Surveillance in England, 1840–1914* (Rochester, NY: University of Rochester Press, 2015); James Hanley, *Healthy Boundaries: Property, Law, and Public Health in England and Wales, 1815–1872* (Rochester, NY: University of Rochester Press, 2016); Tom Crook, *Governing Systems: Modernity and the Making of Public Health in England, 1830–1910* (Oakland: University of California Press,

historiography has firmly situated its development within broader narratives about local politics, government growth, protest literature, and medical controversy. Yet, little attention has been paid in this literature to Britain's participation in the largest transnational scheme for preventative medicine before the formation of the WHO: Mediterranean quarantine.[52]

You are beginning a book in which you will find yourself transported, within a matter of pages, from a Middle Eastern city in the throes of a plague epidemic to a cholera hospital in Britain to a quarantine fortress on an isolated Maltese island. While the *practice* of quarantine mandated detention and delay, the *history* of quarantine is necessarily mobile. The dual lens used here – with interventions in both the history of the Mediterranean and the history of Britain and its Empire – is accompanied by a division of the book into thematic parts within which we move continuously among Britain, Continental Europe, the Middle East, North Africa, and the British Empire.

In Part I, I seek to fix the specificities of universal Mediterranean quarantine both in time and space. Chapter 1 presents the period of the Revolutionary and Napoleonic Wars as a public health crisis during which the modern quarantine system took shape. It investigates the series of plague and yellow fever epidemics that breached the defenses of a string of Mediterranean islands and considers the response of European governments. The frequency with which armies and navies crossed the Mediterranean created a massive augmentation of quarantine traffic just as new epidemic threats challenged the system as never before. Despite wartime debacles that suggested the quarantine system might break down, I demonstrate that it emerged stronger than ever. A conflict that has been called a "total war"[53] actually fostered transnational sanitary cooperation in fundamental ways. Chapter 2 explores the contours of what I call the "British Mediterranean world." This categorization, I argue, applies beyond the nation's formal colonies (Gibraltar, Malta, and the Ionian Islands) to the diverse ensemble of British personnel driven to the Middle Sea by the obligations of military service, by the needs of diplomacy, or by personal inclination. It applies also to the set of concerns, strategies, and transactions

---

2016); Matthew Newsom Kerr, *Contagion, Isolation, and Biopolitics in Victorian London* (New York: Palgrave Macmillan, 2017).

[52] Even among the historians who have studied British quarantine specifically, the focus has been on European comparisons (Baldwin), administrative practice (Booker, McDonald, and Mullett), or the significance of quarantine in Britain itself (Hardy and Maglen). See Peter Baldwin, *Contagion and the State in Europe, 1830–1930* (Cambridge: Cambridge University Press, 1999); C. F. Mullett, "A Century of English Quarantine, 1709–1825," *Bulletin of the History of Medicine* 23 (1949): 527–45; J. McDonald, "The History of Quarantine in Britain during the Nineteenth Century," *Bulletin of the History of Medicine* 25 (1951): 22–44; John Booker, *Maritime Quarantine*; Anne Hardy, "Cholera, Quarantine"; Krista Maglen, *The English System: Quarantine, Immigration and the Making of a Port Sanitary Zone* (Manchester, UK: Manchester University Press, 2014).

[53] See David Bell, *The First Total War* (Boston: Houghton Mifflin, 2007).

that tied metropolitan concerns to Mediterranean events. It is along the routes and patterns of the British Mediterranean that *The Yellow Flag* proceeds.

In Part II, we enter the world of the lazarettos. From huts in the Rothenthurm Pass in the Carpathian Mountains to looming fortresses in Mediterranean ports, these uncanny structures marked out Western Europe's border with points eastern and southern. While other histories of specific sites of quarantine have presented aspects of its practice, the aim of this section of the book is to paint a synthetic picture of nineteenth-century Mediterranean quarantine as a connected system. Chapter 3 offers a social and institutional history of sanitary control from the perspective of employees and administrators across the Mediterranean, emphasizing the continuities in practice among different ports. The chapter considers the administrative logic underlying disinfection practices and the daily scope of board of health activities. Lazarettos comprised a rigid hierarchy of employees, from the "Captain/Prior" in charge of the building, through doctors, to the "guardians" who attended each traveling party and who cycled in and out of quarantine themselves. At the top of the hierarchy, boards of health wielded immense power as they acted as local administrators with a national (even international) remit. I investigate how the lazaretto could simultaneously serve as an economic engine for cities like Marseille and Genoa, a civic institution, and an international space, whose jurisdictional status remained murky. Drawing upon travel narratives as well as administrative records, Chapter 4 shifts the perspective to the travelers, traders, sailors, soldiers, merchants, and missionaries whom quarantine detained. We consider incidents of suspicious deaths in the lazaretto, ghostly experiences that frightened travelers, and the routines developed by those in quarantine to ward off boredom. In this chapter, I also address sanitary crimes – from smuggling to attempted escape.

Having considered the intimate details of fumigation and expurgation in Chapters 3 and 4, the focus broadens in Chapter 5, which studies the transnational cooperation that enabled quarantine to function as a broader network. I show how circuits of exchange among boards of health and European consuls serving in the Middle East fashioned a "European biopolity" that included Britain. The chapter argues that, contrary to scholarship that has depicted quarantine prior to the 1850s as an improvised and irregular precursor to a late-century regime of international health, reciprocal correspondence among boards of health fostered a system that was durable and adaptable. The centerpiece of the chapter focuses on the events surrounding the passage of the 1825 Quarantine Act in Britain, in which an attempt to liberalize quarantine regulations led to a Continent-wide quarantine against British shipping. The spectacle only concluded when the Privy Council backed down. Rather than demonstrating British ambivalence, however, the reaction of the government in London shows how seriously politicians and advocates regarded membership in what one MP called the "family compact" of quarantine.[54]

In Part III, the account moves from the practice of quarantine to the theories, mentalities, and practices it shaped. In Chapter 6 we turn to the ways Ottomans and Europeans residing in the Middle East contended with actual plague epidemics and explore the ways in which Western conceptions of plague informed broader evaluations of the Ottoman Empire. The chapter examines how diplomatic conundrums filtered into the casual discourse of travelers and how closely medical and political evaluations were intertwined. Plague helps open up the Eastern Question by making clear how the political dilemmas it posed were not the exclusive purview of high diplomacy but were deeply implicated in medico-cultural perceptions of the "East."

In Chapter 7, we turn our attention to the centrality of plague and debates about quarantine in the birth of the British public health movement. The chapter makes the case that though it is often thought of as a premodern scourge, the plague's diffuse and dramatic reputation shaped conceptions of other killer diseases of the nineteenth century, such as cholera. I argue that debates surrounding Mediterranean quarantine formed an essential part of the development of British public health reform. Within this wider transnational perspective, I offer a reinterpretation of the much-discussed "contagion debate" between those who believed epidemic disease was communicated by contact and proximity ("contagionists") and those who believed quarantine was useless and that plague spread because of atmospheric factors, such as temperature, winds, marsh exhalations, or putrefying matter ("anticontagionists" or "miasmatists"). This debate has achieved a rather tired reputation in recent historiography, as scholars have cast the arguments of advocates on both sides as simple posturing in the midst of broad agreement. So it may be when looking at cholera. But by focusing on quarantine and plague (which was central to the concerns of medical polemicists), we see a revised picture of a medical argument understood in global, and especially Mediterranean, terms.

Part IV addresses the diffusion of Mediterranean quarantine practice: both around the world (in Chapter 8) and further in time (in Chapter 9). The former chapter considers how imperialism spread quarantine practice to new areas of the globe. It examines British responses to plague epidemics in Malta, Corfu, and India and argues that British use of quarantine in these imperial contexts demonstrates how firmly inflected by Mediterranean practice global quarantine became, even as it was employed only in specific circumstances. Yet, despite its persistence and its wide reach, quarantine did not last forever. One of the leading arguments of Chapter 9 is that its character fundamentally shifted in the 1850s, when the system lost its role as a universal barrier. Though it

---

[54] Joseph Hume, Hansard, House of Commons Debate, July 10, 1823, Vol. 9, c. 1526.

remained a tool within a later medical and political arsenal, it was no longer a universal checkpoint against all arrivals from a specific region of the world. I suggest that it was primarily *after* quarantine lost its universal character that it became more potent as a mechanism to target specific individuals, races, and ethnicities. Chapter 9 further argues that the end of the system of mandatory quarantine had at least as much to do with the decline of plague in the Middle East as it did with the ascent of anticontagionist arguments in London, Madrid, Paris, and Vienna. And such a durable system did not simply vanish without a trace; I show how the systematic structure of Mediterranean quarantine practice determined the shape and scope of the International Sanitary Conferences (precursors to the World Health Organization).

In sum, then, *The Yellow Flag* addresses a discrete period and place that represented the most sustained operation of a universal quarantine system at any time in world history. From the expansion of the system in the late eighteenth century to its demise in the middle of the nineteenth, Mediterranean quarantine imposed a geography that was absolute. Its influence redounded across the world and remains with us more than a century and a half after it became possible to sail from Alexandria to Southampton and disembark freely. In practical and doctrinal origin, quarantine displays a premodern pedigree, but its incontrovertible influence can be felt in the latitudes and longitudes of the modern world.

Part I

Mediterranean Currents

1   Universal Agitation

In 1799, at the height of the Revolutionary and Napoleonic Wars, a rumor spread like wildfire along the coasts of Provence. A pamphlet by Marseille's *Conservateurs de Santé* described a report "that the English and the North Africans are conniving in the atrocious project of introducing the plague on the coasts of France."[1] This unholy alliance may well have been the invention of the *Conservateurs* themselves, who were concerned about the alarming increase in smuggling by sailors from North Africa and eager for any opportunity to remind the public of the importance of the quarantine laws. Cloaking their sanitary task in patriotic terms (under their new, revolutionary letterhead: *liberté, égalité, santé*), the authors of the pamphlet suggested that the rumor should be taken seriously simply because of the well-known "*caractère barbaresque* and *perfidie anglaise*."[2]

The authors emphasize the duplicity of the English by stressing the dubious nature of any alliance with the medically suspect *Barbaresques*. "In France and throughout Europe," they opined, "in league with the pestiferous peoples of the Levant and Barbary, the enemy of *la Grande Nation* provokes unprecedented fears of the terrible plague of evil contagion."[3] Britain is cast as an insidious enemy as much because of the idea that it would ally with "pestiferous peoples" as because their joint plot involved biological warfare. In this way, France could take up the mantle of defending not just its own coasts but "Europe" as a whole from sanitary outsiders. The pamphlet calls the quarantine laws "the protective laws of the general health of Europe," a set of Continent-wide rules that each nation needed to observe.[4] To contravene them meant a conscious decision to endanger the sanitary integrity of Europe.

---

[1] L'Administration Sanitaire de Marseille, *Conservation de la Santé Publique* (Marseille: Bertrand, 1799), 1.

[2] Ibid., 6., It is also possible that the British did indeed contemplate such a plan, though there is scant evidence for this. Using infectious epidemics as a tool of biological warfare was at least contemplated elsewhere in the late eighteenth-century British world. On this phenomenon, see Elizabeth Fenn, "Biological Warfare in Eighteenth-Century North America: Beyond Jeffrey Amherst," *Journal of American History* 86, no. 4 (2000): 1552–80.

[3] *Conservation de la Santé Publique*, 9.   [4] Ibid., 6.

The question of Britain's commitment to quarantine recurs throughout this book. Here, however, it is most important to note that the exigencies of war and the existence of an apparently irreconcilable and perfidious enemy gave the Marseille Board of Health a rationale for redoubling its commitment to quarantine and evangelizing the system to the public (something particularly visible from its reception of French soldiers returning from Napoleon's Egyptian Campaign). As Marseille's *Conservateurs* sought to prepare themselves for the onslaught, they produced a huge handbill describing their plan and justifying quarantine anew to the general public. The occasion provided a chance to offer a forceful description of quarantine's nature and purpose. "There exist countries which present risks to public health," the *Conservateurs* began. These included both "those which are afflicted with the plague" and "those which communicate with these first countries without taking preventative measures."[5]

Such a line evinced a clear logic: failing to quarantine arrivals from a "suspect" country was sufficient justification to detain ships proceeding from a country typically free of the plague. Referring to this group of unfortunate countries failing to see the wisdom of quarantine practice, the *Conservateurs* lamented the "ignorance, despotism, and superstition" that, in their view, magnified the threat of the plague. Maintaining quarantine ports, lazarettos, and health authorities thus constituted a proof of civilized government. Boards of health, the authorities noted, corresponded with each other and maintained their lazarettos as an international system that provided safety against the plague. Across the Mediterranean, protection was mutually assured, and war put that cooperation in jeopardy.

Or did it? The central argument of this introductory chapter is that the Revolutionary and Napoleonic Wars constitute a transformative moment in the history of Mediterranean quarantine. This is not because this period of crisis made systematic quarantine impossible. Somewhat paradoxically, this period (1792–1815) was a moment when nation-states, city-states, and empires across the northern half of the Mediterranean Basin *recommitted* to the universal maintenance of quarantine.[6] The post-Napoleonic system remained mostly intact until the late 1840s, and it constituted the most sustained, extensive, and multipolar application of a quarantine system in world history.

How could a moment of crisis generate such coordination? This chapter suggests several different reasons. First, as we explore below, the late eighteenth and early nineteenth centuries saw a greater number of epidemic

---

[5] Marseille Board of Health, "Proclamation des Conservateurs de la Santé Publique" (Marseille: Elisabeth Martin, 1801). Bill published 28th Fructidor, An 9 (September 15, 1801).

[6] For a recent contrasting view of quarantine chronology, at least in the case of Spain, see Jon Arrizabalaga and Juan Carlos García-Reyes, "Contagion Controversies on Cholera and Yellow Fever in Mid Nineteenth-Century Spain: The Case of Nicasio Landa" in *Mediterranean Quarantines*, ed. Chircop and Martínez, 170–73.

outbreaks. Second, the vituperative rage contained within the pamphlet quoted above shows how easily the fight against the enemy during the total war of 1792–1815 could be portrayed as a fight of civilization against barbarism.[7] This, too, helped shape the practice of quarantine; as the British ostensibly threatened biological warfare, the members of Marseille's Board of Health could portray themselves as the defenders of Europe as a whole. Civilized behavior could be proved and enacted through efficient quarantine practice. Third, the wars themselves provoked an expansion of bureaucracy across many different European states. In particular, the coordination necessary to rapidly expand authority over newly conquered (or reconquered) lands necessitated a new sense of quarantine as a basic set of premises that could (and should) function similarly in any European port. Finally, the period coincided with an information revolution, in which letter writing, newspaper and journal publication, and statistical compilation skyrocketed. Here the propulsive force of greater information (regarding quarantine procedures, lengths of detention, board of health deliberations, and knowledge of foreign epidemics) made coordination among boards of health seem easy to achieve and impossible to exist without. Lives depended on it.

In other words, for a variety of intersecting factors, and in the midst of a brutal and ideological sequence of wars, the coordination of Continent-wide norms came to seem normal and essential among the bureaucrats who composed Mediterranean boards of health. This extraordinary change has largely been missed in the historiography, in part because it involved a change in assumptions rather than in form. Quarantine existed before and after the Revolutionary and Napoleonic Wars. Yet, in the period considered here, it truly became "the sanitary system of Europe" in a new and meaningful sense. The transformation proceeded through the exchange of correspondence among Mediterranean boards of health; Chapter 5 examines the mechanics of that cooperation, but this chapter explores its causes as it investigates the specific moment of its origin in the midst of a continent-wide military conflict. In conducting this examination, a picture emerges of a coevolving consensus in which cooperation on sanitary matters came to be seen not as strategic but as essential.

In this way, the very extremity of the fighting, and, in particular, its wide reach, helped accentuate the growing attraction of a more robust and systematic approach to quarantine even as war pushed the practice to the breaking point. One might expect that scenes like the reception of Napoleon Bonaparte in Fréjus (in violation of the quarantine laws, on his return from the Egyptian Campaign) would have been relatively common in the chaotic era of the

---

[7] On the growth of such ideas during the French revolutionary period, see Dan Edelstein, *The Terror of Natural Right* (Chicago: University of Chicago Press, 2009).

Napoleonic Wars. But as we have seen, many at the time roundly criticized Bonaparte's flagrant challenge to sanitary precedent. And in the wake of the Napoleonic Wars, the window for unpunished evasions of quarantine closed definitively, even for would-be political heroes. In the 1830s, a young Benjamin Disraeli expressed a hope that he could "somehow or other shuffle quarantine" on his return from his travels in the Eastern Mediterranean.[8] Yet, he was detained like the rest.

At the moment when the modern Mediterranean was born, then, the medical boundaries that had characterized its premodern trade were made ever firmer. A recommitment to quarantine occurred alongside the beginnings of mass tourism, steam travel, and expanding British power. This should remind us that Mediterranean change was discontinuous. The Napoleonic Wars upended the states, technologies, and trading patterns that had defined the Middle Sea since the early modern period, while quarantine expanded and intensified.

Epidemic Crises on the Frontiers of Western Europe

It is one thing to note that, after the 1720 plague of Marseille and 1744 plague of Messina, with few exceptions, no Western European city experienced the plague again. But the urgency behind the expansion and regularization of quarantine in the late eighteenth and early nineteenth centuries owed as much to new epidemic threats as it did to confidence in traditional procedures. British, French, and Italian governments enacted, expanded, and regularized quarantine between 1780 and 1820 not out of conservative myopia but as an active and direct response to new outbreaks of disease. This fact has largely been lost on historians, who have tended to portray the survival of quarantine as the consequence of inaction or stasis. Partly, this is because historians who have focused on the history of epidemic disease in the East, such as Daniel Panzac, have ignored the political debates over quarantine in the West. Similarly, Western-oriented scholars have considered the relationship between cholera epidemics and the politics of British and Continental public health reform without reference to the epidemic experience of Europe's southern periphery.[9] The sense of a "crisis" in public health did not begin with cholera in the 1830s, still less with the hungry 1840s. Epidemic diseases threatening Europe's southern coast at the turn of the nineteenth century focused increasing

---

[8] Benjamin Disraeli to Isaac Disraeli, January 11, 1831. Contained in *Lord Beaconsfield's Letters*, ed. Ralph Disraeli (London: John Murray, 1887), 55.

[9] See, for example, Christopher Hamlin, *Public Health and Social Justice*; Margaret Pelling, *Cholera, Fever, and English Medicine*; Peter Baldwin, *Contagion and the State*; David McLean, *Public Health and Politics in the Age of Reform* (New York: Tauris, 2006); R. J. Morris, *Cholera 1832: The Social Response to an Epidemic* (New York: Holmes and Meier, 1976); A. S. Wohl, *Endangered Lives*, chapter 5.

attention on the security of the *cordon sanitaire*, more so by far than did memories of early modern plagues or the Black Death.

Panzac, in particular, has noted that the first quarter of the nineteenth century witnessed a confluence of epidemics. Not only was plague "more active than ever" but other diseases emerged: "at the very moment when yellow fever, until now kept at bay across the Atlantic, began to menace the Old World, it was followed by a growing anxiety over the apparently inevitable progression of a new plague with an origin in the Orient: the cholera."[10] Disease threatened on all sides just as the Napoleonic Wars disrupted shipping patterns and led to an increase in smuggling. In this way, it is possible to see the political and economic upheavals of the period from 1789 to 1815 as constituting a public health crisis: a crisis of knowledge (in which war disrupted communication), a crisis of administration (in which the typical efficacy of boards of health was challenged by unstable and transitory political regimes), a crisis of volume (in which battleships, prisoner-of-war ships, and North African smugglers posed new challenges to boards of health), and a crisis of microbes (in which plague and yellow fever menaced Europe's Mediterranean frontier and occasionally penetrated it).

In 1778, Constantinople suffered one of the worst plague epidemics in its history, losing an estimated 100,000 out of 500,000 inhabitants. Around the time the population had rebounded, in 1812–13, a second devastating plague epidemic hit the Ottoman capital, for which estimates of mortality range as high as 300,000.[11] Certainly for Constantinople, the plagues of 1778 and 1812–13 were the most devastating since at least 1700. Plague outbreaks in Smyrna (in 1784) and Salonika (in 1814) killed fewer in terms of absolute numbers but had similar rates of mortality; each city lost between 16 and 20 percent of its population. Aleppo lost 40,000 citizens out of 100,000 in 1787, a devastating loss of population that was only compounded in future epidemics in 1814 and 1827 (when it lost roughly a quarter of its population in the last major epidemic in Syria).[12] One of Egypt's worst ever plague epidemics would come in the mid-1830s, just at the time when cholera hit western and southern Europe for the first time. These epidemics, it should be noted, do not represent the "normal" state of affairs in the Ottoman Empire at this time. Though isolated plague cases smoldered, and small-sized epidemics often hit individual neighborhoods and towns, mortality on such massive scales was relatively rare in the

---

[10] Daniel Panzac, *La Peste dans L'Empire Ottoman, 1700–1850* (Leuven: Éditions Peeters, 1985), 411. Focusing particularly on the 1820s, Mark Harrison has also noted the conjuncture of outbreaks of these epidemic diseases on the Mediterranean. See *Contagion*, 62–63.

[11] See Donald Quataert, "The Age of Reforms, 1812–1914," in *An Economic and Social History of the Ottoman Empire, 1300–1914*, ed. Halil Inalcik and Donald Quataert (Cambridge: Cambridge University Press, 1994), 787.

[12] Panzac, *Peste*, 359.

nineteenth century, provoking an increasing sense of unease among Western observers when major epidemics occurred.

The disturbing succession of devastating Ottoman epidemics was noted by European consuls, doctors, and travelers resident in the Empire. In particular, as Donald Quataert notes, the period between 1812 and 1818 represents a particular inflection point during a fifty-year period in which plague epidemics affected almost every city in the Ottoman Empire.[13] Most worrisome for European observers (none more so than the British), these epidemics rippled across the Mediterranean. In 1813, plague hit the new British colony of Malta. In 1816, it hit the Ionian Islands at the precise moment the British were seeking to impose a new constitution and entrench their power there. During the 1790s, and then again in 1816 and 1818, plague struck the Dalmatian coast, an advance that was anxiously watched by diplomats across the continent.[14] Mallorca lost more than 2,000 inhabitants in a plague epidemic in 1820. In such a time of upheaval, quarantines constantly shifted. In the course of the 1790s plague epidemics in Dalmatia, for example, Venice instituted, and then suspended, a foul bill regime on all Dalmatian ports at least three times in five years.[15]

A further epidemic merits special attention: the plague of Noja (on the Puglian coast) in 1815. Largely unknown, and more swiftly extinguished, this was actually the last bubonic plague epidemic in history to break out on the Western European mainland. The response to it demonstrates just how seriously governments across Europe took the threat of pestilential importation and how ready they were to respond to an epidemic as the plague spread throughout the Mediterranean in the 1810s.

Noja (today Noicattaro) is a town in Puglia near the port city of Bari, and in the chaotic era of the post-Napoleonic restoration, the area was in a state of political transition. The plague's arrival coincided with turmoil surrounding the demise of the Bonapartist ruler, Joachim Murat, after the Hundred Days (and Bonaparte's final defeat at the Battle of Waterloo); it broke out in the formative months of the Kingdom of the Two Sicilies. Its origin, according to a report conducted by the Board of Health of Naples, was undoubtedly smuggling – in this case from the Ottoman provinces of Dalmatia.[16] Armies were heavy on the ground in southern Italy at this time, and on the declaration that plague had appeared in Noja, a military detachment was immediately sent to form a cordon around the town. To complete this, soldiers erected two concentric quarantine barriers and forced all of the town's inhabitants to take their chances inside

[13] Quataert, "Age of Reforms," 787.
[14] For the French reaction to these Dalmatian epidemics, see AN (Pierrefitte) F/8/10/I/1.
[15] See 1790s correspondence between Venice and Marseille, ASVe Provv. Sanità 551.
[16] See "Prospetto Storico del contagion di Noja," Archivio di Stato di Napoli, Naples (hereafter, ASN) Mag. Salute 194/311.

(though the Neapolitan doctor tasked by the Board of Health with preparing a report on the epidemic noted the necessity of building isolation hospitals in Noja to prevent the total collapse of a city that, in fairness, was "not entirely contaminated").[17] In addition to the thousands of soldiers required to man these lines, a Baltimore newspaper reported that some 10,500 sailors were required to man the 500-mile "sea quarantine" preventing commerce with the eastern Neapolitan littoral during the duration of the plague.[18] The Board of Health's doctor argued that the provision of funds for preventative medicine during the epidemic should be considered "a holy debt" on the fledgling postwar Neapolitan state.[19]

Years later, this extreme reaction was singled out for praise by the American medical textbook author James Wilson. Emphasizing that extreme epidemic conditions justified extreme state responses, he cited two (potentially apocryphal) stories of harsh quarantine justice during this plague. In one, a man who was suffering hallucinations from the plague ran out to the drawbridge over the moat dug around the village, where he was immediately shot. In the other, a citizen of Noja tossed a bored soldier a deck of cards across the moat. Both, Wilson relates, were summarily tried and executed for breaking the quarantine.[20] In the end, the epidemic was contained, with 800 dead (out of a population of just over 5,000). Throughout the episode, all ships arriving at other European ports from the Kingdom of Naples were put under quarantine across Europe (including in Britain). This extreme response to a relatively small epidemic should be seen not simply in isolation but rather as part of the cascade of epidemics around the Mediterranean Basin during the Napoleonic period. The plague writer J. D. Tully specifically singled out the plague of Malta as part of a genealogy of plague fighting that specifically shaped the experience here: "The plague of Malta ... was productive of much good abroad," as it "served as a useful lesson to the health authorities in general, but particularly those of Naples; so much so, that the moment a disease of a malignant nature was announced as having made its appearance at Noia, the suspicion of the latter authorities was at the moment roused."[21]

Across the Mediterranean, then, as the modern era dawned, the plague, that ostensibly premodern scourge, was more threatening than it had seemed for a hundred years. Again, this proliferation of Mediterranean plague coincided

---

[17] Memo by the "Medico Ordinario" of the Naples Board of Health, July 15, 1815, ASN Mag. Salute 194/312.
[18] "Foreign Articles," *Niles' Weekly Register*, June 1, 1816.
[19] Memo by the "Medico Ordinario."
[20] James Wilson, "Plague," in *A System of Practical Medicine*, ed. William Pepper and Louis Starr (Philadelphia: Lea Brothers, 1885), 1:783.
[21] J. D. Tully, *The History of the Plague as It Has Lately Appeared in the Islands of Malta, Gozo, Corfu, Cephalonia, etc.* (London: Longman, Hurst, Rees, Orme, and Brown, 1821), 213.

with the first visitation of yellow fever to the European mainland. This disease, known to doctors and scientists in Britain, France, and Spain for decades (due to their colonial experience in North America), crossed the Atlantic for the first time in the late 1790s. Cadiz and Seville were the first major cities to be hit. At this time, yellow fever's etiology was hotly debated; Benjamin Rush, the influential American physician, had laid down an anticontagionist vision of the disease's transmission (stressing environmental causes rather than person-to-person spread). Indeed, American anticontagionists such as Rush gained numerous European fellow travelers – most notably the energetic French physician Nicolas Chervin.[22]

While this opinion grew in popularity over the early nineteenth century, at least initially, most doctors assumed that yellow fever was contagious. Some even mistook it for plague itself, given its horrific mortality, its fast spread, and its dramatic progression. Though current estimates put the mortality at Cadiz during the epidemic of 1800 at roughly 8,000,[23] contemporaries often wrote hyperbolically of much greater mortality (a British doctor and quarantine official, Francis Millman, put the total at 100,000).[24] In Gibraltar, more than one-third of the population of 15,000 was killed during successive epidemics in these years. At Livorno, normal quarantine procedures were suspended in 1804 when that venerable quarantine port was struck by a yellow fever epidemic that killed roughly 500.[25] Several Spanish port cities were hit before the yellow fever epidemics died down at the end of the 1820s; most notably, in Barcelona, roughly 20,000 people died from a yellow fever epidemic in 1821.[26] In the end, though sporadic cases reached the British coast and the south coast of France, aside from the Tuscan epidemic, yellow fever was mostly confined to Spain. But even so, the huge mortality, the link with American trade, and the apparent vulnerability of the quarantine system generated shock (Figure 1.1).

The link to the plague was crucial in understanding how these yellow fever epidemics were understood at the turn of the nineteenth century. As I argue later in this book, by the late eighteenth century, the plague came to represent an

---

[22] On the controversies generated by American yellow fever epidemics, see Mark Harrison, *Contagion*, 52–55. Also see David Barnes, "Cargo, Infection, and the Logic of Quarantine," *Bulletin of the History of Medicine* 88 (2014): 80–82. On Chervin's assimilation of North American scholarship on yellow fever, see Arner, "Malady of Revolutions," 2.

[23] See George C. Kohn, *Encyclopedia of Plague and Pestilence* (New York: Facts on File, 1995), 44.

[24] Fraser Brockington, "Public Health at the Privy Council, 1805–6," *Medical History* 7, no. 1 (1963): 14.

[25] For mortality figures, see George C. Kohn, *Encyclopedia*, 182. During the fever time, the Livornese Lazzaretto di San Rocco was converted into an isolation hospital and the quarantine Guardians were seconded for the duty of forcibly removing individuals suspected of contagion from their homes and placing them therein. See "Rapporti di Guardiani" in Archivio di Stato di Livorno, Livorno (hereafter ASLi) Sanità 600.

[26] See Kohn, *Encyclopedia*, 24.

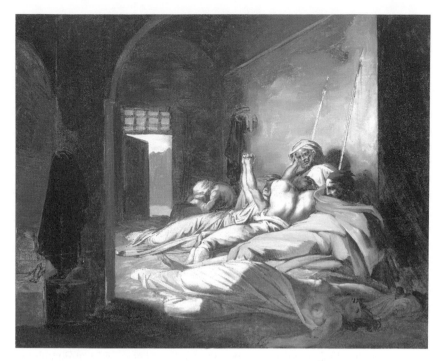

Figure 1.1 Théodore Géricault, *Scene from the Epidemic of Yellow Fever in Cadiz*, c. 1819. Oil on canvas. Virginia Museum of Fine Arts, Richmond. © Virginia Museum of Fine Arts. Adolph and C. Williams Fund. Photograph by Sydney Collins.

epidemic archetype, to which apparently "newer" epidemic diseases were conceptually assimilated. A solemn Genoese proclamation issued by that city's Napoleonic "Commissione Centrale di Sanità" urged redoubled attention to sanitary matters on behalf of the populace:

Citizens! The yellow fever has manifested itself throughout the Kingdom of Spain. This pestilence, undiminished and terrible, has desolated the once beautiful cities of Cadiz and Malaga ... There is little difference between this disease and the true Plague in its effects, it is communicated in the same manner as that disease – by way of contagion. Ignorance, carelessness, and the contravention of the quarantine laws have almost always been the causes that have introduced it to the cities that have become its victims.[27]

This lack of certainty as to the true nature of yellow fever, and its apparent transgression of sanitary barriers, inspired terrified reactions all over Europe.

[27] Leopoldo Olivieri and Domenico Piaggio, "Proclamazione della Commissione Centrale di Sanità," October 17, 1804, ASLi Sanità 627.

So extreme was the reaction of the Russian Tsar Paul I to the yellow fever epidemics of 1800 (he ordered the fumigation of mail from anywhere in Europe) that Western diplomats took it to be evidence of insanity.[28]

In this first epidemic, the most concerned of all, perhaps, were the French, who eyed their Spanish frontier with newfound alarm. "How can we repulse (from our borders and our ports) the unfortunate strangers who seek pure air in our territory?" demanded the Minister of the General Police in a report on how to address the Spanish epidemic. The minister suggested that French frontier communities were in "a state of siege" provoked by fleeing yellow fever victims. He argued that all individuals who attempted to enter France without rigorous quarantine should be "condemned to death," given that "the dying man stops only at death itself."[29]

For the French, the frequency with which this "new" disease crossed the Atlantic to Spain during the waning years of the Spanish Empire led to a growing sense that the Pyrenees represented not simply a physical frontier, but a significant sanitary border. When the disease appeared in Barcelona from 1819 to 1821, France's Restoration government assembled a huge military detachment to enforce a quarantine against Spain – a detachment so large it was able to intervene in the Spanish political struggles of the 1820s on behalf of Spanish conservatives. Such an event demonstrates the extent to which the medical and the political could blend together when it came to the epidemic threat. In this case, the connection was made even clearer because the liberal *Cortes* had delayed the enactment of its own sanitary law, thereby allowing the radical anticontagionist Charles Maclean to proclaim that the liberal regime in Spain (in power from 1820 to 1823) was a test case for his revolutionary theories.[30] When, with French assistance, Spain's liberal government was suppressed, the restored King Ferdinand VII canceled any moves toward reform.[31] The entire episode shows why European reformers who had felt some affinity with Spain's brief liberal experiment might come to resent the logic of quarantine itself along with the French intervention.

As the French reaction to Spanish yellow fever helps to show, the post-1815 hardening of borders among European nation-states was occurring in an era of sanitary siege. That such a state of crisis was felt can be seen from the correspondence of quarantine bureaucrats and government ministers across the Continent. On top of these epidemics I have already described, *rumors* of

---

[28] Hugh Ragsdale, *Tsar Paul and the Question of Madness* (New York: Greenwood, 1988), 105–7.

[29] Undated report by the Minister of the General Police (given the dossier's date range, almost certainly 1800–1801), AN (Pierrefitte) F/8/1, Dossier VII.

[30] On this episode, see Mark Harrison, *Contagion*, 65–67, and Erwin Ackerknecht, "Anticontagionism between 1821 and 1867," *Bulletin of the History of Medicine* 22 (1948): 572.

[31] See Arrizabalaga and García-Reyes, "Case of Nicasio Landa," 172.

epidemics (that eventually proved false) also troubled their lives. For example, when yellow fever arrived in Spain in 1818, the French government received reports that it was plague itself and treated it as such.[32] Suspicious fevers, smallpox epidemics with grossly inflated mortality rates, and typhus fevers accompanied by buboes created a specter of plague that loomed larger than the real threat and made determining suitable quarantines difficult throughout this period. Boards were often obliged to act on scant information and then later reduce their quarantines on the receipt of fuller intelligence.

Between rumors and false reports, real episodes of plague and yellow fever, the later appearance of cholera, and the arrival, every few years, of a plague ship in at least one Mediterranean quarantine port, there was never a time during the last half-century of universal quarantine when it was thought of as simply routine. The sense one gets from much of the secondary literature is that quarantine lingered for decades after its apparent usefulness ended, that the epidemic threat it was created to address was a thing of the past. In fact, quarantine lasted almost exactly as long as epidemic threats impinged on the European frontier. At all times during the system's existence, members of boards of health were confronted by apparent examples of what might happen were attention to be diverted or quarantine's severity reduced.

Quarantine in the Napoleonic Wars

The Revolutionary and Napoleonic Wars were not simply part of the background as the quarantine system faced epidemic stresses in the 1790s, 1800s, and 1810s. Then, and later, the fighting itself could push the limits of the system and create further bureaucratic challenges. After 1800, for example, it became possible for the first time ever for North African merchants to ship goods directly to Europe. Piracy (often carried out by individuals who also ran legitimate ships) also found more avenues to Europe's south coast at this time.[33] This was a brief window of opportunity opened by the war; traffic from North Africa precipitously declined after 1815. Nevertheless, such innovations were what made the war so unpredictable for sanitary officials. After 1807, and the introduction of Napoleon's Continental System, British blockade-runners further complicated the lives of sanitary bureaucrats who saw accurate knowledge about the arrival of every ship as fundamental to their work. Smuggling was directly blamed for such concerning events as the

---

[32] See "Plague in Galicia," AN (Pierrefitte) F/8/10/I/3.

[33] See Daniel Panzac, *Les Corsaires Barbaresques: La Fin d'une Épopée* (Paris: CNRS Editions, 1999), 140–42. See also a letter from Famin, the Agent of the Foreign Affairs Ministry at Marseille, in which he notes with concern the rise in ships from Algeria and elsewhere in North Africa and attempted to compile statistics about them: Famin to the Duc de Vienne, October 20, 1813, AN (Paris) AE/B/III/220.

plagues of Malta and Noja. If customs services and marine patrols were incapable of enforcing the maritime border at a time of war, each board worried the city it represented could be next. The Provençal historian J. P. Papon, for example, gave a stern warning on the risks of the war:

In an ordinary time, the precautions taken in Mediterranean ports to save us from the plague are enough to reassure even the most cautious individuals. However, the current war puts Europe and a part of Africa and Asia in a ferment, which could trouble the harmony of our customary general police and render useless the sanitary laws on which the health of nations rests; it would be imprudent to rely on a false sense of security. It is possible that in the midst of the universal agitation in which we live, the plague might creep into Europe in more than one way.[34]

Quarantine depended on knowledge, while blockade running and piracy relied on obfuscation. Quarantine rested on regular and predictable patterns of shipping; war made this impossible. Aside from Bonaparte's irregular landing in France on his return from the Egyptian Campaign (discussed in the Introduction), there are a few other scattered examples of the chaos of war allowing individuals to return to Europe without quarantine; in October 1798, a courier sent by Bonaparte from Egypt to Italy was permitted to disembark at Ancona without quarantine. So incensed were the Boards of Health of Marseille and Toulon that they not only quarantined all ships from southern Italy but also pressured all other northern Italian boards of health to follow suit.[35] Yet, as with the future Emperor himself, the robust responses to these irregularities set an enduring precedent. Aside from the plague of Noja, the plague did not penetrate the European mainland. Blind luck and enhanced vigilance by board members appear to have filled the gap.

Perhaps the biggest strain war imposed on the quarantine system was simply the increased traffic. Military conflicts in Egypt and Syria resulted in more individuals traveling back and forth across the *cordon sanitaire*. Planning the necessary quarantines for such a large number of soldiers and sailors was a highly complex undertaking, and managing the logistics of these military quarantines mobilized officials both in national capitals and in port cities. Should an entire army return at once, the resulting undertaking was comparable in scale to government efforts against cholera in a mid-size city. Military quarantines remain largely understudied, but the bureaucratic expertise gained by boards of health during such events clearly impinged directly on the history of quarantine during peacetime. If, as Catherine Kelly suggests, military medicine drove medical reform and professionalization in the early nineteenth century,[36] it

---

[34] Jean-Pierre Papon, *De la Peste*, 1:i–ii.

[35] Conservateurs de Santé to Talleyrand, 7 Brumaire, An 7 (October 28, 1798), AN (Paris) AE/B/ III/211.

[36] See Catherine Kelly, *War and the Militarization of British Army Medicine* (London: Pickering and Chatto, 2011).

is unsurprising that the experience of coordinating military quarantines forced sanitary administrations to reform timeworn early modern procedures. In the wake of the war, Mediterranean boards of health began to compromise on quarantine lengths, to reform the rotation system for sanitary guardians, and to reconceive the assignment of space in an era of expanded numbers. Military quarantines during and after the Napoleonic Wars helped administrators anticipate the dramatic increases in quarantine traffic that would come during the 1830s and 1840s.

Encounters between military and sanitary bureaucrats had ramifications for the rancorous contagion debate of the 1820s and 1830s. Though many ex-military men urged reform during these decades, in Britain at least, three of quarantine's most influential defenders were Sir Gilbert Blane, Sir James McGrigor, and Colin Chisholm, the head of the Navy Medical Board, the head of the newly formed Army Medical Board, and the military's one-time Inspector-General of Hospitals in the West Indies, respectively.[37] Military men featured prominently among those testifying before a Parliamentary Select Committee appointed to settle the contagion question in 1819. The precise details of plague epidemics experienced by British and French armies during campaigns in Egypt and Syria in the 1790s remained at the center of treatises about the plague throughout the nineteenth century.

The extraordinary volume of quarantine traffic experienced in the course of the Napoleonic Wars was not limited to ports like Marseille, which received an entire returning army. Ships often needed to perform (usually short) quarantines wherever convenient, meaning some very small ports might find themselves ministering to men-of-war docked nearby. Naval letters and records throughout the war contain frequent mentions of such quarantines.[38] Even after the war, the large number of soldiers present in the Mediterranean augmented quarantine traffic. Genoa's lazarettos, for example, normally handled only 200 to 400 people each year but, on one occasion in 1816, some 539 British servicemen sailing from Corfu performed quarantine there together during one particularly busy month.[39]

News of plague and outbreaks of ophthalmia among soldiers returning from the Egyptian Campaign led to fears of a more amorphous kind of contamination. "At present," observed the poet Robert Southey in 1807, "as the soldiers from Egypt have brought home with them broken limbs and ophthalmia, they carry an arm in a sling, or walk the streets with a green shade over their eyes." This invasion of Egyptian disease, he goes on to say, coincided with the popular

[37] See Harrison, *Contagion*, 57–58.
[38] For an example of such a letter, see Bob Hollowell to the Earl of Egmont, January 29, 1808, National Maritime Museum Archive, London, PER/1/56.
[39] William Keer Brown to the President of the Sanità, Genoa, October 16, 1816, ASGe Sanità 1365.

rage for Egyptian aesthetics and antiquities – Egyptomania. "Every thing [*sic*] must now be Egyptian: the ladies wear crocodile ornaments, and you sit upon a sphinx in a room hung round with mummies, and with the long black lean-armed long-nosed hieroglyphical men, who are enough to make the children afraid to go to bed."[40] Illness, here, is the flipside of Egyptian aesthetics – a connection that we will return to later. For now, it is sufficient to recognize the sense to which, in the 1800s, it seemed truly possible that the diseases of the "East" might invade and take root in Western Europe.

In the spirit of the 1820s, the threat posed by epidemic disease was a conceptual equivalent to the other dangers to European security that the Congress system sought to prevent. During the Napoleonic Wars, the threat of plague and the threat of military invasion were conceptually linked. In the pamphlet already discussed in which Marseille's Board of Health suggested the British planned to introduce the plague, the comparison is made explicit. "It is to be feared," they suggest, "that the irreconcilable enemy of France, from the depths of despair where it must be thanks to the failure of all its efforts against her, has conceived the diabolical stratagem of introducing on our territory the only plague which could defeat us."[41] Without the same explicit rumor at its base, the French mandate that all ships from British ports be treated as sanitarily suspect was based on identical logic; pathogenic and military threats to state security ran together.

In Britain, a similar line of thinking is evident in the work of the 1805 Board of Health (discussed below). This board acknowledged that the war was making Britain more vulnerable than ever to the importation of disease. It essentially suggested that the only way an epidemic could be defeated would be to turn lazaretto administration outward onto the entirety of Britain. In this way, they proposed the division of the country into districts (in the event of an epidemic), each patrolled by constables reporting to civil and military authorities.[42] Members of the recently suppressed radical London Corresponding Society would have been quick to sense a whiff of Pittite repression behind these proposals. Again, the Napoleonic Wars made it easy for regimes, fearing their own vulnerability, to assimilate political and medical threats.

This orientation, shared among all major European powers, was shaped by the real threats of disease that unfolded during the wars and the sense that the Mediterranean was a clear conduit through which epidemics could reach the European continent. In Britain itself, ships from anywhere in the Mediterranean (above all ones carrying enumerated goods) remained subject to the quarantine

---

[40] Quoted in Nigel Leask, *British Romantic Writers and the East* (Cambridge: Cambridge University Press, 1992), 1.
[41] *Conservation de la Santé Publique*, 4.   [42] *First Report of the Board of Health*, 10–11.

laws in the wake of the conflict. Opponents of the quarantine system liked to suggest that quarantine itself was imposed on Britain solely because of the dictates of Mediterranean commerce. Though this was part of the story, so too was a lingering sense well after the Napoleonic Wars that the Mediterranean itself was a risky sanitary zone.

Other legacies from that conflict also affected quarantine practice – the extension of French control, for example, down the entire northern Mediterranean coast (from the Pyrenees to Corfu) was accompanied by numerous temporary boards of health that sprung up in ports under French control. Like so many facets of Napoleon's administrative program, the quarantine laws were seen as an importable commodity in newly occupied territories – hence General Vaubois's declaration as the Governor of French Malta in 1798 that "the sanitary laws of Malta shall be neither more nor less rigorous than at Marseille."[43] French control facilitated standardization of procedures in the ports where it operated. Furthermore, the new boards set up in these ports were often composed of native quarantine officials who were assimilated into the new French sanitary administration and had access to French consular reports from across the Ottoman Empire. We could consider the case of Giovanni Vordoni, both a representative of the Greek Community in Trieste and a member of the Napoleonic *Conseil Central de Santé Maritime Séant à Trieste*, who kept the *Préfet* of Livorno apprised of a series of sanitary reform initiatives being undertaken in Ottoman Thessaly.[44] In other words, a Greek doctor and sometime Austrian quarantine official, served on a French board, received epidemic intelligence from a French consul in Greece, and sent it to an Italian official, also serving the French, in the once and future state of Tuscany. Many officials who conducted similar correspondence often remained in service when boards reverted out of French control. In the post-Napoleonic context they were endowed with a greater sense of the power of sharing information and contacts across the Mediterranean.

It is worth remembering that the unprecedented logistical, financial, and military demands of the Napoleonic Wars generated a spirit of bureaucratic experimentation – from new schemes of disbursing prize money, to new welfare systems for the wives of naval officers, to novel forms of taxation. It was during the wars, in 1800 and 1805, that the British government committed some £95,000 to building a lazaretto at Chetney Hill, in Kent, and allowed ships with foul bills of health to perform quarantine in Britain for the first time. It was also during the wars that an unprecedented expansion of smuggling by North Africans generated a coordinated sanitary response across southern European ports. Between 1800 and 1840, the number of quarantine ports across Europe

---

[43] Quoted in Panzac, *Quarantaines et Lazarets*, 170.
[44] See the Trieste correspondence in ASLi Sanità 594.

expanded dramatically. In this way, then, although lazarettos across Europe began to be dismantled in the late 1840s and early 1850s, the system was at its greatest extent just before its precipitous demise. The Revolutionary and Napoleonic Wars were the catalyst for this period of growth.

A Case Study of Epidemic Response: Britain's 1799 and 1805 Quarantine Committees

This phenomenon takes on greater meaning if we examine a clear trajectory in Britain, in which the epidemic threats of this era gave rise to urgent bureaucratic innovation. Twice during the Napoleonic Wars, governments controlled by William Pitt the Younger (responsible in so many other ways for the growth of the British state) convened extraordinary, national boards of health composed of eminent doctors and officials. The plans for sanitary security these committees advanced, though not fully put into action, set precedents for later efforts at disease control. They even provided blueprints for aspects of public health reform in the 1840s. In this way, the military-medical milieu of the Napoleonic Wars clearly influenced public health policy more than a generation later; the military context in 1799 and 1805 infuses the urgency and stringency of both boards' reports.

As we proceed, it will become obvious that quarantine administration in Britain was somewhat anomalous compared to Continental norms, though often this meant greater stringency, not the comparative lack of severity other historians have assumed. Here, for example, it is important to recall that, while most Mediterranean ports consigned their quarantine operations to a local board of health, in Britain, the Customs Service administered quarantine (again, under the ultimate direction of the Privy Council). For much of the nineteenth century, a Superintendent of Quarantine helped to coordinate the service at the different quarantine ports, but it was nevertheless the PC's ultimate responsibility to set quarantine lengths and admit ships to pratique. Though meeting registers demonstrate that quarantine was often discussed by Privy Councilors, this rigid national structure meant that, when specific threats emerged, Britain was particularly likely to rely on extraordinary or ad hoc committees to make recommendations to preoccupied politicians. At times, as we will see, Britain was forced to integrate its own procedures with Mediterranean norms, just as its citizens served on foreign boards of health (such as Genoa's), and its colonial administrators ran such boards in Gibraltar, Malta, and the Ionian Islands. At the turn of the nineteenth century, even in Britain itself, the traditional role of the PC did not appear suited to the new threats emerging from Spain, North Africa, and the Ottoman Empire. Consequently, in the first quarter of the century, no fewer than six extraordinary committees, parliamentary select committees, and delegations of the Royal

College of Physicians considered the issues of epidemic disease, contagion, and quarantine. The PC responded to such advice, though councilors were careful to retain their monopoly over more quotidian quarantine administration.

By the 1790s, the exigencies of commerce and war meant that it became a pressing need for Britain to come up with some way to avoid "double quarantine" by permitting ships with foul bills of health to perform a single quarantine in Britain (without an initial expurgation at a Mediterranean lazaretto). To facilitate this, Pitt finally convened a "Quarantine Committee" in 1799. This commission was chaired by Patrick Russell, who had served for eighteen years as a doctor at the British Factory in Aleppo and published the influential *Treatise of the Plague* (1791). Russell was joined by two elite doctors (one of them physician to the king), two representatives from the Levant Company, two Customs Commissioners, and Stephen Cottrell, the PC clerk. Thus, the membership of the Committee reflected the emerging view that quarantine was too diverse for one field of expertise. It depended on close coordination between merchants, doctors, bureaucrats, and politicians.

The Committee (assuming tasks conventionally within the purview of the PC) set the quarantine procedures for ships with foul bills whose captains had applied to land on the British coast. But it also conducted a wide-ranging inquiry of all realms of quarantine practice. Despite the ongoing war with France, the Committee cited procedures and traditions from Marseille approvingly in an effort to describe how Britain might create a permanent lazaretto of its own. Patrick Russell recommended that the British government dispatch two teams of investigators to further improve the workings of quarantine in British harbors – one team to the lazarettos of Livorno, where they could serve as temporary employees and bring back an intimate knowledge of procedure in one of the largest Mediterranean quarantine facilities, and another team to Constantinople, where they might observe the plague in its supposed home.[45]

Despite the concentration of elite doctors and bureaucrats among its membership, this Committee was clearly willing to think creatively and eager to align British practice with Mediterranean precedents. Even in the context of a consuming European war, the expansion and solidification of Britain's sanitary defenses demanded further integration and coordination with European countries. Furthermore, at a time when finances were being stretched for all activities other than the fighting, the commissioners continued to view quarantine as a legitimate object for the expenditure of relatively large sums of public money. The final recommendation of the Committee resulted in the 1800 Quarantine Act, which appropriated some £65,000 for a permanent lazaretto in Britain (to be built at Chetney Hill in

---

[45] Patrick Russell, "Report of the Quarantine Committee," April 2, 1800, British Library, London (henceforth, BL) Add. Ms. 38234, ff. 36–43.

Kent).[46] Indeed, perhaps this action set a precedent; whether or not the French government was conscious of the equivalence of its expenditures, in the face of new fears of yellow fever importation from Spain or across the Atlantic, it appropriated a roughly equivalent sum of 1.5 million francs (about £60,000)[47] for new lazarettos and sanitary improvements in its 1822 Quarantine Act.[48] On both sides of the Channel, then, the new epidemic challenges warranted a new kind of response.

At no time was this clearer than in the 1799 Quarantine Committee's most famous action: the reception of three ships from Mogador – the *Mentor*, the *Lark*, and the *Aurora*. Mogador, a port city in modern-day Morocco, had a reputation for being one of the unhealthiest ports on the North African coast.[49] It was well known that a plague had been raging there when the three ships departed, and though their crew members were all healthy, their cargoes included inward-facing goatskins, considered to be one of the goods most capable of harboring contagion.[50] Even unrolling the cargo to investigate further appeared dangerous, and the Quarantine Committee, after much discussion and consultation, issued an opinion that said the health of the realm depended on the complete destruction of the three ships. In January 1800, the PC acceded to this request and ordered that the *Mentor*, the *Lark*, and the *Aurora* "be forthwith carried out to sea, and there sunk in deep water, under the Direction and Inspection of one of His Majesty's Ships of War."[51] This was a drastic and controversial action; though specific elements of cargoes were occasionally burned when considered impossible to fumigate, to burn an entire ship was exceedingly rare. The episode was still debated decades later.[52] But whatever the merits of the decision, it is clear that quarantine had achieved so great a level of prestige that British commerce could tolerate such a controversial gesture. In a wartime era of irregular shipping patterns, it was necessary to project an air of sanitary invulnerability

---

[46] A further £30,000 was appropriated a few years later. Although the Chetney Hill Lazaretto it was supposed to fund was never completed, this meant that as early as 1805, Parliament had appropriated close to £100,000 for a quarantine institution. See C. F. Mullett, "A Century of English Quarantine, 1709–1825," *Bulletin of the History of Medicine* 23 (1949): 27.

[47] For an approximate conversion, I consulted Rodney Edvinsson's historical currency converter. See www.historicalstatistics.org/Currencyconverter.html (accessed February 12, 2019).

[48] Pierre-Louis Laget, "Les lazarets et l'émergence de nouvelles maladies pestilentielles au XIXᵉ et au début du XXᵉ siècle," *In Situ* 2 (2002): 6.

[49] See Booker, *Maritime Quarantine*, 273.

[50] Fibrous substances (like cotton, rugs, and fur) were always considered difficult to clean, but the skins surrounding the goat hairs appeared to make this cargo even more contagious as it was thought they could lock contagion inside the merchandise.

[51] Order in Council, Privy Council Meeting of January 7, 1800, TNA PC 2/154.

[52] See James Laidlaw, "Report on the Contagion of the Plague," *Edinburgh Medical and Surgical Journal* 68 (1847): 356.

and capability. The Committee specifically discussed the idea of maintaining public confidence in the quarantine system as a central reason for such drastic actions.

Despite the wishes of its members to retain the 1799 Committee as a permanent British Board of Health, the PC ordered its disbandment once the 1800 Quarantine Act had been set in motion. Only a few years later, however, Privy Councilors found themselves completely unprepared for the growing fears of yellow fever importation. As would be the case again in the 1830s, when an epidemic threat (in the form of cholera) challenged the status quo, councilors were pushed toward further experimentation.

In 1805, yellow fever hit the British colony of Gibraltar after five years in which tens of thousands had died in nearby Spanish ports. There were more reasons for concern about the importation of epidemic disease. Again, the venerable quarantine port of Livorno succumbed to yellow fever in 1804, and British troops continued to return from Egypt bearing tales of the plague. The conventional sanitary geography of Europe was thus being challenged in a way it had not been for decades. Extraordinary moments generated extraordinary responses, and it was against this background that the PC again convened a special board of health.[53]

This board was charged with producing a report on what to do should an epidemic ever breach British quarantine defenses and invade the metropole. There were grave doubts throughout the 1805 Gibraltar epidemic that it was indeed yellow fever and not a manifestation of plague from the Middle East. Also, a rise in the number of smugglers and privateers during the Napoleonic Wars gave the sense that many ships might evade quarantine and import an epidemic to Britain. Notwithstanding the passage of the 1800 Quarantine Act, Britons felt unprepared for these threats. Despite receiving more funds through another Quarantine Act in 1805, the promised lazaretto at Chetney Hill showed no signs of imminent completion – abandoned a few years later, the unfinished building would languish in the Kentish mud.

Facing this uncertainty, the board proposed a draconian program that would immediately go into effect should an epidemic ever breach Britain's borders. Set down at the height of the War of the Third Coalition, its plan clearly drew from precedents within military administration. On the declaration of an epidemic, Britain would be divided into "districts," each categorized as "sound" or "unsound." A team of three magistrates in each district would receive information from constables and watchmen who would be posted permanently at the doors of all infected houses and would patrol the neighborhood to detect new cases. Carriages and carts would be commandeered by constables and put to the

[53] On the summoning of this board, see Fraser Brockington, "Public Health at the Privy Council, 1805–6," *Medical History* 7, no. 1 (1963): 14–17.

use of transporting the dead and dying.[54] Mandatory fumigations and ventilations of infected houses would become routine.[55]

The Board acknowledged that these procedures might sound draconian, but in a lengthy disquisition, members suggested the public would eventually support them because they would allow anyone stricken with an illness to receive palliative care from the state (an important signal of an argument we explore further later in this book – concern about foreign epidemics was a central, and neglected, progenitor of public health reform). Yet, the Board expected something in return: convalescent patients would be expected to join the vast bureaucracy required by the new sanitary system (by driving carts, fumigating homes, and caring for patients) – a novel social contract of the plague in which private property and private interest would be surrendered to the public good. The PC endorsed the vast majority of the Board's recommendations and forwarded copies of them to British magistrates and to a number of colonial governors.[56] This report may have been nothing more than a thought experiment, but it helped formulate an administrative repertoire that would prove long-lasting.

Epidemic diseases were hotly debated and poorly understood. The 1805 Board's reports offered a frank acknowledgment of the problem of operating in a state of sanitary ignorance. The science behind fumigation, members conceded, was murky at best. Each procedure had its defenders. Given this, board members recommended a mixture of washing, airing, and disinfecting that, one way or another, would "clean" infected rooms. In this way, board members were relying on both "anticontagionist/miasmatist" and "contagionist/quarantinist" impulses in their set of prescriptions.[57] Most importantly, given that the very identity of the disease that might hit Britain remained unknown, the Board devised a novel solution. "It should be observed," they began their *First Report*:

That the following regulations are founded chiefly on experience in what has been called the Plague, by way of pre-eminence, or the Plague of the Levant. But as no disease can be said to equal, still less to exceed this, in its infectious and fatal nature; it is not unreasonable to presume, that the precautions, which have been found sufficient to guard against that, would likewise be effectual against … any other contagious and mortal distemper.[58]

Here, the Board was responding to the confusion of the beginning of the Napoleonic crisis of public health. The plague itself was poorly known given

---

[54] *First Report of the Board of Health* (London: William Bulmer, 1805), 10–11.
[55] *Second Report of the Board of Health* (London: William Bulmer, 1805), 4–7.
[56] Booker, *Maritime Quarantine*, 299.
[57] And thus, prefiguring a pattern that Peter Baldwin demonstrates was adopted by European governments during the cholera epidemics. See Baldwin, *Contagion and the State*, chapter 3.
[58] *First Report*, 2.

that its etiology was a subject of contestation, its symptoms differed among those stricken, and its nature remained obscure to most British doctors. But, as the most basic form of pestilence, it offered a set of precedents that were very well known. This is an illustration of how, around the turn of the nineteenth century, epidemic diseases came to be consolidated into a general type – a fast-spreading, devastating, atypical sort of illness. Not least because of historical experience, it was a genre that many associated with the plague.[59] Here, then, as elsewhere, the Napoleonic public health crisis helped reaffirm and reinvigorate the sanitary practices of the previous century in a new context.

The continuing importance of the plague explains why plague-based Mediterranean quarantine retained such influence on the development of public health policies in Europe for the next half-century. The continuation of epidemic threats over the next three decades ensured that the 1805 Board's vision retained influential power even though it was never fully put into action. In 1831, when a Central Board of Health was created to organize the British response to cholera, the 1805 Board was named as the specific inspiration.[60] The early nineteenth-century public health crisis inspired bureaucratic experimentation and set lasting precedents.

If the Revolutionary and Napoleonic Wars were the "first total war," it should not surprise us that the Marseille Board of Health could cast France's military antagonists as literally "pestiferous," as they did in the pamphlet with which this chapter began. And yet, even as the conflict drove European nations apart, it simultaneously unleashed subterranean moves toward integration, particularly when it came to quarantine practice. Modern quarantine took shape in an era when the state began to expand dramatically and when novel bureaucracies emerged in response to the exigencies of war and epidemic crisis. Though in form and substance it resembled what had come before, it operated according to new assumptions and in response to new threats. It functioned as a system, in which different authorities agreed to operate according to shared standards, to make order out of chaos, without an external dictate. The "universal agitation" of the first fifteen years of the nineteenth century helped transform quarantine into a cohesive system after the peace.

---

[59] On the assimilation of yellow fever and plague as a means of making quarantine practice more global, see Arner, "Making Commerce Global," 788–92. On the uses of the conflation of these two diseases in American medical argument, see Thomas Apel, *Feverish Bodies, Enlightened Minds: Science and the Yellow Fever Controversy in the Early American Republic* (Stanford, CA: Stanford University Press, 2016), 55–59.

[60] Brockington, "Public Health," 13.

In an era when international law barely existed, when "free-born Englishmen" proudly proclaimed their distinction from those held in the thrall of Continental officialdom, precisely six administrative bodies run by European governments were given the power of life and death over British subjects. These were the lazaretto staff members and boards of health at the quarantine ports of Malta, Venice, Messina, Livorno, Genoa, and Marseille. Again, the British Quarantine Act of 1753 set out the unusual situation in which ships with foul bills of health were subject to a "double quarantine" of initial purification in the Mediterranean and final expurgation on the British coast. The law reveals a growing sense of implicit trust among sanitary bureaucrats based in rival nations. The sign-off of a French, Maltese, or Italian quarantine official was thus an essential document for a ship subject to this law, and British medical officers accepted the word of their Mediterranean colleagues without question. Even in a period of recurrent wars, then, trust was sufficient that officials at these ports would operate according to transnational understandings of prophylactic rigor.

In Chapter 1, we explored how the period around the turn of the nineteenth century was marked simultaneously by tremendous Mediterranean upheaval *and* the remarkable durability of long-standing systems such as quarantine. The 1790s and 1800s also represented a significant increase in British involvement in the Middle Sea. If the animating concern of this book is the relationship between a robust quarantine system and an expanding imperial power, Chapter 2 seeks to give shape to the plane on which that relationship transpired. This was a "British Mediterranean world," a space that had both a cartographical reality and an imaginative geography. The notion of such a world began to form in the eighteenth century,[1] but it took on its most robust form in the time period considered by this book. It was not an exclusively imperial space; in addition to colonies, it encompassed trade routes, communication networks, and long-standing expatriate communities. Quarantine helps to reveal the contours of

---

[1] See Tristan Stein, "Passes and Protection in the Making of a British Mediterranean," *Journal of British Studies* 54, no. 3 (2015): 602–31.

this politico-economic-diplomatic entity. After all, to the extent that the Mediterranean retained regional coherence in the nineteenth century, it is because the sea was so often crossed. As a barrier that mediated such crossings, quarantine was deeply implicated in the diplomatic, military, and political realities of the early nineteenth-century Mediterranean world.

As the anthropologist Naor Ben-Yahoyada has noted, "Mediterranean modernity" can seem like a contradiction in terms with typical hallmarks of a shared Mediterranean culture seen as emphatically premodern.[2] Certainly the growing political and economic inequalities between northern and southern coasts of the Middle Sea in the nineteenth century challenge the sense that it consisted of a unified region of world history. Yet, in this chapter, I demonstrate how the idea of the "British Mediterranean" elucidates the persistence of Mediterranean dynamism and interchange in an era simultaneously marked by nationalism and imperial exploitation. Throughout this book, the cacophonous exchange among Mediterranean diplomats, travelers, health boards, and ship captains of different flags resembles the metaphor of "frogs round a pond," which Plato ascribed to Socrates, and which Peregrine Horden and Nicholas Purcell use to encapsulate the persistent urge to portray the Mediterranean as a unity.[3] In considering a "British Mediterranean," however, rather than simply discussing the British *in* the Mediterranean, I am suggesting not only that the region came to be seen as a particular sphere within the broader British world, but also that it existed alongside an acknowledgment that success in the Mediterranean depended on adaptation and coexistence.[4]

Especially in the first half of the nineteenth century, the period at the heart of this book, Britons accommodated themselves to Mediterranean patterns even as they hoped for vast gains. In increasing numbers, British merchants expected abundant return from untapped markets, British radicals and liberals flocked to Mediterranean causes, Anglican divines sought inspiration from the Holy Land, and travelers of all sorts, who had the means, embraced the convenience, warmth, and exoticism of travel to the Middle Sea.[5] Well aware of its Latin meaning as the "center of the world," British thinkers recognized its pivotal position among intersecting networks of imperial concern. Yet, in a region where their power was comparative, rather than absolute, British strategists

---

[2] See Naor Ben-Yahoyada, "Mediterranean Modernity," in *A Companion to Mediterranean History*, ed. Peregrine Horden and Sharon Kinoshita (Hoboken, NJ: Wiley-Blackwell, 2014), 107–21.

[3] Horden and Purcell, *Corrupting Sea*, part 1.

[4] Indeed, in her analysis of British Mediterranean trade during the Napoleonic Era, Katerina Galani deems "successful adaptation" as the key source for economic success. See Galani, *British Shipping in the Mediterranean during the Napoleonic Wars* (Leiden, Netherlands: Brill, 2017).

[5] On the growing attraction of travel across the Mediterranean travel during the nineteenth century, see John Pemble, *The Mediterranean Passion* (Oxford: Clarendon Press, 1987).

envisioned Mediterranean gains that would require multilingual, multiconfessional negotiation.

Many of the great characters in Braudel's portrait of the dynamic early modern Mediterranean had a long senescence and a sudden finale. One can certainly speak of the "decline of Venice" in the seventeenth century,[6] but that Mediterranean superpower persisted as a venerable political entity until the storm of Napoleon's march across Italy in 1797. So, too, the Serene Republic of Genoa, which was destined first to become a French province under the First Empire and then a second city to Turin in the newly expanded post-1815 buffer state of Piedmont-Sardinia. Malta, famous for its impregnable resistance against the Ottoman Fleet in 1565, remained under the control of the Knights of St. John for hundreds of years, but succumbed to Napoleon's forces in 1798 without much of a fight.

Into the new Mediterranean order stepped the British, returning to shores whose commercial possibilities had long been known. English merchant communities in cities such as Livorno were long-standing, and the Levant Company, which had rivaled the East India Company in the seventeenth century, still trundled along, despite a dramatic decline in its trading volume. The picture changed from the onset of the Revolutionary Wars. Well before the outbreak of hostilities in 1792, Levant Company members were attuned to the possibility that a European war might restore the seventeenth-century strength their organization had once enjoyed. Indeed, the collapse of the French carrying trade and the extension of the British Empire in the Mediterranean over the course of the broader 1792–1815 conflict captivated the attention of diplomats, politicians, and strategists. It continued to do so after the Congress of Vienna. In a post-1815 map of Europe where conservative stasis threatened to entrench regimes across the Continent, the Mediterranean (on all of its coasts) remained in flux.

Britain became a Mediterranean superpower in the nineteenth century, but preponderance in Mediterranean trade, politics, and diplomatic heft did not mean dominance. This was a unique zone of British power, and as we will see in this chapter, the equivocal nature of British gains served as grist for the mill of even greater expectations. At the same time, the Mediterranean's historical associations (to the world of the Bible and that of Greece and Rome) inspired a set of cultural fantasies that became nineteenth-century fads. It is instructive to note just how many nineteenth-century cultural preoccupations were linked to Mediterranean locales: philhellenism, Egyptomania, a growing preoccupation with the Holy Land, neoclassicism, Orientalist painting, and political movements from Garibaldism to Urquhartism. Concurrent with new

---

[6] See, for example, Alberto Tenenti, *Piracy and the Decline of Venice, 1580–1615*, trans. Janet and Brian Pullan (Berkeley: University of California Press, 1967).

assessments of their potential centrality in future Mediterranean developments, then, Britons of all kinds ventured southward and eastward: diplomats, imperial officials, artists, writers, commercial strategists, merchants, doctors, speculators, missionaries, and engineers. Alongside British imperial subjects on Mediterranean islands (Maltese, Gibraltairians, and Ionian Greeks in the period considered here), these constitute the personnel of what I am calling the "British Mediterranean world."

It was a cohesive world, but one with a diverse coterie of inhabitants. A liberal philhellenist drawn to the Mediterranean during the Greek War of Independence (1821–29) may have shared little with a military Governor of Corfu; an emissary of the Church Missionary Society was cut from different cloth than a radical doctor performing experiments in Constantinople. Yet, there were simultaneously ties that bound the British Mediterranean together. One was an expatriate sensibility developed from engagement with the same sources and deference to the same authorities (long-established diplomats in Mediterranean ports and well-known merchant houses). British travelers in the Mediterranean were largely within reach of *Galignani's Messenger*, an English language newspaper published twice daily in Paris with excerpts of news stories from around the Continent. Mail from home arrived in a few short weeks.

Furthermore, the British Mediterranean was a united conceptual web because dreams hatched in and around the Middle Sea shared similar structures. Connectivity itself united different genres of thought about the region. The Mediterranean sat in the geographic center of the British imperial world; a midpoint in Britain's "swing to the East," situated halfway between North America and India. As a potential strategic bridge, it united different regions of acute commercial, strategic, and imaginative concern. Symbolism accrued easily to Mediterranean events, due to Biblical legacies and historical resonance. In this chapter, we consider the motivations behind outward journeys and also how the Mediterranean was consumed back home. It is the substance of journeys to the Middle Sea, plans hatched surrounding it, and connections forged therein that defined the British Mediterranean World and it is here, by way of quarantine, that we explore its contours. Though quarantine is the leitmotif of the chapter, it is so in no small part because of the imbrication of its own history with the history of broader British ambitions in the Middle Sea.

Quarantine, Strategy, and the Post-Napoleonic Mediterranean Order

Over the course of the eighteenth century, the British presence in the Mediterranean had waxed until it waned. Gibraltar had been a British colony since the Peace of Utrecht in 1713 and Menorca fell successively into and out of

British control until 1802. But the dominance of the French Navy and merchant marine in the Middle Sea limited British political and commercial penetration. The Worshipful Company of Merchants Trading to the Levant Seas (better known as the Levant Company) had been founded in 1586, but its seventeenth-century gains dwindled after 1700 thanks to French advances and the collapse of the Persian silk trade.

Despite a meager volume of trade and a Mediterranean Empire limited to the far western part of the Middle Sea, British strategists in the 1760s and 1770s dreamed big. One anonymous author imagined a large merchant marine fleet in the Mediterranean as an essential "nursery" for naval power that could be projected around the world. Writing in 1766, he noted how French dominance of the carrying trade and overwhelming advantage in the number of cross-Mediterranean traders had made their position nearly unassailable. "Perhaps a new war only," the author mulled, could reduce the French advantage to a point where the British could take advantage.[7] In fact, soon after war broke out between Britain and Revolutionary France in 1792, Lord Hawkesbury (President of the Board of Trade and the future first Lord Liverpool) initiated an inquiry into the nature of the decline of Britain's Levant trade, perhaps with new confidence that the war might bring a reconfiguration to Britain's benefit. The records of the same inquiry show that Hawkesbury paid significant attention to quarantine as he considered Britain's cross-Mediterranean trade. He focused on complaints from Levant Company merchants that British quarantine laws exposed their ships to lengthy delays and that Britain's lack of a major land-based lazaretto capable of receiving ships with foul bills of health put them at a disadvantage compared to other Mediterranean powers (a moment of political attention that was part of the build up to Britain's major Quarantine Act of 1800).[8] At this early stage, then, official thought dedicated to Mediterranean mobility intersected with official thought dedicated to quarantine. Understanding the system that mediated Mediterranean contact was essential to broader Mediterranean strategy.

Many recognized that the Napoleonic Wars offered the British suggestive opportunities for new projects of colonization as well as commerce. In 1796 and 1798, Mark Wood (a "nabob" enriched by his time as a surveyor and landowner in India and now an MP for the rotten borough of Gatton) wrote to Prime Minister William Pitt and War Secretary Henry Dundas alerting them to "the importance of Malta."[9] As a surveyor, Wood emphasized the geographical ties that bound the Empire together, and in Malta, he recognized a territory (and a region) with outsized importance due to its "middle" situation between

[7] Anonymous, *Considerations on the Nurseries for British Seamen* [1766], 10–11.
[8] Charles Jenkinson, "Causes of Decline of the Turkey Trade," BL Add. Ms. 38353 f. 84.
[9] Mark Wood, *The Importance of Malta Considered in the Years 1796 and 1798* (London: John Stockdale, 1803).

Europe and imperial spheres of power in India. British control of the islands, he predicted, "would give us completely the command of the Levant."[10] It was "another Gibraltar," one aimed eastward rather than westward, and the key to naval greatness far beyond Mediterranean shores.[11] When, during the abortive Peace of Amiens (1802–3), the British government promised to relinquish control of Malta,[12] Wood expostulated by publishing his letters for the broader public.

Wood's thinking was shared by a generation of diverse strategists. After hostilities resumed, with Malta still in British hands, the author and government clerk Granville Penn argued that an expanded Mediterranean Fleet based at Malta would be "guarding the whole of the Levant, and effectually controlling the naval movements of France."[13] Perhaps the most significant argument for Malta's contribution to the Empire came from the commercial writer John Galt. Writing in 1812, as British fortunes turned in the Peninsular War and further Mediterranean power seemed assured, Galt suggested that "in Malta ... we may be said to possess a fulcrum, on which we might construct engines sufficient to move the whole Mahomedan world."[14] Beyond the political and commercial effects along the Mediterranean coastline, others argued that new colonies might mitigate threats to Britain's growing Empire in South Asia. Admiral Nelson was widely quoted as remarking that Malta constituted an ideal "outwork to India," a lynchpin within a global network.[15]

Just as fantasies of global connection grew around the colonial acquisition of Malta, as we know from the last chapter, a major revision to the quarantine laws occurred in the pivotal years of 1799 and 1800. After years of debate, the "floating lazaretto" (consisting of decommissioned Royal Navy ships) at Stangate Creek was finally designated a "foul bill" station, capable of receiving ships coming from Mediterranean ports where plague epidemics raged.[16] The entire Mediterranean Basin was left within the zone of suspicion, given that ships from Southern Europe were still (for the most part) required to undergo quarantine. Again, until this rule changed in 1827, Britain's quarantine regulations were harsher than those of most Continental powers. While deviations from the letter of

---

[10] Ibid., 7.   [11] Ibid., 5–6.

[12] This was a promise that was not kept and one of the reasons for the resumption of hostilities in May 1803.

[13] Granville Penn, *The Policy and Interest of Great Britain with Respect to Malta, Summarily Considered* (London: J. Brettell, 1805), 16.

[14] John Galt, *Voyages and Travels in the Years 1809, 1810, and 1811* (London: T. Cadell and W. Davies, 1812), 121.

[15] Quoted in C. A. Bayly, *Imperial Meridian: The British Empire and the World, 1780–1830* (New York: Longman, 1989), 103.

[16] John Booker provides a lengthy history of the debates surrounding this policy in his chapter on "the foul bill dilemma." See Booker, *Maritime Quarantine*, chapter 8.

the law exempted some ships,[17] especially in the midst of the Napoleonic public health crisis, the Mediterranean as a whole continued to appear medically threatening (a reputation it had gained in the eighteenth century thanks to the memory of the plague of Marseille). The 1799 and 1800 Acts were passed at a time of real fear that epidemic disease (plague or yellow fever) could reach Britain from the south and east. These laws were designed both to manage a future in which more and more ships reached Britain from the Middle Sea and to level the playing field for British merchants who envied Continental competitors' access to more convenient quarantine facilities.

The Napoleonic Wars set a pattern in which the Mediterranean loomed more centrally within British military strategy. Beyond major victories at the Battle of the Aboukir Bay (1799) and the Battle of Trafalgar (1805), the British were impelled toward the Mediterranean (in particular, its eastern edge) as a means of evading Napoleon's commercial blockade. When the dust settled after 1815, a new insular empire began to take shape, with crucial nodes in Malta and Corfu. It was from such places, strategists hoped, that broader projections of power might be possible (Figure 2.1). Indeed, even beyond the 1815 settlement, the Napoleonic conflict had revealed tantalizing glimpses of even greater power. Had events turned out differently, the short-lived "Anglo-Corsican Kingdom" might have been a permanent feature of imperial maps.[18] Almost two decades later, Sir William Bentinck's occupation of Sicily (1806–14) inspired numerous British enthusiasts with the hope that that island, too, could be a permanent seat of British power.[19] The potential colony, enthused the military traveler George Cockburn, was "worth six West Indies islands."[20]

After 1815, new British gains may have been limited to Malta and the Ionian Islands, but in contrast to the rest of Europe, where borders were tightened during the conservative reaction, upheavals in the Mediterranean roused the imaginations of authors, diplomats, and strategists. This unsettled situation further captivated liberals and radicals already drawn to the area for its historic and Romantic associations. From Spain's Liberal Triennium of 1820–23, to the

---

[17] For evidence of deviation from the letter of the Quarantine Act of 1800, see the testimony of Charles Saunders before the 1824 Select Committee. 1824 Select Committee, *Report on the Foreign Trade of the Country: Quarantine*, 56.

[18] This entity was founded due to cooperation between the Corsican leader Pasquale Paoli and the Royal Navy and was headed by the Scottish politician and future Governor General of India, Sir Gilbert Elliot. It collapsed after the British withdrawal in October 1796.

[19] Edward Blaquiere envisioned an "intimate alliance" rather than a formal colonial relationship. See Blaquiere, *Letters from the Mediterranean* (London: Henry Colburn, 1813), 2:122. Bentinck himself called his vision of British colonization of Sicily a "philosophic dream." See Lucy Riall, *Under the Volcano: Revolution in a Sicilian Town* (Oxford: Oxford University Press, 2013), 48.

[20] George Cockburn, *A Voyage to Cadiz and Gibraltar, up the Mediterranean to Sicily and Malta, in 1810 & 11* (London: J. Harding, 1815), 1:vi.

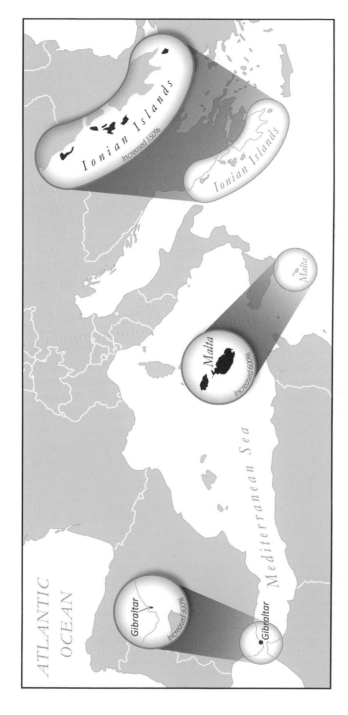

Figure 2.1 Britain's Mediterranean Empire, 1814–64. Map designed by the University of Wisconsin–Madison Cartography Lab.

first stirrings of the Greek War of Independence, radical thinkers such as Edward Blaquiere and the Benthamite John Bowring became entrenched in Mediterranean causes. It should not be at all surprising that a man such as Bowring, whose political career began with a fascination for Mediterranean politics, became the chief antagonist of the quarantine laws in Parliament in the 1830s and 1840s.

Opponents of quarantine, both in the nineteenth century and in more recent historiography, have been accused of basing their opposition on an instinctive defense of commerce and a support for free trade. For some, this holds true, yet in many cases, such explanations are limited. Quarantine practice was under-girded by the traditions and administrative practices of the Old Regime; in many cases, liberals and revolutionaries were opposing the very governments dedicated to enforcing the system. The instinctive sense that quarantine offended a nebulous concept of "English freedom" was at least partially informed and enhanced by the ubiquity of quarantine practice in France, Spain, Austria, and the Italian states. This should help us understand the evident anti-Catholicism inherent in many tracts written to oppose quarantine and the doctrine of epidemic contagion.[21]

Napoleon's Continental System, never very effective in halting British trade with the Continent, actually had a salutary effect on the fortunes of the Levant traders. Until 1808, as one official noted, the Levant Company had depended on a government subsidy, so slim were its profits. After that year, a sustained increase in trade made the subsidy unnecessary; Company accounts achieved a surplus ("a desideratum never before accomplished").[22] The spike in income continued, even accelerated, after the peace of 1815 (notwithstanding a brief dip during the postwar contraction). According to figures from a Company official, by 1822 the value of British exports to the Levant totaled some £972,000, a figure that rose to £1.4 million in 1824. The cotton trade had ballooned from a few hundred thousand pounds (in weight) of imports in the

---

[21] Charles Maclean echoed a long-standing anticontagionist canard that the Pope (with the assistance of the doctor Fracastorius) had invented the doctrine of contagion to frighten the Council of Trent. After its invention in the sixteenth century, he wrote, it was "maintained, by the influence of the oligarchs, to cover the disastrous effects of their own ascendancy, in the nineteenth." Maclean, *Specimens of Systematic Misrule: Or, Immense Sums Annually Expended in Upholding a Single Imposture, Discoveries of the Highest Importance to All Mankind Smothered, and Injustice Perpetrated, for Reasons of State* (London: H. Hay, 1820), xxix and xxxv. On the eighteenth-century origins of this idea, see Catherine Kelly, "'Not from the College, but through the Public and the Legislature': Charles Maclean and the Relocation of Medical Debate in the Early Nineteenth Century," *Bulletin of the History of Medicine* 82, no. 3 (2008): 555–56. For an example of a treatise by a less polemic writer repeating Maclean's assertion, see T. Forster, *Essay on the Origin, Symptoms, and Treatment of Cholera Morbus, and of Other Epidemic Disorders, with a View to the Improvement of Sanitary Regulations* (London: Keating and Brown, 1831), 28.

[22] Memorandum of George Liddell, BL Add. Ms. 59266, ff. 110–17.

immediate aftermath of the Napoleonic Wars to 1.2 million lbs. in 1823 and 7.9 million in 1824.[23]

The immediate prelude to the revocation of the Levant Company's charter in 1825, then, was a period of growth and optimism. While some scholars have interpreted its extinction as a long-delayed consequence of eighteenth-century decline, the Company was clearly a victim of its own success.[24] Foreign Secretary George Canning embraced the possibilities for expanded commercial interaction that an "open" trade would represent and considered the end of the Levant Company as part of a "complete change of system" for Britain's engagement with the Middle East.[25]

An essential part of that new system was a reformed organization of quarantine. The expanded possibilities for trade in this period of Mediterranean flux, along with the efforts of the radical doctor Charles Maclean at publicizing anticontagionist etiology (of which more below) lay behind Parliament's decision to appoint select committees in 1819 and 1824 to examine the doctrine of contagion, the quarantine laws, and their relation to trade with the Middle East. In his testimony to the 1824 Committee, the Levant Company merchant Samuel Briggs fervently emphasized his belief that a reduction of quarantine rates paired with a diminution in the mandated number of days of detention would dramatically augment the already surging Levant trade. This would be the opportunity, he confirmed to Parliament, both to invest in quarantine infrastructure and reform the procedures required.[26] Testimony of this kind was persuasive; in 1825, less than three decades since the last major reforms to quarantine, a major, new Quarantine Act was passed that remained on the books until the 1890s. In the wake of its passing, the Privy Council exempted French, Italian, Spanish, and Maltese ports from quarantine. The PC was granted the authority to abrogate quarantine for ships coming from "Turkey or Barbary" with clean bills of health, if it chose. More significantly still, the government assumed the exorbitant cost of paying the quarantine dues required of ships on arrival in British ports.[27] This was a notable expense and

---

[23] Figures derived from Levant Company, *Proceedings Respecting the Surrender of Their Charters* (London: J. Darling, 1825).

[24] Here I am referring in particular to Ralph Davis's assessment that the late eighteenth century represented the Company's "final plunge to insignificance." See Davis, *Aleppo and Devonshire Square: English Traders in the Levant in the Eighteenth Century* (London: Macmillan, 1967), 22. More dynamic visions of the institutions of the Levant Company in its later period are presented in Ina S. Russell, "The Later History of the Levant Company, 1753–1825," PhD diss., Manchester University, 1935, and more recently, Despina Vlami, *Trading with the Ottomans: The Levant Company in the Middle East* (New York: I. B. Tauris, 2014).

[25] See G. Liddell to Lord Grenville, April 18, 1824, BL Add. Ms. 59266.

[26] 1824 *Select Committee Report*, 27.

[27] For a more detailed summary of the content of this law and the Order in Council in which it was implemented, see Booker, *Maritime Quarantine*, 401–3 and 442–43.

represented a clear government commitment not only to the provision of a form of public health but also to the continued success of the Levant trade.

If the twin actions, however, of revising the quarantine laws and opening up the Levant trade seemed like a new beginning in 1825, it quickly became clear that expectations would have to be tempered. Despite the changes, less cotton was imported at the end of the 1820s than had been at that decade's beginning. In 1826, only a year after promising a "complete change of system," George Canning confronted the complex web of British consuls and vice-consuls serving in Middle Eastern cities and threw up his hands at the jumble. His instructions, according to the Foreign Office's John Bidwell, were that "for the present, the whole of the Establishment in the Levant should continue on the same footing on which it had been maintained, and with the same Jurisdiction which it had enjoyed under the late Levant Company."[28] Though the consular system was eventually revised, here and at other times, the kind of root and branch reforms imagined by Mediterranean strategists rarely unfolded as grandly as they were conceived. So, too, with quarantine. After Britain was hit with retaliatory quarantines in Continental Europe, the PC indefinitely tabled the most ambitious reform of the 1825 Act, which could have exempted all ships with clean bills of health from quarantine.

Despite growing disenchantment with quarantine across Europe (due to its failure to stop the cholera epidemics of the 1830s), it was not until the end of the 1830s that a serious effort emerged to challenge the status quo. In the summer of 1838, France attempted to organize an international conference to standardize and reduce quarantine lengths.[29] Though the proposed sanitary conference did not take place at this time, it gained the tentative support of both the Austrian and British governments. The proposal inaugurated a twelve-year period during which both France and Britain gradually reduced their quarantine requirements, now sure that, given Austrian Chancellor Klemens von Metternich's approval and an apparent change of heart among the governments of Italy, there would be no more retaliatory quarantines. More significant for the argument of this chapter is the fact that this renewed attempt to reduce the burden of quarantine occurred in the midst of new Mediterranean upheaval and the region's growing importance in new global networks of communication. Seen in this light, Britain's reformist stance in sanitary diplomacy depended far more on contemporaneous attention to Mediterranean strategy than it did on ideology.[30] This is an important distinction. Historians have (almost

---

[28] John Bidwell to John Cartwright, April 20, 1826, TNA SP 105/343.

[29] On this initiative, see F. J. Martínez, "International or French? The Early International Sanitary Conferences and France's Struggle for Hegemony in the Mid-Nineteenth Century Mediterranean," *French History* 30, no. 1 (2016): 82.

[30] Here, in particular, I am questioning John Booker's interpretation that British zeal to pursue such an international conference owed primarily to the advance of anticontagionism, the

universally) argued that British liberalism created a national predisposition against the maintenance or expansion of quarantine requirements. While liberal imperatives *did* impel certain doctors and politicians to oppose quarantine, the political energy required to actually change policy came about primarily during occasions when a potential strategic imperative in the Mediterranean inspired a sense that a reform of cross-Mediterranean trade was especially desirable.

The "Eastern Question" is habitually defined as an anxiety, in British political and diplomatic circles, that the Ottoman Empire could disintegrate to the advantage of the Russians. It is a long-standing shorthand for the variety of concerns British diplomats felt about engagement in the Eastern Mediterranean, yet in the late 1830s, the "question of the Orient" was a more dominant phrase. This referred to the aggressive posture taken by the Pasha of Egypt (Mohammed Ali), and the possibility that he might establish his Ottoman province as an independent state that would supplant the remainder of the Ottoman Empire as the dominant regional power. Between 1831 and 1839, Ali's son Ibrahim Pasha had established Egyptian control over the Ottoman provinces of Syria and Lebanon and was threatening to invade Anatolia. Ministers of France's July Monarchy vaunted the prospects of Ali and encouraged Britain's Whigs to think similarly.[31] With Britain in a position to ally decisively with either side (given its Mediterranean Fleet conveniently located at Malta), it finally seemed that an insular Mediterranean Empire might pay off in strategic dividends, that partnership with the victorious party could result in a lucrative trade deal and economic partnership. And who should then emerge on the scene but John Bowring – dogged advocate of quarantine reform in Parliament, veteran of Mediterranean causes in the 1820s, and now Foreign Secretary Lord Palmerston's personal envoy to Egypt.[32]

Bowring was immediately taken with Mohammed Ali. To Palmerston, he referred to him as "him of the eye of lion – the voice of music – the beard of snow."[33] Captivated by Ali's industrial reforms and efforts to modernize state administration, Bowring was bitterly disappointed by Palmerston's decision to back up the Sultan. At the same time, Palmerston himself was clearly intrigued by the promise of Ottoman renewal and a believer in the possibility that the

impending imposition of quarantine in Ottoman ports, and fears that renewed plague epidemics in the Black Sea region would result in harsher quarantine everywhere. See Booker, *Maritime Quarantine*, chapter 15.

[31] P. E. Caquet has recently suggested that French enthusiasm for Ali derived from his "Napoleonic" character and a series of unresolved legacies of the Egyptian Campaign. See Caquet, "The Napoleonic Legend and the War Scare of 1840," *International History Review* 35, no. 4 (2013): 702–22.

[32] On Bowring's mission, see G. F. Bartle, "Bowring and the Near Eastern Crisis of 1838–1840," *English Historical Review* 79, no. 313 (1964): 761–74.

[33] Bowring to Palmerston, November 28, 1837, TNA FO 78/373.

Tanzimat reforms (initiated in 1839) would lead to a positive restructuring of the Ottoman state.

In this way, at the precise occasion when Britain and France were discussing the initiative to have an international sanitary conference, both nations were positioning themselves at the center of major political upheaval in the Middle East. Furthermore, British strategists were renewing arguments that the Eastern Mediterranean was a crucial zone through which Britain's expanding empire could be drawn together. Thomas Waghorn, a retired Lieutenant from the Royal Navy, devoted several years spent in the Egyptian desert in the mid-1830s to organizing the so-called Overland Route.[34] This system, operational from 1837, enabled travelers and letters from India to reach Britain via the overland transit of Egypt. Waghorn set up a circuit of coaches, horses, and resting stops between Suez and Cairo, onward travel to Alexandria, and then a cross-Mediterranean trip crossing back to England either by sea voyage or across the European continent. Compared with a retrospective evaluation of its merits, the import of Waghorn's system lay more in anticipation, on the way it looked on a map. In its original instantiation, it ran only until 1842. Nevertheless, in promising to convert the typical 16,000 mile journey around the Cape of Good Hope to a shorter trip of 6,000 miles, the Overland Route proved one more way the Mediterranean served as a mid-imperial hub, capable of linking British worlds together (Figure 2.2). Such a system made the gratuitous length of quarantine even more provoking to policy makers. I explore the end of universal quarantine in more detail in Chapter 9, but for now, readers should note that, yet again in the 1840s, pressure toward reform coincided with strategic and commercial imperatives in the Mediterranean.

The Colonial Mediterranean (and Beyond)

Thus far, we have seen how momentum for revising the laws of quarantine occurred at moments of Mediterranean upheaval. In most of these examples, Britain pushed for a reformist approach that would make quarantine shorter. It is equally important to note that, particularly prior to the 1850s, sometimes the currents of the British Mediterranean pushed the other way: toward greater severity. In quarantine matters and beyond, officials posted to Mediterranean colonies recognized the potential for dramatic gains, but realized simultaneously that they were constrained by the region's rules.

[34] Waghorn's Overland Route became active only in the late 1830s, but consular records suggest that the East India Company considered opening such a route considerably earlier. In 1829, for example, the Foreign Office contacted all British consuls in the Middle East to alert them that the EIC would be conducting an inquiry in the hope of establishing such a route themselves. See John Bidwell to Peter Abbott, December 29, 1829, TNA FO 78/185, f. 246.

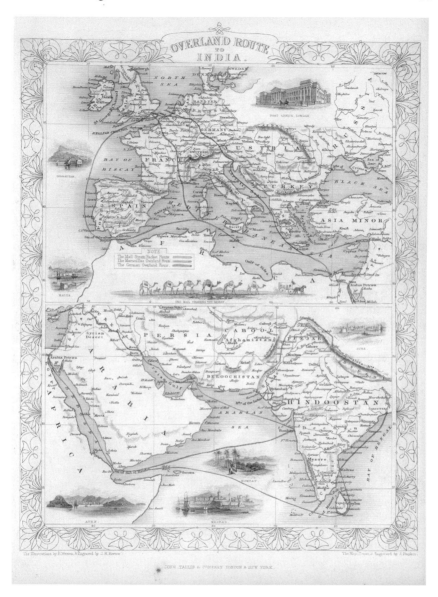

Figure 2.2 The Overland Route from R. M. Martin and J. and F. Tallis's 1851 *Illustrated Atlas*. This map was drawn, engraved, and illustrated by H. Warren, J. Kernot, and J. Rapkin. Courtesy of the David Rumsey Collection.

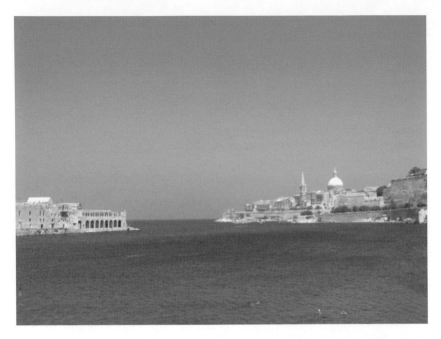

Figure 2.3 The Lazaretto of Malta (on the left) as it stands today. Photograph by the author.

The assumption of colonial power in Malta meant that Britons now controlled what became the most frequented lazaretto in Europe (Figure 2.3). And in administering Malta's imposing lazaretto and the more limited quarantine establishments in Gibraltar and the Ionian Islands, officials faced formidable demands. They struggled to balance the imperial requirements of the military, the comfort of British travelers, the necessities of public safety, and the needs of Maltese merchants. Trade with other European states, and thus, assimilated quarantine procedures, were crucial to the development of Malta as a commercial *entrepôt*. The British desire to secure "free pratique" for ships from Malta in European ports required Malta to adopt stricter quarantine rules for British men-of-war (a policy bitterly opposed by the Admiralty).[35] Ships

---

[35] On the development of this dispute, see Booker, *Maritime Quarantine*, 444. Defenders of the policy did not argue solely based on military necessity but also insisted that men-of-war featured better hygiene than merchant or passenger ships. In response to a critical statement in Parliament that this policy damaged Maltese commerce, Sir Wilmot Horton defended it on the grounds that, unlike other ships, men-of-war practiced the "fumigation" and "expurgation" of quarantine "all the while they were at sea." Hansard, House of Commons Debate, July 10, 1823, Vol. 9, c. 1529. On the importance of the idea of a hygienically sound, "sweet" ship among

from other British Mediterranean colonies, such as Corfu, continued to be subjected to quarantine in Malta. Finally, even as steamship routes resulted in an ever greater number of wealthy travelers subjected to delay and disruption, administrators refused to reduce the required number of days of detention beyond European norms.

Malta's status as quarantine port of choice helped the local economy, and its colonial government recognized the Quarantine Department to be a vital piece of the island's administration. In 1837, Sir Hector Greig, the longtime Superintendent of Quarantine, was promoted to the powerful position of Chief Secretary to the government: a recognition of the administrative skill required to oversee quarantine practice. The balance between revenue and expenses at Malta's lazaretto varied in the course of the 1820s and 1830s, but overall, quarantine came close to paying for itself through fees alone. Furthermore, the presence of quarantine facilities widely reputed to be among the best in the Mediterranean clearly drove shipping to Malta that might have proceeded to another European port. Malta's location as a quarantine port struck the French contagionist Arsène Bulard as so convenient, that he argued in an address to the Imperial Medical Society of Vienna that it should replace all other lazarettos in Europe as a central place of disinfection for the Continent. Apparently, the British and French governments briefly considered this proposal in the 1830s.[36]

After 1826, Maltese ships began to be freely admitted to ports across the Mediterranean – a hard-won victory of British quarantine diplomacy and a result of the harmonization of Malta's rules with those of other Continental powers. In this way, the British government's attitude to quarantine (though ever tied to strategic imperatives) was subject to multiple and shifting considerations. At any moment, it simultaneously suited British administrators in Malta (and Maltese merchants) to advocate for increased severity, British officials at Corfu to hope for a diminution of quarantine, and British diplomats in London to be responsive to attitudes in other European countries as well as the interests of British merchants.

Especially at Malta, the concession that ships of the Royal Navy should receive increased quarantine is evidence of how important quarantine regulation was to imperial government in the Mediterranean. Not for nothing had Lord Byron called Malta a "little military hothouse."[37] It had taken years for the islands to be granted a civil governor, with the first one being Sir Thomas

Royal Navy captains, and its relevance for quarantine debates later in the century, see Rosner, "Policing Boundaries," 130.

[36] Giovanni Bussolin, *Delle istituzioni de sanità marittima nel bacino del Mediterraneo: Studio comparativo* (Trieste: Lod. Herrmanstorfer, 1881), 268. On this proposal, see also Annibale Omodei, "Sulla peste orientale," *Annali universali di medicina* 89 (1839): 455.

[37] Quoted in Albert Smith, *A Hand-book to Mr. Smith's Entertainment* (London, 1850), 34.

Maitland, a military man himself. In 1824, 17 out of a total 110 battalions of the British Army were stationed in Britain's three Mediterranean colonies: Gibraltar, Malta, and the Ionian Islands. This is a total not so far off the twenty-three battalions in all of North America and the Caribbean and the thirty in what Bruce Collins calls "the Indian sphere" – Cape Town to Calcutta.[38] Furthermore, Malta became the center of the Royal Navy's Mediterranean Fleet, which used the islands as a staging ground for a series of major interventions across the Middle Sea in the course of the nineteenth century. Per capita, Britain's imperial subjects in the Mediterranean saw the heaviest concentration of military power of any part of the imperial world.

Despite this serious investment of military power, and given the hopes for dramatic improvements to the Levant trade explored in the previous section, British power to influence Mediterranean events was far from absolute. We can use Katerina Galani's conception of British Mediterranean power as a "successful adaptation" not only to test British recovery after the Napoleonic Wars (as Galani does) but also to characterize a British administrative inclination to accommodate Mediterranean precedents.[39] British colonial officials in the Mediterranean corresponded fluently in French and Italian, they interacted with bureaucrats and officials of other Mediterranean powers (both Christian and Islamic) at a variety of levels, and they tempered their expectations of further gains again and again as cycles of Mediterranean strategic ambitions repeated themselves. Quarantine helps make all of these patterns visible, just as the concept of the British Mediterranean world helps us understand how events, precedents, and arguments centered in the Middle Sea impinged on metropolitan consciousness.

One of the central reasons they did so was the large volume of publications (from travel narratives, to political treatises, to commercial writing, to the records of imperial administration) regarding Mediterranean themes published in Britain. British Mediterraneans themselves were a heterogeneous crew, but overall, they shared a loquacity and a proximity to the metropole that amplified their preoccupations (something that mattered enormously in the course of British debates about quarantine in the 1820s, 1830s, and 1840s). Furthermore, there was greater visibility in greater numbers, and from the act of acquiring new colonial subjects alone, the number of residents of the British Mediterranean expanded enormously at the turn of the nineteenth century. As Britain's imperial footprint increased throughout the region, the Mediterranean became an increasingly prominent site of diplomatic and military postings. Leisure travel to the area, increasingly accessible to a variety of (still relatively

---

[38] These figures are quoted in Bruce Collins, "The Limits of British Power: Intervention in Portugal, 1820–30," *International History Review* 35, no. 4 (2013): 746.

[39] See Galani, *British Shipping in the Mediterranean*.

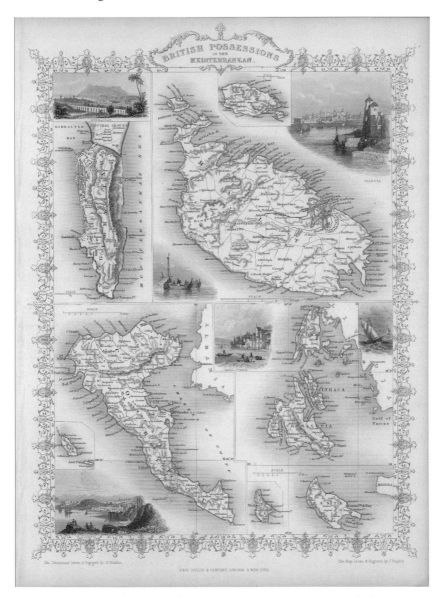

Figure 2.4 The imaginative coherence of Britain's Mediterranean colonies as a single insular system is visible in this image from R. M. Martin and J.&F. Tallis's 1851 *Illustrated Atlas*. J. Rapkin and H. Winkles, "British Possessions in the Mediterranean." Courtesy of the David Rumsey Collection.

elite) Britons, expanded dramatically in the immediate aftermath of the Napoleonic Wars (Figure 2.4).

Yet despite the new ubiquity of British subjects across the Middle Sea, one of the salient features of imperial British Mediterranean spaces was how integrated they were into preexisting Mediterranean configurations. Malta and Gibraltar, in particular, not only had diverse populations, but an itinerant set of temporary residents. Quarantine helps make this apparent; an examination of Malta's lazaretto records reveals that both Britons and Maltese were dwarfed by the large number of "foreigners" performing quarantine there. In the year 1831, for example, there were 2,631 Maltese detained in quarantine against 586 Britons and 4,102 "foreigners."[40] In few other spaces in Britain's imperial world were Britons dwarfed by *both* colonial subjects *and* a large set of others (in this case, mostly Europeans). In turn, the inhabitants of the colonial Mediterranean ranged more broadly than the contours of the British Empire itself. Maltese, Gibraltairians, and Ionians all traveled back and forth across the Mediterranean, spending significant time in North African cities such as Tunis and Alexandria as seasonal workers, servants, cooks, thieves, and small-time shopkeepers.[41]

Compared to subjects of imperial colonies, most elite British travelers felt they had more in common with a similarly elite Western European community of "Franks" – a term appropriated from the era of the Crusades that marked out a community of expatriates whose affiliation was made particularly tangible in times of plague (as Chapter 6 demonstrates). Yet, despite this apparent closing of ranks among Western Europeans, expatriate life around the British Mediterranean (in spaces both imperial and not) cultivated a kind of marginality. Later in the century, for example, various anarchist and radical groups found colonial Mediterranean cities a convenient place to lie low.[42] In the 1820s, the doctor R. R. Madden sarcastically evoked the "select" company of a "Frank" party in precolonial Egypt that included "nine fraudulent bankrupts, thirteen republican outlaws, five avowed atheists, four physicians who had never studied physic, one who had escaped from the galleys at Genoa ... another who had poisoned his confrere, and another who had done as much for his wife."[43] Even among the law-abiding, outsized ambition and, often, an equivocal social position at home impelled careers toward the Middle Sea.

---

[40] See NLM LIBR 812/I.

[41] On this phenomenon, see Clancy-Smith, *Mediterraneans,* and Will Hanley, *Identifying with Nationality: Europeans, Ottomans, and Egyptians in Alexandria* (New York: Columbia University Press, 2017).

[42] Lucia Carminati, "Alexandria, 1898: Nodes, Networks, and Scales in Nineteenth-Century Egypt and the Mediterranean," *Comparative Studies in Society and History* 59, no. 1 (2017): 127–53.

[43] R. R. Madden, *Travels in Turkey, Egypt, Nubia, and Palestine, in 1824, 1825, 1826, and 1827* (London: Henry Colburn, 1829), 1:290–91.

A large proportion of "British Mediterraneans" regularly experienced quarantine themselves, and the centrality of the system to the regular operation of trade, travel, and migration in the Middle Sea created a locus of expertise on quarantine matters for the entire British world. As debates about quarantine accelerated in Britain itself, Mediterranean experience mattered. This section has cataloged the diversity of Britain's Mediterranean commitments, but in so doing, it has also evoked the various milieux from which opinions about Mediterranean quarantine were derived. One final category of British Mediterranean remains to be investigated. Like the merchants, travelers, artists, enthusiasts, colonial subjects, and other Britons who resided in or traveled through the region, most British doctors serving there were preoccupied by the plague. From the 1810s through the 1840s, they formed an influential contingent in British debates about epidemic contagion, public health, and the validity of quarantine.

The Doctor's Mediterranean

As a medical landscape, the Mediterranean offered doctors and medical travelers the nearest examples of exotic maladies; it became an essential zone of research for polemicists invested in a bitter argument (from the 1810s to the 1840s) about the etiology of epidemic diseases. Plague sat at the center of medical debates surrounding epidemic contagion, and it is unsurprising that service and research in the Mediterranean should have furnished Western European doctors with a way to enhance their professional credibility. In the event, there were numerous reasons why the increase in British Mediterranean power around the turn of the nineteenth century meant there were far more British doctors in the area than at any time previously: British doctors affiliated with the military served throughout the Mediterranean battles of the Napoleonic Wars, and the Levant Company retained a doctor on its staff, as did the British Embassy in Constantinople. Other British doctors spent part of their careers across the Mediterranean, catering, for example, to the merchant community at Livorno, or to the travelers, merchants, and speculators inhabiting Alexandria. Finally, as we have already seen, doctors were prolific Mediterranean travelers, and the authors of some of the most evocative narratives published on their return to Britain.

Mediterranean medicine gained additional prestige from debates surrounding quarantine in the wake of the Napoleonic Wars. A slow-burning eighteenth-century debate over the origin of epidemic disease flamed more brightly as the quarantine system was attacked in increasingly public venues. Leading the charge were doctors who believed that atmosphere, environment, and individual predisposition determined who would catch the plague rather than contagion (thus, these were the "anticontagionists"). These new challenges to quarantine's utility had a special salience in Britain because many radical anticontagionists connected quarantine to a distinctively Continental "despotism" (and to Catholicism). As emphasized above, criticisms of the power wielded by boards of health, which cast quarantine as overlaid with paranoia and ritualism, were potent to many Britons at a time when resentment of the Holy Alliance was strong.

The first half of the nineteenth century saw a transition for the British medical profession in which elite doctors retained significant power in the Royal Colleges even as new claims to professional status were being advanced through alternative venues. The power of publications like the *Lancet* and the influence of doctors and campaigners from atypical medical backgrounds in the Health of Towns Associations, and (post-1848 Public Health Act) local boards of health, are clear. Concurrently, the aftermath of the Napoleonic Wars witnessed both a new prestige for military medicine and a rise in the status of imperial medical practice.[44] The threat of cholera, for example, gave new credibility to British doctors who had practiced in Bengal and treated cholera patients there in the epidemic of the 1810s. The search for new evidence to fuel arguments about quarantine policy and the etiology of the plague played the same role for Mediterranean medicine.

Through at least half a dozen inquiries – some conducted by parliamentary select committees, some on the initiative of the Foreign Office – the British government attempted to catalog and synthesize the opinions of doctors who had treated plague victims around the Mediterranean and Black Sea. Bureaucrats and quarantine reformers throughout the 1820s, 1830s, and 1840s continued to believe that contested questions about plague could be resolved through a canvas of medical opinion in the British Mediterranean. Could the plague be spread through contact with infected persons or trade goods? If so, what was its incubation period? Frustratingly for all, even in the 1830s and 1840s, when reduction in quarantine lengths became conventional wisdom for policy makers, doctors continued to differ on these basic questions.

The theater of exchange in the vituperative contagion debate attracted a large but recurring cast of characters – medical writers, polemic journalists, MPs, and sanitary reformers – many of whom will impel narrative in the coming pages. Emphatic among these voices were doctors who had practiced in the Mediterranean. One Dr. Whyte, martyr to the cause of anticontagionism, was so intent on proving the incapacity of pestiferous matter to transmit the disease that he injected himself with the blood of a plague victim in January 1801 in Egypt. He promptly died. Contagionists took Whyte's death as *prima facie* proof of contagion, while their opponents emphasized that an individual in Egypt in winter 1801 was prone to an epidemic atmosphere regardless of any

---

[44] See Kelly, *War and the Militarization of British Army Medicine.*

inoculations she or he might have attempted.[45] The case was debated for decades, despite the dry notation of a medical writer in the 1840s that "there can be no fear that the mass of a population will ever allow themselves to be inoculated with the plague."[46]

Other doctors associated with the Mediterranean contributed prolifically to the debate surrounding epidemic contagion. Augustus Bozzi Granville, a society doctor and contagionist defender of quarantine, came to England after receiving an MD in Pavia and after having served as embassy doctor in Constantinople (where he caught and survived the plague).[47] William Pym served early in his career as Superintendent of Quarantine at Malta and was rapidly promoted to the role of Superintendent of Quarantine for the entire UK (a position which seems to have gained enhanced authority at the time of Pym's appointment). Among many other examples of doctors whose service in the Mediterranean preceded successful London careers (and significant involvement in debates surrounding quarantine), a final case that bears mentioning is that of James Johnson, who had served as a military doctor during British campaigns in Egypt and India before becoming physician extraordinary to the future William IV. Like others working in the British Mediterranean, doctors there benefited from their proximity to the metropole. They socialized with Grand Tourists and other elite travelers, and they were immersed in medical communities alongside doctors from other European nations, many of whom became famous medical polemicists in their own right. Service as a physician in the Mediterranean highlights that region's status as the "near abroad" – prestige gained and connections formed through Mediterranean practice were particularly easy to turn into success and influence in the metropole.

The career of the anticontagionist Charles Maclean, the single most influential medical writer on quarantine in our period, is an excellent case study of medical influence derived from experience in the British Mediterranean. An irascible and intemperate man, who began his medical career in Scotland, Maclean would hardly have wielded the influence he did had it not been for a career that carried him across the world. Though he briefly served in the

---

[45] For a contagionist's interpretation of the Dr. Whyte story, see Robert Gooch, "Plague, a Contagious Disease," *Quarterly Review* 33 (1825): 237–38. The arch-anticontagionist Charles Maclean claimed that Whyte (here, spelled White) had already survived two auto-inoculations, so his death from the third must be considered inconclusive. See Charles Maclean, "Communication from Dr. Maclean as to His Experiments on the Plague at Constantinople," *Literary Gazette*, January 25, 1817, 210. Joseph Adam stressed that Whyte's death occurred during an epidemic: Adam, *An Inquiry into the Laws of Different Epidemic Diseases, with the View to Determine the Means of Preserving Individuals and Communities from Each* (London: W. Thorne, 1809), 205–6.

[46] Gavin Milroy, *Quarantine and the Plague* (London: S. Highley, 1846), 38.

[47] On Granville's career, see A. Sakula, "Augustus Bozzi Granville (1783–1872): London Physician-Accoucheur and Italian Patriot," *Journal of the Royal Society of Medicine* 76, no. 10 (1983): 876–82.

Caribbean and, for a time, in Calcutta, his later life was shaped by his experience treating and researching the plague in Constantinople. A socially marginal figure, who died in poverty in 1829, he nevertheless acquired political influence and polemical advantage from both his encounters with disease and his association with the Levant Company. His windy voice and stormy pen propelled the question of the contagiousness of the plague from Ottoman ports to the heart of the British state.

Having absconded from service as a naval surgeon, Maclean launched his career at the head of a practice in Calcutta. After a brief period, he was expelled from India by Lord Wellesley (having apparently abandoned his wife) for his intemperate attack on a local magistrate. Returning to England around the turn of the nineteenth century, he formulated plans to study epidemic disease systematically and in situ. Indeed, though it has been suggested that Maclean's intense focus on quarantine dates mostly from the 1810s,[48] his interest in epidemic disease was clearly long-standing. By 1801 he was calling research on epidemic transmission "my particular study."[49]

En route to the Levant, however, he was detained by Bonaparte's imprisonment of all English still in France at the resumption of hostilities after the Peace of Amiens. Between his antagonists in medical debates, the Marquess Wellesley, and the Emperor Napoleon himself, Maclean would later muse that "it has been the singularity of my fate to have been in collision with almost every species of despotism" possible to imagine.[50] Despotism itself, alongside plague, quarantine, and corruption in pre-Reform British politics, clearly came to be interchangeable ideas in Maclean's medico-philosophical imagination. In 1814, he obtained Levant Company backing for his long-held ambition of conducting research that could vanquish two conceptual despots he abhorred: universal quarantine and the plague itself. Now able to travel to the Mediterranean without impediment, he proceeded to Constantinople to undertake the study he had long anticipated.

To the doctor himself, what followed was the glorious vindication of his hypotheses. Others remained unconvinced, an early collision that came to reinforce Maclean's position as an outsider, even as he retained support from Levant Company President Lord Grenville and numerous Company members. Some of his early patrons had glimpsed the challenges that this energetic anticontagionist might create. At the outset of his travels, Jacob Bosanquet, the Levant Company's Deputy Governor, warned that Maclean's self-importance and the

---

[48] See Harrison, *Contagion*, 61.
[49] See Maclean to the Duke of Portland, May 3, 1801. Quoted in Charles Maclean, *An Excursion in France, and Other Parts of the Continent of Europe* (London: T. N. Longman and C. Rees, 1804), 5.
[50] Quoted in "Censorship of the Press in India," *Oriental Herald* 17 (1827): 52.

apparent patronage of Lord Grenville might lead him "to entertain expectations which may not be realized."[51] This, it turned out, was a colossal understatement.

Maclean arrived in Constantinople carrying Grenville's reference to Robert Liston, the British ambassador. Liston subsequently arranged with the Ottoman authorities for Maclean to take up residence in the Greek-run plague hospital at the Seven Towers. After the medical employees were placed under Maclean's direction, the ambitious doctor launched his new program of treatments for the many plague victims lying before him: a vigorous (and, to modern eyes, highly poisonous) regimen of calomel, mercury, and opium. Maclean estimated that his cure was successful for a rate of "forty in the hundred," and that, if not for the intrigues of the hospital's servants, the rate could double with a larger staff and better facilities. He predicted confidently that his methods would eventually provide an established template, which even individuals with no medical training could use with the "certainty of effecting a cure."[52]

Maclean viewed his treatments as effectively proved by what he considered his trump card: the fact that during this residency in this hospital, he himself caught the plague and survived. As he wrote it in his memorial to Lord Grenville, in favor of his theory of treatment he could "cite the attack of the disease, and the speedy removal of it, in my own person."[53] Grenville, at this stage, was impressed by Maclean, communicating his support to the doctor and stimulating great expectations. Maclean returned to England with blooming optimism. Armed with testimonials from the ambassador and several members of the Levant Company, he expected confirmation, celebrity, and money. After all, he noted, in the *one* case of plague where he could rigorously administer treatment of mercury, calomel, and opium, and where he could be independent of pernicious attendants, he had achieved an incontestable cure. "My own case," Maclean wrote, "was the only one . . . in which I could be assured that my principles were correctly applied to practice."[54]

The consequence for quarantine was quickly drawn. Maclean depicted it as a vastly expensive and unnecessary encumbrance relying on a model of contagion that both his medical theories and personal experiences refuted. In his *Evils of Quarantine* (1824), Maclean declaimed in characteristic tones that:

Had I perished in the course of my experiments in the Levant, it might with some plausibility have been said of me . . . that I fell victim to my want of belief in the contagion of the plague; [my opponents] would have been credited by the multitude; and epidemic diseases might have remained contagious . . . But "I survive/To

---

[51] Bosquanet to Lord Grenville, January 12, 1814, BL Add. Ms. 59265.
[52] Charles Maclean, *Practical Illustrations of the Progress of Medical Improvement, for the Last Thirty Years* (London, 1818), 226.
[53] Maclean's "Report," February 14, 1816, Section II, BL Add. Ms. 59265.
[54] Maclean to Lord Grenville, February 14, 1816. Quoted in Maclean's "Report," section IV.

mock the expectations of the world/To frustrate prophecies, and to raze out/Rotten opinion."[55]

In this work, Maclean insisted that quarantine ("a melancholy delusion") was supported "by faith, dread, and fiction only."[56] It was the ludicrous legacy of a ruse perpetrated by Pope Paul III to induce the members of the Council of Trent to move their meeting site. From this "Papal stratagem," Britain had suffered "the destruction of lives, and the detriment to health, morals, medicine, commerce, navigation, the intercourse of nations, individual freedom, military operations, the general consumer, and the public revenues."[57] The quarantine laws were "the most gigantic, extraordinary, and mischievous superstructure, that has ever been raised by man, upon a purely imaginary foundation."[58] They were worse than useless. In fact, some "fifteen-sixteenths" of the deaths attributed to plague, were actually "occasioned by the consequences of the belief in contagion." Quarantine, according to Maclean's arithmetic, killed precisely 937,500 people each year.[59]

Presumably because of Lord Grenville's advocacy, Maclean's efforts and publications pushed Parliament, for the first time, to take upon itself a medical argument when it convened a select committee to investigate the contagiousness of plague in 1819. Maclean testified before this committee twice, but its eventual rejection of his ideas turned him once again to a searing rejection of the British polity as irredeemably corrupt and a further attempt to find glory through Mediterranean practice (this time in Barcelona during a yellow fever epidemic). Maclean had argued for years that the British government owed him thousands of pounds for his "proofs" of the invalidity of quarantine. When he died in 1829, the only official recognition he received was a grant to his widow from the Literary Fund – a fair recognition that the polemical power of his writing was his most durable legacy. Though the prediction of the Radical MP John Cam Hobhouse that Maclean would be one "to whom the finger of the historian would point, as one of the greatest benefactors of his species" never came true,[60] the very fact that Maclean continued to be lauded in Parliament by ideological fellow travelers points to his staying power. As we will see in Chapter 7, his ideas, his zeal, and his conflation of questions moral and medical would be taken up by a later generation of anticontagionist doctors.

---

[55] Charles Maclean, *Evils of Quarantine Laws and Non-Existence of Pestilential Contagion* (London: Thomas and George Underwood, 1824), 382. Here he is quoting from Shakespeare's *Henry IV*, part II.

[56] Charles Maclean, *Suggestions for the Prevention and Mitigation of Epidemic and Pestilential Diseases* (London: T. and G. Underwood 1817), 17.

[57] Ibid., 18.

[58] Charles Maclean, *Remarks on the British Quarantine Laws, and the So-Called Sanitary Laws of the Continental Nations of Europe, Especially Those of Spain* (London, 1823), 2.

[59] Maclean, *Suggestions*, 27.

[60] Hansard, House of Commons Debate, March 30, 1825, Vol. 12, c. 1324.

Maclean's work injected a jolt of energy into the anticontagionist position that gave it a greater polemic edge as the nineteenth century unfolded. This came from his sense of self-righteousness derived from the practical and intimate experience of having endured Mediterranean quarantine practice and survived Mediterranean plague. If anticontagionists could position their largely Hippocratic worldview as a modern theory at the vanguard of reform, they could do so primarily because doctors who practiced in the Middle Sea mobilized their experience so eloquently. Maclean, for example, took advantage of the ability to move quickly back and forth between Britain and the Mediterranean by literally haunting the offices of the Levant Company. "Dr. McLean was sitting here as I finished my letter," wrote an exhausted Levant Company Secretary in 1819, "he is evidently feverish."[61]

Though Maclean's choleric sensibility may have stunted his own career, it fostered a generation of "Macleanites."[62] As one British doctor who went to Constantinople in the mid-1820s wrote, he left Britain "with a firm belief in the doctrines of Dr. M'Lean; they were plausible; and the very violence with which they were urged had something to recommend them to a young man."[63] The Doctor's Mediterranean made room for audacious polemics and for discoveries of elusive cures for dread diseases. Its bald certainties and dramatic declarations mirrored political and diplomatic optimism for a new Mediterranean order post-1815. It exerted a draw for practitioners of all kinds throughout the nineteenth century, and it lapped as far as Britain itself as it formed the churning heart of the debate about contagion.

---

[61] George Liddell to Lord Grenville, undated; from context, it is clear it is from June 1819, BL Add. Ms. 59266.
[62] Francis Adams, *The Medical Works of Paulus Aegineta* (London: J. Welsh, 1834), 1:211.
[63] Madden, *Travels*, 260.

Part II

Lazarettos, Health Boards, and the Building
of a Biopolity

3   Governing Quarantine

The lazaretto was a murky world and an extraordinary institution. Isolation was its purpose, but it did not *exist* in isolation. Too many histories of Mediterranean quarantine present each port city, each site of land-based quarantine as a space with a unique history. These individual stories are worth retelling, but the most remarkable thing about quarantine was its scale and its systematic operation. This book argues that boards of health – collectively, not individually – built a cohesive system that endured thanks to its own momentum. In Chapter 5, the mechanics of the cooperation that enabled that system to emerge are explored in detail. Here and in Chapter 4, my aim is to present a history of quarantine from a new perspective – a synthetic one, which highlights the extent to which the patterns of governing it and the texture of experiencing it were phenomena shared across Western European ports. Boards of health in different ports and within different nations shared similar problems and conducted equivalent practices. In the era between 1780 and 1850, quarantine was simultaneously multipolar and unitary; its precedents evolved over centuries, and coordination among boards of health had its own momentum. Essential in propelling this system forward was a sense that plague was a unique threat and that the lazaretto was an extraordinary environment, too important to interpret solely within the context of one port city, or one nation. Plague did not respect national borders, and neither could quarantine.

Gravely and proudly, the Marseille *Intendance* termed the lazaretto a "terrible place" beyond the reach of the law. To many, however, it was simultaneously extreme and ordinary. Travelers, perhaps, felt this sense, as they neared the ends of their prescribed terms of detention – we examine their experiences in the next chapter. No one felt it more, however, than the hundreds of porters, guardians, servants, casual laborers, restaurateurs, chaplains, and bureaucrats for whom the lazaretto was a place of daily work, even a permanent home. Governing this world was a complex dance between enforcing the rigid laws of quarantine and also managing the complex interactions among lazaretto employees, diplomats, and national governments that allowed quarantine to function. In this chapter, through a variety of case studies, I expose recurrent patterns that help us understand how the government of quarantine depended on a constant negotiation among the local, the national, and the transnational.

This chapter explores events both extraordinary (the arrival of ships with the plague actually on board) and quotidian (dealing with fractious consuls and impatient ministers in national capitals). It retains a synoptic focus across different Mediterranean port cities and explores the ways in which the political and economic connections between the Middle Sea and the Northern European powers extended "Mediterranean quarantine" as a phenomenon across Western Europe. The tasks that boards performed and the considerations they balanced were so similar that a member of Livorno's *Sanità* would have found it extraordinarily easy to work on secondment, for a stretch, with the Marseille *Intendance*.

Introducing Boards of Health

Mediterranean boards of health were the ultimate arbiter of quarantine questions in their ports – their sanction was needed for even the most uncontroversial ship to be granted pratique, their suspicion could land arrivals from a particular foreign port in quarantine. Though they met outside the gates of the lazaretto, board members needed to give explicit approval for numerous lazaretto procedures. Their intercession with government ministers was key to the seamless operation of quarantine. But much of their work was oriented outward to foreign boards of health; the maintenance of free pratique among Western European quarantine ports depended on it.

Boards of health met frequently (sometimes daily, sometimes weekly). Members could expect a regular and extensive commitment of time and effort. They headed a vast sanitary bureaucracy – from the secretaries who wrote their letters, to the lazaretto captains who executed their commands, to the guardians and porters who practiced the procedures they set down. Who composed their membership? Though board members were never drawn from the working classes, their social milieu was different in each European port. But everywhere, the composition of boards reflected the idea that quarantine matters were a hybrid subject that demanded input from a variety of civic actors. While their size could vary (from a minimum of six to a maximum around twenty), their members represented a cohesive set of interests.

The features that made boards of health resemble each other are more extensive than those that differed according to locality; the variation that did exist tended to be reduced as the nineteenth century went on. In Malta, uniquely, a "Superintendent of Quarantine" decided most quarantine matters. In 1826, however, it was decided that a board was necessary, if only for the appearance of assimilating to Mediterranean norms. This modern assembly of a board (others took on their form in the seventeenth and eighteenth centuries) gives us a window into the kinds of interests it was felt most boards should represent. Malta's new board, then, consisted of the Governor and the Chief Secretary to the Government (there to represent the broader interests of the colony in quarantine matters), the Superintendent of Quarantine (the bureaucrat *par excellence* with experience running the system), the Maltese aristocrat Baron Pasquale Trigona (a local grandee included to help legitimize it to the Maltese whose border it regulated), and the doctor Stefano Grillet (present to offer medical advice).[1] Quarantine was to be governed as a matter of politics and administration influenced by medicine rather than the other way around. Finally, not only can we see the composition of this board as an exercise of conciliating different Maltese interests, but it was also a statement for foreign boards of health that Malta would adopt their forms and share their principles of quarantine administration.

Elsewhere, the interests represented on boards of health were similar. As in Malta, Livorno's *Consiglio di Sanità* was headed by the Governor of the city. After the suppression of the 1814 Genoese republic, the *Magistrato di Sanità* was reconstituted under the Sardinian monarchy and put under the charge of the Marchesa di Pallavicini – a scion of one of the oldest aristocratic families in Liguria. In Marseille, though the precise nomination procedure changed in the late eighteenth century to give more power to Parisian ministers, *Intendants* were chosen by the Prefect and the responsible minister (the Interior Minister before the July Monarchy, then the Minister of Commerce) from a list proposed by the Mayor of Marseille. Nominated members were drawn from the ranks of Marseille's commercial elite, and experience conducting business in the Levant was considered a distinct advantage. Despite variation, then, in every major quarantine port, quarantine was in the hands of a group steeped in administration, commerce, and civic authority – well versed in the ways of Mediterranean trade and well integrated in local power structures.

Francoise Hildesheimer has suggested that by the mid-eighteenth century, the members of Marseille's Board of Health were ridiculed for being drawn solely from inexperienced civic elites – who rotated between the Chamber of Commerce, the City Council, and other influential Marseillaise establishments.[2] In certain cases, this was undoubtedly the case. Yet, as late as the post-1815 Restoration, it seems clear that service in the Levant still seemed to be a vital requirement for most members of the *Intendance Sanitaire*. On one occasion in 1818, the sole change (made by the Prefect and Minister) to the Mayor of Marseille's *Intendance* nominations was the replacement of a prospective *Intendant* who had simply served in various roles of urban

---

[1] See Circular Letter of April 6, 1826 (announcing the formation of the Maltese Board of Health), NAM CSG 03/71.

[2] Françoise Hildesheimer, *Le Bureau de la Santé de Marseille sous l'Ancien Régime* (Marseille: Fédération historique de Provence, 1980), 29–30.

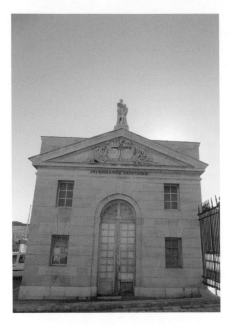

Figure 3.1 The former offices of Marseille's Intendance Sanitaire, close to
city's Vieux Port. Courtesy of baladedunemarseillaise.com.

administration with another prospective candidate who had lived in the
Ottoman Empire and engaged with the Levant trade. The Prefect cited this as
indispensable experience for anyone on the board, and indeed, all four of the
Intendants named on this occasion had conducted commerce in the Levant.[3]

Marseille's *Intendance*, as a corporate body, was arguably the most influential board of health in the Mediterranean (Figure 3.1). As merchants engaged in
the Levant trade dominated its membership, it would be reasonable to assume
that *Intendants* used their position to encourage reform as pressure on quarantine grew in the 1830s and 1840s. In fact, the opposite is true. Marseille's
Intendance serves as a useful counterexample to Mark Harrison's contention
that the quarantine debate pitted commerce against the interests of public
health.[4] By the 1840s (when, as we shall see, the reformist instincts of the
Minister of Commerce prompted the entire *Intendance* to resign), the two
medical members were the most open to change while all of the members

---

[3] Prefect of the Bouches-du-Rhône Department to the Minister of the Interior, October 27, 1818,
AN F/8/28/II/ "Personnel – 1819." See also Extract from the Registers of the Délibérations of the
Municipal Council of Marseille, October 21, 1818 (same file), for the original recommendation.
[4] See Harrison, *Contagion*.

who were ex-Levantine *commerçants* insisted that any dismantling of quarantine would be an unmitigated disaster. The weight of procedure and custom, and the influential position Marseille had achieved due to its sanitary severity, were more than enough to persuade even commercial men that the hurdles that quarantine represented were but a small price to pay for the preservation of public health.

Boards of health were often criticized for their reliance on tradition and routine.[5] In part, this sense of their conservatism was due to the unique stability they experienced even during a period of extreme political upheaval. Marseille's Board is a good example. Though the *Intendants* of the Old Regime's *Bureau de Santé* saw themselves transformed into *Conservateurs* in the course of the Revolution, and though their titles would be changed yet again by the Restoration, the actual membership does not appear to have changed substantially in the course of the power struggles and regime changes their country experienced between 1789 and 1815. Most members of the Old Regime *Bureau* served into the Revolutionary period and most Napoleonic *Conservateurs* became Restoration *Intendants de Santé* after 1815. The precise designation changed – the individuals, mostly, did not.[6] After the apparent abolition of the quarantine laws by the National Assembly in 1792 led to a widespread outcry and immediate back-tracking, quarantine became one of the few areas of national law where even Robespierre's Committee of Public Safety was willing to let the Old Regime's dictates stand.

In Venice, too, the quarantine administration saw great continuity of personnel during an era of political crisis. In 1796, the last year of the *Serenissima* as a fully independent state, one Antonio Buffetti was singled out for praise by Niccolò Vendramin, president of the Board of Health, for his performance as Prior of the Lazaretto Vecchio.[7] It is clear from the Austrian almanac for the Venetian province in 1822 that Buffetti was still serving as Prior some twenty-six years, and several regime changes, later.[8] He appears to have been ceremonially reelected each year by the Venetian Senate; such reelections, in Buffetti's case, span the period from Venice's pre-1797 independence, the first French military government, the first Austrian period, the Napoleonic Kingdom of Italy, and the post-1814 period of renewed Austrian domination. In Malta, until Captain Pulis of the lazaretto was forced to resign in 1831 in a wheat-smuggling scandal, he served the British in a role his father had filled under

---

[5] See, for example, Louis Aubert-Roche, *De la réforme des quarantaines et des lois sanitaires de la peste* (Paris: Juste-Rouvier, 1843), 3.
[6] This observation is based on diverse material from the "Personnel" file of the *Intendance*. See ADBR 200 E 18.
[7] Niccolò Vendramin to Antonio Buffetti, Venice, December 29, 1796, ASVe. Provv. Sanità 204.
[8] *Almanacco per le Province dell'IR Governo di Venezia per 1822* (Venice: Andreola, 1822), ASVe. Bib. Leg., 216.

the Knights (i.e., before 1798). As late as 1829, Hector Greig (as Superintendent of Quarantine) was making serious efforts to convince the colonial government to honor promises the Knights had given to Pulis's father some fifty years earlier by giving his son a raise.[9]

In Genoa, the officials at the *Sanità* did serve over several changes of regime, though we have seen that the post-1815 settlement did mark the beginning of more aristocratic leadership. Political upheaval never resulted in substantial changes to quarantine procedure, but nor were Genoa's quarantine officials immune to the vicissitudes of Napoleonic-Era politics. Genoa's relations with Marseille in the course of the Wars also present an interesting case of the impact of political change on quarantine administration. In 1807, roughly at the time Genoa was made a Department of France itself, the Genoa board seems to have been put under the control of Marseille's *Conservateurs*. Letters from the Genoese to the Marseille Board of Health switched, in this year, from the Italian to the French language, and Genoa was forced to subscribe to the French policy that all ships from powers doing business with Britain should be treated as sanitary threats. In 1814, with the advent of the Genoese Republic, correspondence in Italian was immediately resumed, and the same Sanità President, Vice-President, and Executive Secretary who had served under French domination immediately proclaimed that "the *Sanità*, having been restored to its former rights, has cancelled the state of quarantine that it has had to impose on countries that were not sanitarily suspicious, except for the commerce they had with Britain."[10] Having heard this news, Marseille promptly placed Genoa and the Ligurian littoral under a severe quarantine, prompting the Genoese to remonstrate in May of that year that "political barriers" had no place in sanitary decision-making.[11] Clearly, the Genoese were attached to the idea that the patterns of quarantine were more fundamental than the exigencies of European wars, and that the original French quarantine against nations trading with Britain was itself illegitimate.[12] Indeed, though Mark Harrison has cast early nineteenth-century quarantine as an arbitrary and politicized institution,[13] it is clear from episodes like this that periods when international disputes shaped sanitary decision-making were aberrant and that independence from politics was seen to be the norm.

[9] Hector Greig to Sir Frederick Hankey, November 14, 1829, NAM CUST 04/1.
[10] Mongiardini to the *Intendants de Marseille,* April 30, 1814, ADBR 200 E 423.
[11] Unsigned Genoese quarantine official to *Intendants de Marseille*, May 21, 1814, ADBR 200 E 423.
[12] It should be noted that British authorities in Malta had ordered a retaliatory quarantine of a more limited variety on ships from Marseille, on the grounds that France had (as part of its general quarantine on enemy shipping) begun to detain Maltese ships in Marseille. Thus, the French ship that brought news of the Peace of Amiens to Malta in 1802 was immediately put in quarantine on its arrival. See "Malta," *Caledonian Mercury*, February 10, 1806.
[13] Harrison, *Contagion*, chapter 3.

Managing the Local

Thus far, we have explored the economic and social milieu from which board of health members were drawn, the different structures for sanitary government that existed in Mediterranean ports, and the extent to which, nearly everywhere, board members and quarantine bureaucrats managed to stay in their jobs during periods of political turmoil. Here, we examine the substance of their activities, noting the distinct unity of practice at different Mediterranean ports.

A meeting of Genoa's *Magistrato di Sanità* typically featured the reading of correspondence, the approval of correspondence to be written, and a series of "deliberations" – decisions made by the *Magistrato*, usually about five to ten at each meeting.[14] Such a pattern, both in terms of the substance of individual meetings and the number of board members present, was common across the Mediterranean. Boards ruled on the fate of individual ships, on proposals to raise or lower the quarantine on arrivals from specific areas of the world based on foreign intelligence, and on requests from foreign consuls. Each decision generated orders, letters, and minute-book records. Such records point us to the diversity of issues boards considered – they synthesized material gleaned from abroad and from national governments even as they gave direction to hundreds of employees in the lazaretto and set the quarantines of individual ships. But, though much about quarantine was set by international understanding and shared standards, there was ambiguity around the edges. Serving on a board of health required tact, patience, and finesse.

For example, though each port produced a standard table of quarantine lengths, special circumstances meant that each ship's bill of health and the answers the captain gave to quarantine questions had to be examined in detail (had the captain called at another port? had he completed any term of quarantine elsewhere in the Mediterranean? had someone been taken on board from a suspect ship?). In Genoa, where the Black Sea trade was especially important, some 74 ships arrived from Odessa (out of 108 total) in a four-month period in the winter and spring of 1828. Seventy-two of them had a standard quarantine length of thirty-five days. The remaining two served completely different lengths of time, probably because they had completed partial quarantines abroad. Furthermore, at Genoa, the standard quarantine time for arrivals from Gibraltar in the late 1820s appears to have been seventeen days, though one ship was given a twenty-day detention, and several more a detention of fifteen days.[15] During the same period, the quarantine lengths applied to passengers in the lazaretto was even more irregular.[16] All of these matters were debated and

---

[14] See ASGe Sanità 543 and 544, which are the minutes of *Magistrato di Sanità* negotiations from July 1835 to November 1839.

[15] ASGe Sanità 1671 (data for January 27–April 27, 1828).

[16] See ASGe Sanità 1707 (data for February 12–April 28, 1828).

ruled on by the *Magistrato* based on specific information about the health of the crew. At Marseille, the progress of each ship through the various stages of quarantine (its arrival, the formal ruling of its detention period, its admission to the final phase of detention, and its release) was discussed and approved by the *Intendance Sanitaire*. If any event intervened (an illness, a sanitary infraction, or the receipt of information from abroad that revised the sanitary picture of the port of departure), the length of detention could change.

There were rules, but there was also a point to sanitary lobbying. Consuls regularly wrote to the local board of health in the city they served and asked for leniency for ships arriving under the flag of their home nations. Captains themselves occasionally wrote to request special treatment (in terms of quarantine length) due to the good health of their crew. In 1824, for example, the captain of a British frigate wrote a hopeful letter to the President of Genoa's *Sanità* asking for pratique to be granted "immediately." Charles Harting, the British consul at Genoa, massaged this impossible demand to a request for pratique to be granted "as soon as possible" in the letter he attached.[17] Harting was a frequent correspondent with the Genoese *Sanità*, well versed in the language of sanitary diplomacy. He felt able to ask for frequent small favors and indulgences. In August 1824, for example, he registered an (apparently successful) request to move the pratique-granting of a British ship from "after lunch" to noon because he was busy in the afternoon and wanted to attend.[18]

Foreign consuls were clearly frequent attendants at quarantine harbors. At Genoa, the Ottoman Consul, Niccolò Petrococchino, wrote in November 1815 to protest "a fact which I saw yesterday" in the quarantine harbor, where a Greek captain had been given unfair treatment by sanitary authorities.[19] Boards of health responded to these sorts of requests patiently and in detail, though they were loath to grant unusual liberality in quarantine matters. Nevertheless, they often needed to adjudicate among the demands of competing foreign powers for special treatment in terms of quarantine lengths. Henry Veith, British Consul-General to Madeira, arrived in the quarantine harbor of Genoa in August 1824 and was told he needed to wait for approval from the *Magistrato* before he could land. On seeing a Sardinian ship from the same point of origin admitted to pratique immediately, Veith wrote a letter to Pallavicini, expressing outrage at "the unjust preference that has been given to the Sardinian Flag (in a matter of Health which hitherto in all civilized nations has never at the least been acknowledged to admit of exceptions) and to the disgrace of the British Flag."[20] Veith's outrage was aggravated by an

[17] Charles Harting to Marchesa di Pallavicini, October 31, 1824, ASGe Sanità 1365.
[18] Charles Harting to Marchesa di Pallavicini, August 18, 1824, ASGe Sanità 1365.
[19] Niccolò Petrococchino to the Magistrati di Sanità Sedente a Genova, November 16, 1815, ASGe Sanità 1365.
[20] Henry Veith to the Marchesa di Pallavicini, August 9, 1824, ASGe Sanità 1365.

unusual quarantine, but he probably would not have been surprised to discover that foreign consuls in Malta in the early 1820s complained incessantly at the perceived preference given there to British warships. Yet there, Maltese administrators were constantly involved in a delicate negotiation with the Admiralty to ensure that the quarantine for warships was not too out of line with the treatment of other European ships. Again, changing the rules so that warships performed the same quarantine as other ships was essential to Malta's victory in 1826 in persuading other European boards of health to grant ships from the island's harbors free pratique in their ports.

Given that a large percentage of foreigners (and foreign goods) who entered a port came by way of the lazaretto or quarantine harbor, it is unsurprising that consuls engaged so frequently with boards of health – more often, indeed, than they would have engaged most other local authorities. Boards of health were part of the urban administration, but unlike typical civic bodies, they adjudicated diplomatic incidents alongside local matters. Their authority, in fact, extended far beyond the traditional confines of the city in which they were located. Marseille's *Intendance*, responsible until the 1830s for every civilian arrival from the Levant in France, had a national role, as well as a local one. The Mayor of Marseille may have been an "*Intendant né*" of the *Intendance Sanitaire*,[21] but if he chose to exercise his rights, he would have found the matters the board discussed far removed from traditional matters of local administration.

This hybrid nature of the board – a local authority with an international remit – can be seen most clearly in the oldest boards of health, like Venice's, which addressed wide varieties of local health concerns.[22] In a name that reveals the board's premodern pedigree, members of Venice's Board were technically denominated the *Provveditori e Sopraprovveditori alla Sanità*. The registers of their declarations reveal that there were usually several meetings each week with between three and five *Provveditori* typically in attendance at the more routine gatherings. Into the nineteenth century, when the board's traditional role was changing, it still prepared a *Necrologia* each year, which recorded the death of every Venetian – not simply those in quarantine. The list of *Terminazioni* for the year 1796 (the last year of uninterrupted existence for the Old Regime *Sanità*) reveals 462 separate matters on which rulings were issued. Most concerned grants of money – particularly to Venetian charities and to elderly lazaretto employees. Others involved efforts to stop the

---

[21] AN (Pierrefitte) F/8/28/II/1819. This makes clear that by the Restoration, the Mayor was considered an Intendant (*ex officio*), though the material from this Personnel folder suggests the Mayor rarely exercised the privileges that would have gone along with that designation.

[22] Junko Takeda discusses this hybrid nature of boards of health in *Between Crown and Commerce*, 116. Her interest, however, is primarily in early modern contestation between the monarchy and local authorities in the governance of quarantine.

clandestine arrival of cattle during a time when Verona was suffering from a cattle plague.[23] All of these rulings came *on top* of the onerous duties of traditional quarantine government. The *Provveditori* were responsible for the government of two enormous lazarettos, and (before 1797) they commanded respect throughout the Mediterranean as the most senior and eminent board of health still in continuous operation.

As modern boards were reconstituted across Europe in the wake of the Napoleonic Wars many of these more local functions were set aside; boards of health became more oriented toward the lazaretto and across the sea rather than inward toward the cities in which they sat. Nevertheless, even in the modern era, boards retained a responsibility for superintending local health – albeit in a way that was primarily about securing a sanitary border. The *Magistrato* at Genoa superintended the work of smaller boards at La Spezia, Rapallo, Portofino, and Savona (among other small ports) and frequently loaned sanitary personnel to these local boards. The *Magistrato* regularly considered the apparently small-bore matters of the Ligurian littoral alongside more typical quarantine concerns. In 1822, for example, it was asked to rule on the question of whether the tiny seaside village of San Pier d'Anna should allow fishermen to dock at night, or whether daylight was needed to ensure they were not smuggling quarantined items in some way.[24] Through such an incident, we see how quarantine caught up individuals, events, and procedures seemingly unrelated to trade with the Middle East. Shipwrecks, for example, were a major source of concern, particularly if a possibility existed that a wrecked ship washed up with any goods connected to the Ottoman Empire.[25] Local boards peppered Genoa's *Magistrato* with questions about such events, and the care shown by its members in each case shows the centrality of the belief that in episodes of uncertainty, quarantine had to remain watertight.[26]

In all of these ways, despite their comparatively modest situation, the boards of health of Mediterranean ports performed similar functions. While often grounded in local concerns, they should be seen as more analogous to a national ministry than a municipal agency. No nation, Britain included, had more than a few fully operational quarantine facilities. Between them, the three *Magistrati* of Genoa, Nice, and Cagliari were charged with superintending the security of the entire coastal border of the Kingdom of Piedmont-Sardinia. The

---

[23] ASVe Provv. Sanità 788. See in particular No. 204, July 21, 1796.
[24] S. Cubino of the San Pier d'Anna Sanità to the Genoa Magistrato, February 2, 1822, ASGe Sanità 1213.
[25] The archives of Naples's *Magistrato di Salute*, for example, contain some fifteen volumes devoted to shipwrecks occurring between 1769 and 1869.
[26] For an example of the Genoa *Magistrato's* involvement in shipwrecks along the Ligurian coast, see Vigo, President of the Board of Health of Voltri, to the Magistrato di Genova, September 3, 1822, ASGe Sanità 1213.

boards of health at Ancona and Civitavecchia were in charge of the coastal health of the Papal Sates, while Livorno's *Consiglio* was granted the sole responsibility for guaranteeing the maritime sanitary security of the Grand Duchy of Tuscany. In the early nineteenth century, Port Mahon and Barcelona were the only Spanish Mediterranean quarantine ports typically capable of receiving traffic from the Middle East. Similarly, in France, until 1835, the ports of Toulon (for warships) and Marseille had a monopoly over all ships arriving in France from the Middle East and North Africa, a fact that justified the legal change in 1805 that gave Paris a veto over nominations to the *Intendance Sanitaire* of Marseille and (presumably) lay behind the unique presence in Marseille of a permanent "Agency" of France's Foreign Affairs Ministry. Finally, the *Provveditori* at Venice were in charge of a vast set of subsidiary health boards in the eighteenth century, and though Venice was subordinated to Trieste after the Austrian conquest, it remained one of the four largest sites of quarantine in the Habsburg Empire. In sum, in a variety of different polities, individual boards of health had enormous, statewide influence.

Negotiating the National

Boards of health were bodies with nation-level stature. But in the eyes of board members, this position needed to be constantly maintained. Some called their domination of quarantine policy a monopoly – mostly the critics of the system. In one of his most ringing indictments of the quarantine system, the Radical MP John Bowring declared that, "far mightier" than other reasons for quarantine's existence, "pecuniary interests, and other interests of place and power" prevented reform.[27] The allegation about "pecuniary interests" was common to critiques of quarantine. But though boards of health often made a profit in a given year, the sum was deposited in account for years when quarantine operations might incur a deficit – it was certainly not pocketed by board members, who were rarely paid for their service.[28]

Boards of health and governments often operated together uneasily. Particularly during France's July Monarchy, it is clear that the *Intendance*

---

[27] John Bowring, *Speech of Dr. John Bowring, M.P., on Submitting His Resolution Relating to Quarantine Laws and Regulations* (London: Hansard, 1844), 3.

[28] It is not true, however, that board of health members never sought to take advantage of their position. The Intendants of Marseille made an attempt during the Directory to argue that they should be exempted from the *patente* tax on the grounds that their role was analogous to "health officers attached to armies, hospitals, or care of paupers." They were unsuccessful; an inquiry of the Interior Ministry's Commercial Office concluded that though an analogy existed between the roles, the Intendants were not themselves involved in medical care and should receive no exemption. Report of the Bureau de Commerce, Interior Ministry, Paris. 16 Vendémiaire, An IX (October 8, 1800), AN (Pierrefitte) F/8/29 Dossier III.

Sanitaire in Marseille and the responsible minister in Paris (the Minister of Commerce and Industry) were often operating at cross-purposes. When they were not being pushed to reform, other boards of health seem to have operated more seamlessly with their national governments – the correspondence between Niccolò Corsini, the Tuscan minister responsible for overseeing the Livorno *Sanità*, and the Governor of Livorno, its president, evinces a sense of cooperation and mutual reliance. Corsini, in fact, refers to Livorno's *Sanità* as the *Dipartimento Sanitario*, as if it were a division of the national government.[29] Elsewhere in Italy, sanitary bureaucrats seem to have enjoyed similarly good relations with ministers, while in Malta, the Quarantine Department was actually a discrete division of the colonial administration, with the Governor himself as the nominal head (after 1826) of the Board of Health. This pattern of integration between quarantine officials and the national government was also common in Northern Europe. In both Britain and Holland, quarantine was linked to the Customs Service and directly super-intended from London and Amsterdam, respectively.

Again, Britain's Privy Council persistently sought to defend its role as the sole progenitor of quarantine rules in the UK, and even as the laws were gradually liberalized, it continued to be mandated that PC approval was necessary before many ships could be granted pratique. The archival remains of British quarantine practice show how unclear it was to many captains and merchants with questions and complaints that the Privy Council was the source of quarantine administration. And yet, on many days, quarantine correspondence would have been the primary activity of the Council's secretary. Minute questions relating to breaches of the rules and requests from localities for new sanitary outposts and "floating lazarettos" were regular items on the Council's docket.[30] Their Lordships in Council were consulted on such issues as the repatriation of the corpses of Britons who died in the East, the correct procedure for sorting quarantined mail, and best practices for airing rags.[31] This shows how extensively many political luminaries must have understood quarantine's particularities.

In sum, then, though Marseille's *Intendants* liked to see themselves as the leaders of Mediterranean boards of health, their relationship with their national government was anomalous – particularly after 1830. As we will see in Chapter 9, this created embarrassing problems for Marseille in the 1840s as it attempted to remain in sync with Italian ports at a time when Parisian ministers had entirely different priorities. Although British zeal for reform in the 1830s and 1840s mirrored the French, the firm location of quarantine administration at the

[29] ASLi Sanità 37.
[30] For examples of all of these items and more from the early 1840s, see, for example, TNA PC 1/4531.
[31] See TNA PC 7/5.

heart of government meant that debates about quarantine and evolving policies did not involve the same kind of disputes and discontinuities experienced across the Channel.

Another source of ambiguity and contestation between boards of health and national ministers concerned the status of the lazaretto. As the point of contact between zones of health and suspicion, the lazaretto was the locus of decontamination. As such, it was not fully inside the conceptual zone of European security – access to it was very strictly regulated. A Marseille *Intendant* insisted that he could not bring even his own parent into the building during an inspection. For him, the space was cordoned off by a principle that transcended regulation or national legislation: "an inviolable law which no reason whatsoever might abrogate."[32] Across diverse sources, the practices of quarantine were undergirded by an abstract notion of "sanitary laws," which were shared by all "civilized" ports of the Mediterranean. So considered, the lazaretto takes on Continental, and even global, dimensions that show its ambiguous status as a physical institution. The rules and procedures of any one lazaretto were determined more by custom, agreement, and cross-Mediterranean negotiation than they were by national legislation. Theoretically, the whims of a board of health could shape quarantine practice in any direction, but in practice, whims were constrained by traditions, and sanitary bureaucrats behaved similarly across the Mediterranean.

The very question of whether lazarettos were under the jurisdiction of one locality or subject to a broader and more nebulous international jurisdiction was put under the consideration of a French court in 1818, when an inspector for the *Octroi* (local tax) of Marseille seized some wine from the stores of one Sieur Poucel, the lazaretto restaurateur. The subsequent dispute went as far as France's Interior Minister and Minister of Finances; Marseille's *Intendance* used the occasion to vigorously (and apparently successfully) insist that the institution they oversaw could not come under the remit of local laws and regulations.[33] The lazaretto, insisted the *Intendants*, was effectively not in Marseille at all, because its purpose transcended the local sphere: "To speak properly, the lazaretto belongs to the domain of all nations, diverse subjects of which come within its bosom, to purge themselves of the contagion they might well be carrying."[34]

And yet, to the cities that housed them, the presence of a lazaretto was a boon to the local economy (whether its employees paid taxes or not). Marseille's *Intendants* might have argued that their lazaretto belonged to all nations, but in other contexts they would have conceded that it was a key part of the city of

---

[32] Conservateurs de Santé de Marseille to the Minister of the Interior, 15 Thermidor, An XII (August 3, 1804), AN (Pierrefitte) F/8/29 Dossier VI.
[33] See AN (Pierrefitte-sur-Seine) F/8/28/I/4.   [34] Procès de Sieur Poucel, ADBR 200 E 18.

Marseille's significant investment in Levantine trade. Again, the *Intendants* themselves were largely drawn from the ranks of the city's merchants who had traded to the Levant. Many were also associated, then, with the Marseille Chamber of Commerce – a body whose title conceals a truly international remit. Indeed, the Chamber of Commerce, through its associates in the *échelles* of the Levant, conducted operations with the Middle East that far exceeded the scope and scale of the British Levant Company. Until 1834, it was entitled to a two percent levy on all proceeds made from the Levant trade. Unsurprisingly, then, it was a repository for information about Ottoman commercial policy that surpassed that of the French government. Correspondence between the Chamber of Commerce and the Foreign Ministry shows the extent to which Marseille merchants were habitually the first to know about issues relating to Ottoman commerce, though Marseillaise commercial agents and national diplomats operated in close harmony.[35] Marseille's status as the only port allowed to undertake commerce with the Levant (a right that expired around the same time as the Chamber of Commerce's right to two percent), required the presence of France's largest lazaretto. Lazaretto, *Intendance*, Chamber of Commerce, and the establishments of Marseillaise merchants in the Levant were thus a symbiotic medico-mercantile system. Protecting the sanitary monopoly alongside the commercial one was essential to the city's prestige.

That this conferred a significant boost to the local economy of Marseille to the detriment of other port cities is clear from the complaints of merchants from northern France. Although during the debates over France's 1822 Quarantine Law, an ambitious plan was discussed for a nationwide system of lazarettos, those eventually established in the North and West of the country remained limited to the produce, passengers, and ships of the Americas while all Levantine goods were still required to pass through Marseille. An exasperated merchant from St. Quentin lamented the vast expense that Northern textile factory owners incurred if they attempted to import cotton from Egypt. Transshipping fees, lazaretto fees, and other commissions all accrued, complained the merchant, to the benefit of the Marseillaise, all because Dunkirk was not permitted to receive ships from the Levant.[36] Over the strenuous protests of Marseille's *Intendants*,[37] the rules changed in the mid-1830s – a clear sign that

---

[35] This dynamic is visible throughout the letters at the National Archives containing correspondence between the Foreign Ministry and the Marseille Chamber of Commerce. See AN (Pierrefitte) F/12/7593.

[36] "A Merchant of St. Quentin" to the Minister of Commerce, July 8, 1834, AN (Pierrefitte) F/12/7593.

[37] In 1820, for example, a request to the Intendants to supply its rules and a plan of its lazaretto to authorities in Bordeaux and Rouen immediately raised suspicions in Marseille. The Intendants found obscure administrative rules they said prohibited them from helping the other cities. They ominously warned the Interior Minister of "the dangers to which the multiplication of lazarettos would expose France, if it were a question of admitting ships coming from the Levant or

the government recognized the benefits that a lazaretto could bring to the local economy.

These anecdotes point to the vast, ancillary world of quarantine's beneficiaries that extended far beyond the august halls of chambers of commerce to trans-shippers and to hundreds of local merchants and suppliers (who catered to a captive market of passengers detained in lazarettos). Smugglers, too, could benefit from the concentration of ships quarantine provided. As we will see in Chapter 8, one of the most plausible explanations for the origin of the 1813–14 plague of Malta involved a smuggling operation carried out by local shoemaker. The lazaretto may have been an institution abstracted from the city itself, but it generated a local world of legitimate and criminal businesses that was invested in the status quo.

Plague Ships: An International Problem

There were many benefits, then, to residing in a quarantine port, depending on one's profession. At the same time, the regular appearance of ships actually carrying the plague (in the form of stricken sailors) in European ports could create local panic. Such plague ships created tremors throughout the quarantine system and inspired the anxious exchange of letters among boards of health. Most ships had clean bills of health and most ships with foul bills had simply proceeded from a port where reports of plague existed (they did not include sailors or passengers actually suffering from the plague). Yet, the most intense period of quarantine management occurred when a ship with plague actually on board arrived. According to the statistics collected by the anticontagionist (and former chief doctor of the Egyptian Medical Service) Louis Aubert-Roche, some forty-eight plague ships arrived at Western European ports between 1784 and 1841.[38] If one were to add plague ships in quarantine harbors of the Russian Empire in the Black Sea and the arrival of plague victims at land-based quarantine posts along the Ottoman-Habsburg frontier, this total would be even larger. Rarely did more than a year or two pass without a plague ship somewhere in Southern Europe, and the arrival of such a ship was an event that generated repercussions across Mediterranean Europe. At times, the threat must have seemed overwhelming; during the major Egyptian plague epidemic in 1835, for example, five different plague ships docked at four Southern European quarantine ports (Marseille, Malta,

---

Barbary." See Intendants to the Interior Minister, February 29, 1820, AN (Pierrefitte) F/8/29, Dossier I.

[38] Aubert-Roche, *Réforme des Quarantaines*, 73–74. Daniel Panzac counts thirty-two ships between 1815 and 1845, though his data differ from Aubert-Roche's, given that, for example, he enumerates only four plague ships at Marseille, while Aubert-Roche counts twelve. See Panzac, *Quarantaines et Lazarets*, 85.

Livorno, and Genoa).[39] Some years earlier, in 1819, just as preparations for a centenary commemoration of the 1720 plague of Marseille were being made, a plague ship arrived to perform quarantine in that city's lazaretto (an event so fraught with symbolism and anxiety that the entire *Intendance* received medals in its wake).[40]

Indeed, part of the reason that the arrival of a plague ship seemed like such a fraught event was that the origins of both the Marseille and Malta plagues have traditionally been linked to the arrival of particular infected ships. With such dire potential consequences, members of health boards knew every action they made could condemn them to historical infamy if any aspect of quarantine was compromised. Both for an internal audience and for the benefit of foreign boards of health, scrupulous adherence to standard practices was on show when a plague ship arrived, and constant communication was vital. Some of these events must have seemed quite likely to result in an epidemic – in 1821, for example, a Maltese brig carrying a crew of fourteen in addition to eight passengers suffered an outbreak of plague in the quarantine harbor. Fourteen individuals were struck while in quarantine at the lazaretto, and twelve of these died. A crew of five was sent out by the quarantine office to undertake fumigation and depuration of the ship (two guardians were normally allocated to each ship). Of these five expurgators, two subsequently caught the plague, though both survived.[41] When an event like this occurred, it was crucial to send circular letters with thorough details to foreign boards (a timeline of events, a list of casualties, and details of extraordinary fumigation procedures applied) – both to demonstrate local efficiency and to warn them of the pestilential threat.

In this way, the arrival of a plague ship could trouble local bureaucrats, national ministers, and foreign boards of health for months. The *Leonidas* episode provides a clear example. In early July 1837, the *Leonidas* (a French packet boat) left Constantinople bound for Marseille. Soon after its arrival, the Foreign Affairs Ministry's agent in Marseille reported that "the death of two persons who were part of the crew of the Leonidas, who, it is certain, evinced the symptoms of plague, has required the *Intendance Sanitaire* to take the most severe measures to avoid the propagation of contagion."[42] Marseille immediately informed foreign boards of health – the Minutes from Genoa's *Magistrato* show that a letter about the *Leonidas* was read at a meeting held on July 24. At the next meeting, five days later, the *Magistrato* ruled that all arrivals from

---

[39] Aubert-Roche, *Réforme des Quarantaines*, 74. In 1837, four more plague ships arrived.
[40] Prefect of the Bouches-du-Rhône Department to the Interior Minister, March 9, 1821, AN (Pierrefitte) F/8/28/I/5.
[41] Milroy, *Quarantine and the Plague*, 64.
[42] Constantin Guys to Comte Molé, July 19, 1837, Archives Nationales, C.A.R.A.N., Paris, henceforth AN, Paris, AE/B/III/226.

Marseille would be subjected to a ten-day quarantine of observation.[43] Meanwhile, in Marseille, as the Marseille Agent of the Foreign Affairs Ministry wrote to the Minister in Paris, "the quarantine for the *Leonidas* passengers was just fixed at eighty-five days, which is very disagreeable for them. The decision depends on an ancient rule, a bit too severe, but under which their sentence was required to be passed."[44] Severe or not, Genoa's *Magistrato* expanded its quarantine to include "the Mediterranean Coasts of France, Marseille included," and only ended the suspension of free pratique for southern French ships on October 25.[45] Perhaps this grand display of cautiousness was due to the fact that Genoa's *own* ships had been quarantined at Civitavecchia the preceding spring on rumors of plague in one of Genoa's lazarettos.[46] In this way, the reception of individual plague ships provoked quarantines that could ensnare hundreds of other ships over a period of several months.

Incidents such as this reveal how extensively rigorous quarantine practices begat more of the same in an era when every event in a quarantine port was made for the consumption of a Continent-wide audience. No board of health was immune to criticism that, at some point in the past, it had acted rashly and potentially compromised public health. As Junko Takeda has shown, the consequences of the inattentiveness of the Marseille Board of Health (i.e., the plague of 1720), was understood as a moral condemnation of the dangers of unrestrained commerce from which the city needed to redeem itself with a new model of virtuous commerce.[47] The members of the Marseille Board, no doubt, saw rigorous adherence to the norms of quarantine as a crucial civic obligation.

Even when inattentiveness did *not* produce dire consequences (like the plague of Marseille), boards of health caught relaxing quarantine requirements for particularly prominent individuals or unduly favoring ships of a particular flag were very anxious to restore their sanitary bona fides by excessive (and well publicized) procedures or by "tattling" on other powers. As we will see later, it is no accident that Britain's decision to admit some Egyptian cotton without quarantine in 1825 was broadcast around the Mediterranean by the Board of Health at Trieste (which was, at the time, experiencing blowback for its decision to admit a British diplomat arriving from Constantinople after a dubiously brief quarantine).

---

[43] Deliberations of July 24 and July 29, 1837, ASGe Sanità 544.

[44] Constantin Guys to Comte Molé, August 16, 1837, AN (Paris) AE/B/III/226.

[45] Deliberations of October 25, 1837, ASGe Sanità 544. That said, given the fact that other quarantines were lifted on that date because of signs the cholera epidemic was abating, it is possible Marseille's quarantine had lasted so long because it coincided with concerns about cholera.

[46] Constantin Guys to Comte Molé, April 19, 1837, AN (Paris) AE/B/III/226.

[47] Takeda, *Between Crown and Commerce*, 180–83.

Boards of health needed to be constantly on guard – both out of genuine worry surrounding imported epidemics and also about making a thoughtless decision that would later elicit repercussions from foreign boards. Even without a plague ship or news of an Ottoman epidemic, epidemic disease could feel perilously close. Rumors of plagues exceeded outbreaks, and when individuals died in the lazaretto without a clear diagnosis, the plague was always a possibility. Given the improvements to communication, and the regularization of reciprocal correspondence among boards of health, it became feasible to attempt efforts to get a handle on what threats *might* be in the offing. Just so, in 1816, both the British Military Secretary at Malta and the British Consul at Genoa forwarded to the Genoa *Magistrato* a warning they had received from Admiral Penrose (the Commander-in-Chief of the Royal Navy's Mediterranean Fleet) that a mysterious three-masted sailing ship with a lion's head mast had "carried the plague" from Smyrna to Tripoli and might attempt to call at Genoa.[48] Indeed, Tripoli suffered from a particularly destructive plague just after this letter was received. That such a naval eminence as Penrose should issue this kind of a warning shows the extent to which each plague ship was both a serious threat to European sanitary security and a critical subject within international diplomacy.

The potential need to fumigate a ship with the plague onboard must have been the most dramatic and frightening moment in the routine of service as a lazaretto guardian. As we have seen, some guardians were infected in the course of these events, and a few died. Experiencing a lazaretto around the time of a plague ship's arrival must also have been terrifying for the sailors and passengers involved, not solely those on the ship itself, but those in the lazaretto at the same time or soon after. As we will see in the next chapter, the specter of plague seemed to hang over much inside lazaretto walls, and the reach of the disease extended further than the number of plague ships might suggest. Though boards of health may have been stuck in their routines of disinfection, little about quarantine would have felt routine, even for those who experienced it regularly. That plague ships continued to arrive in Western European ports into the 1840s helps confirm the sense that universal quarantine existed just as long as plague remained over the water or just across the Ottoman frontier.

---

[48] Frederick Hankey to the Marchesa di Pallavicini, November 4, 1816, and Harting to Pallavicini, November 27, 1816, ASGe Sanità 1365.

4   "A Sort of Hospital-Prison"

The Reverend Robert Walsh, a Levant Company chaplain, returned to Britain from Constantinople over land. Some days after his departure, he reached the frontier of Western Europe – the Rothenthurm Pass, which marked the border between the Austrian and Ottoman Empires. Here, at a small station maintained by the Habsburg government, Walsh was required to perform his quarantine before he could reenter the West. After a dismal twenty-one days of detention in freezing temperatures, Walsh waited with eagerness for the morning of his release. If his quarantine had been unpleasant so far, Walsh's experience during its final hours struck him as the most bizarre experience yet.

> The last day of three weeks' detention at length passed over, and the next I was informed I was at liberty to depart. The doctor came by candle-light in the morning; his man brought a pan of charcoal, on which he threw a few pinches of nitre; he then walked round me in a circle like a magician, and so I was purified.[1]

This ceremony marked the moment at which Walsh was free to leave and mix with Westerners once again. Walsh lambasted the flaws of his quarantine experience, but he recognized that rituals like this appeared to contain enormous symbolic power. More than a literal purification, quarantine forced each traveler to confront him or herself as a foreign body.

Quarantine looked different depending on where it was experienced. A small hut or an open piece of fenced-in grass could have been your quarantine quarters in freezing Galatz (on the Ottoman-Russian frontier), or a drafty, stone-floored room in Malta's huge lazaretto, or a cabin on a ship docked off a coast in a specially marked quarantine harbor, yellow flag flying from the rigging. Passengers on a ship about to dock at a quarantine port would not have known whether to expect lenient treatment or a rigorous smoking of their clothes and bodies and a prolonged detention.

---

[1] Robert Walsh, *Narrative of a Journey from Constantinople to England* (London: Frederick Wesley and A. H. Davis, 1831), 264.

In common parlance, quarantine was something individuals were obliged to "perform" and also something boards of health "performed" for each other. The present chapter develops the notion of "performative sanitation" as a way to illuminate the ritualistic character of the purification of suspect people and things. I employ the concept in two senses. The first is consonant with Judith Butler's sense of "performativity," in which repetitive practices give shape and meaning to constructed realities, but also inevitably prepare the unsettlement of the concepts they build. Central to Butler's conception is that the performance is accomplished without intent or planning, which is not precisely true within lazaretto practice. Yet, the designation of individuals as "dangerous/contaminated" and "healthy/purified" proceeded seamlessly and impersonally at each stage of quarantine, governed simply by the passage of time. Sailors, passengers, and other travelers were precisely as "dangerous" or "clean" as the quarantine calendar indicated. Boards of health mandated procedures and guardians followed them, not because of a belief in this or that scientific doctrine, but because repetitive accumulated practice had divided the Mediterranean world into zones of health and contamination. The lazaretto doctor at the Rothenthurm Pass might have thought his charcoal/niter/circling ceremony as absurd as Robert Walsh thought it, and yet, according to the laws and logics that governed quarantine, Walsh was purified when it concluded. No longer would guardians shy away if he approached, no longer would merchants dip his money in pots of vinegar if he made a purchase. As long as quarantine lasted, the weight of its rituals and the letter of the law ensured sanitation had been dutifully performed after a certain duration of time and certain acts of expurgation, independent of the state of body or mind.

"Performative sanitation" has a second and more overt meaning here. The efficient performance of quarantine was explicitly, sometimes theatrically, exchanged among boards of health. Phenomena such as efficient communication, rigid emphasis on correct procedure, and frankness about any unusual events in quarantine were generally oriented outward. Board members performed these tasks for the gaze of inquiring consuls from other powers, or to craft a future anecdote of correct quarantine practice for foreign boards of health. Some of this we have seen already, through such practices as the regular exchange of quarantine rules and the frequent writing of circular letters during the quarantine of a plague ship. Universal quarantine could only sustain itself if its discomforts were acknowledged as normative. The quarantine of royals and other dignitaries traveling across the Mediterranean was designed (and publicized) to make the point that the system truly applied to all. In this respect, even as travelers railed against their experience, they were helping to give the system meaning and to keep it alive.

While quarantine sites and particular boards of health have been studied by other scholars, the *experience* of quarantine, accessed through travel narratives and archival records, has been largely ignored by existing scholarship. This chapter investigates precisely that experience, alongside the processes and ideas that underlay the rituals of decontamination. As Britons negotiated the patterns of Mediterranean lazarettos, they assimilated themselves with a Continental system and came to acknowledge quarantine as a kind of homecoming (albeit an unpleasant one). Many thought quarantine was ridiculous, but the boredom, terror, and anticipation it created left a lasting mark. Quarantine provided the most significant border-crossing experience in the eighteenth- and nineteenth-century world; this chapter is about how it accrued significance in the minds of those it ensnared.

The Idea of a Lazaretto

The Scottish poet and traveler Thomas Campbell described the Lazaretto of Toulon as "a sort of hospital-prison."[2] Indeed, quarantine could undergird a sense that a return to Europe meant a return to a harsher disciplinary regime. Disease was only one element of disorder this border was meant to suppress. On reaching the Russo-Turkish frontier at Galatz, Edmund Spenser "first beheld, since I left Asia, the stars which herald in the dawn of European civilization, in the form of custom-house officers, sanitary officers, police officers, &c."[3] The artist Francis Hervé wryly noted that his attendant was "called the guardian, but answers also for the purposes of gaoler, or turnkey."[4] For Sir Walter Scott, the most "unpleasant" thing about performing quarantine at Malta was "to be thought so very unclean and capable of poisoning a whole city."[5] Others put the same feeling of vague guilt still more explicitly. The doctor William Macmichael called quarantine at the Russian frontier a term of "penance or probation" meted out to "those whom business or curiosity may tempt to leave the healthy regions."[6] The military man C. Rochfort Scott, quarantined in Malta, called the entire experience "a fortnight's moral burking."[7] Quarantine seemed to invert common standards of guilt and

---

[2] Thomas Campbell to Alexander Campbell, May 22, 1835, Glasgow University Ms. Gen. 1662/16, Item 5.

[3] Quoted in V. Denis Vandervelde, "Russia: The River Danube Quarantine Stations," *Pratique: The Journal of the Disinfected Mail Study Circle* 21, no. 2 (1996): 45.

[4] Francis Hervé, *A Residence in Greece and Turkey* (London: Whittaker and Co., 1837), 2:325.

[5] Sir Walter Scott, *The Journal of Sir Walter Scott, 1825–1832: From the Original Manuscript at Abbottsford* (Edinburgh: David Douglas, 1891), 859. Journal Entry for November 25–30, 1831.

[6] William Macmichael, *A Journey from Moscow to Constantinople* (London: John Murray, 1819), 62.

[7] C. Rochfort Scott, *Rambles in Egypt and Candia* (London: Henry Colburn, 1837), 1:2–3. "Burking," here, signifies murder, referring as it does to the Burke and Hare "anatomy murders" in Edinburgh in 1828.

innocence, to expose individuals to punishment for crimes they had never committed.[8] It carried a note of accusation.

The contrast between the light, sun, and drama of a Mediterranean port often seemed a particularly cruel irony to those "honorable prisoners" in quarantine.[9] The English traveler Mrs. Griffith described "seeing a bright-looking spot" in the distance, through an accidentally opened lazaretto door, and feeling "an indescribable wish to go there."[10] The sense of confinement within the lazaretto was made worse by a strict code of segregation within its walls. It disoriented those who experienced it. "My fortnight's imprisonment within the bars of the quarantine, made me feel like a captive bird escaped from its cage," wrote Charles Terry. "I hardly knew what to make of freedom at first, so much does habit grow upon us."[11] The lazaretto experience was hard to shake; quarantine could leave a sense of its awesome power long after the individuals it detained were granted free pratique. The disciplinary mechanisms at work within it suggested a return to hygienic and imaginative conformity.

The French Quarantine Law of 1822 formally defined the lazaretto as a *lieu réservé*.[12] This applied not simply because access to it was limited, but because the rules that reigned within the lazaretto constituted a distinct legal regime. The doctor Patrick Russell argued that,

> The common law cannot be allowed the least pretext for its exercise within the walls, such as seizure of Goods or Persons, or the discipline that it may be necessary to enforce, in the due performance of the rules of the Health Office. The general safety of the state is in this case considered as the supreme law.[13]

In this way, despite the relatively rare appearance of the plague, the lazaretto operated in a permanent state of emergency. If Michel Foucault considered the "plague stricken town" to be a "limited and temporary" antecedent to the modern prison, in the lazaretto we could consider the constant potential of the plague to have enabled perhaps the first institution in which the impulses of

---

[8] Occasionally, however, the lazaretto functioned as an *actual* prison. See Henry Dyer to the Chief Secretary, March 28, 1827, NAM CSG 03/97. Dyer, a British captain, asked for permission from the Maltese authorities to imprison sixteen captured pirates in the lazaretto. Other records from Malta indicate that refractory guardians could be imprisoned in Fort Manoel (which had been annexed to the lazaretto) to serve sentences meted out by sanitary authorities. See Charles Tucker to Richard Plaskett, June 17, 1817, NLM LIBR 843.

[9] Sarah Haight, *Over the Ocean, or, Glimpses of Travel in Many Lands* (New York: Paine and Burgess, 1846), 139.

[10] Major and Mrs. George Darby Griffith, *A Journey across the Desert from Ceylon to Marseille* (London: Henry Colburn, 1845), 2: 94.

[11] Charles Terry, *Scenes and Thoughts in Foreign Lands* (London: William Pickering, 1848), 257.

[12] This piece of Restoration legislation was drafted with heavy involvement by the Marseille Intendance. See the drafts of the law and assorted comments in ADBR 200 E 343.

[13] Patrick Russell, from a Report of the Quarantine Committee, BL Add. Ms. 38234.

the modern prison were permanently enacted.[14] And yet, it was a site of exceptional justice, subject to transnational norms and assumptions rather than local or national control. The obligation to perform sanitation to an external audience encoded within it an exemption from typical forms of national regulation. In this way, we can also see the lazaretto as a permanent locus of Giorgio Agamben's "state of exception." If the "state of exception" is a quasi-legal, quasi-political form of emergency operation, which Agamben sees as having gradually been made permanent in the course of the twentieth and twenty-first centuries,[15] the lazaretto is an early space where this form of irregular jurisdiction was granted ongoing operation. The stark drama of plague prevention, in fact, undermined the stability of "common law," at least in Russell's conception, by showing it to be incapable of contending with the existential threat of pestilential disease. The hypothetical emergency represented by an epidemic justified a "supreme law" that transcended rights and traditions. Whatever your skeptical sensibilities, warned the English traveler A. W. Kinglake, "if you dare to break the laws of the quarantine, you will find yourself carefully shot, and carelessly buried in the ground of the lazaretto."[16] Seen thus, the nineteenth-century lazaretto appears as a harbinger, not an anachronism.

Quarantine's Scope and Demographics

Who were the individuals forced to spend so many weeks and months detained by quarantine? And how many of them were there? Both questions, unsurprisingly, are impossible to answer with absolute certainty. Nomenclatures of sailors and passengers in quarantine, as well as any remarks about their professions, have been preserved only in a haphazard way or not at all. Records of bills of health, medical visits, and customs declarations provide tantalizing glimpses of individual ships in quarantine, but comparing any of these sets of records even for the same year usually reveals glaring inconsistencies. Caveats aside, in most ways, the archives of Mediterranean boards of health are well preserved (less so the materials retained from land quarantines, or "floating lazarettos" off the coast of Britain). It is possible to arrive at some conclusions by using representative years with good documentation and by comparing different kinds of sources (from registers of incoming ships, to

---

[14] Michel Foucault, *Discipline and Punish*, trans. Alan Sheridan (New York: Random House, 1977), 209. In a different context, this point has been recognized in Takeda, *Between Crown and Commerce*, 117.

[15] Giorgio Agamben, *State of Exception*, trans. Kevin Attell (Chicago: University of Chicago Press, 2005).

[16] Alexander Kinglake, *Eothen, or, Traces of Travel in the East* (New York: Wiley and Putnam, 1845), 1–2.

declarations of captains, to reports of quarantine doctors and guardians). In some years, wars or epidemic disease outbreaks dramatically augmented quarantine traffic. But even without such stresses and strains, the system ensnared tens of thousands annually.

Livorno was one of the most cosmopolitan quarantine ports in the Mediterranean, with the vast majority of its quarantined arrivals captained by non-Tuscans (Figure 4.1). It had three major lazarettos in continuous usage – the fortresses of San Rocco, San Leopoldo, and San Jacopo – more impressive sanitary infrastructure than in most other ports. In terms of the total volume of quarantined shipping, Livorno was one of the busiest quarantine ports, alongside Marseille and Malta (though its traffic would fall compared to the latter between 1825 and 1845). The records of its *Consiglio di Sanità* (board of health) are comparatively complete. Livorno's quarantine statistics thus give a fairly representative sense of a bustling quarantine port at the center of Mediterranean shipping.

In 1830, 642 ships performed quarantine at Livorno.[17] An analysis of the medical reports contained for this year reveals that the average crew size of

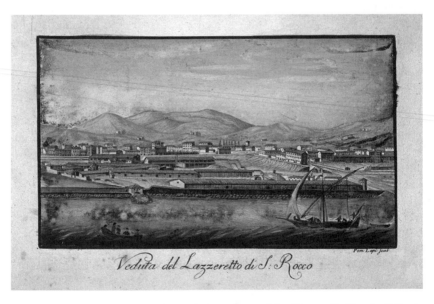

Veduta del Lazzeretto di S. Rocco

Figure 4.1 View of Livorno's Lazzaretto of San Rocco. Etching by P. Lapi. Courtesy of the Wellcome Library. (CC BY license)

[17] Total derived from ASLi Sanità 722. Using only the ships for which medical reports were generated (ASLi Sanità 208), the total is considerably lower (512). The discrepancy is probably due to some ships with short quarantines avoiding medical inspection.

ships performing quarantine at Livorno hovered just over fourteen men per ship.[18] This suggests a rough total of 9,000 crew members performing quarantine onboard ship at Livorno. The data for the lazarettos for that year are incomplete, as the records from the San Jacopo lazaretto only begin in September. Even so, there are records of 38 individuals performing quarantine at this lazaretto, with 101 listed individuals at San Leopoldo, and 165 at San Rocco.[19] Genoa, which also had multiple lazarettos (Foce and Varignano being the largest), also seems to have averaged just over one hundred passengers per year in each around this time.[20] As will be seen below, these totals of a few hundred individuals a year performing quarantine in the lazaretto were far less than the norm at Malta. Still, in total, Livorno posted impressive quarantine traffic. Counting the passengers in the lazaretto and the guardians assigned to these ships (as well as the crew members discussed above), the total number of individuals experiencing quarantine at Livorno in the year 1830 was probably just under 10,000.

The number of individuals in quarantine grew throughout the 1830s and early 1840s before it began to fall as quarantine regulations were curtailed or eliminated. Even so, the total number of ships at Livorno in 1835, 1,171, is exceptionally high.[21] A look at the provenances of most of these ships helps explain the mystery – the mid-1830s marked the arrival of cholera in Mediterranean Europe and the institution of intra-European quarantines as a result. The most common point of origin for quarantined ships that year was Marseille, followed by Genoa and other major Italian ports. The massive spike in quarantine and the consequent fact that about 15,000 individuals probably experienced quarantine at Livorno this year shows the disruptions that could happen when ships from other Mediterranean ports were refused free pratique. Similar increases were visible across the Mediterranean. In 1845, the last year for which I have analyzed the number of arrivals at Livorno and during which the periods of detention had already been curtailed, there were 678 ships performing quarantine: more than in 1830, but lower than during the peak period of the mid- and late 1830s.[22]

Marseille, with its extensive sanitary bureaucracy, its energetic *Intendance Sanitaire*, and its reliable set of contacts with French consuls and agents throughout the Middle East, was a central hub of quarantine throughout this period. We have already seen how the Lazaretto of Arenc occasionally housed

---

[18] Data derived from the first half of 1830 by counting up crew members listed on medical reports contained in ASLi 208.

[19] Data derived from the lazaretto files contained in ASLi Sanità 208.

[20] The passenger data at Genoa are partial, but that is certainly the impression one gets from consulting ASGe Sanità 1707, which contains passenger data for the Lazaretto della Foce between 1828 and 1832.

[21] Total derived from ASLi Sanità 727.   [22] Total derived from ASLi Sanità 739.

entire armies. That said, it appears to have had smaller numbers of paying passengers performing quarantine than Malta, though probably more than most Italian ports. Between 1815 and 1833, the average number of such passengers was just over 330 each year, though the number declined from a post-Napoleonic high in the course of the 1820s before picking up again after 1830.[23] This makes sense, given the comparative abatement of Franco-Ottoman commerce after the Napoleonic Wars and its gradual rebirth. But there is also the likelihood that the Marseille data do not represent the true total because of the categories into which passengers were separated; ordinary passengers were counted separately from "military passengers," who often constituted a huge portion of those undergoing quarantine at Marseille. By the 1840s, it appeared traffic declined again (only 149 and 231 individual passengers are listed for 1842 and 1843, respectively). Not only did fewer epidemic scares in the late 1830s and early 1840s mean more ships approached with clean bills of health, but Marseille had lost its status (in the mid-1830s) as the only French port allowed to admit ships from the Levant and North Africa; a handful of western and northern port cities were granted the same privilege by the Commerce Minister over the strong objections of the *Intendance Sanitaire*.[24]

In Malta, detailed data on quarantined shipping survive from 1831 onward. In that year (as compared with 642 ships in 1830 at Livorno), 560 ships performed quarantine at Malta.[25] In 1835, the total rose to 801 ships performing quarantine at Malta and a total of 12,932 individuals.[26] In contrast with Livorno, however, far more individuals are marked as having performed quarantine at the lazaretto than onboard ship. In a report prepared by Emanuele Bonavia (Captain of the Lazaretto 1832–37, Superintendent of Quarantine thereafter), some 1,629 individuals performed quarantine in the lazaretto in 1835.[27] On average, by comparing this report and the lazaretto register to the register of ships in quarantine, it appears that passengers in the lazaretto made up between 10 and 15 percent of all quarantine traffic.[28] In

---

[23] Average calculated based on passenger data contained in ADBR 200 E 875.

[24] See Dominique Bon, "Cholera Epidemics, Local Politics, and Nationalism in the Province of Nice during the First Half of the Nineteenth Century," in Chircop and Martínez, *Mediterranean Quarantines,* 50.

[25] In all the registers of Maltese quarantine, "Men-of-War" are treated as a single entry each month, so the real totals of ships, no doubt, are somewhat higher than those given above. Nevertheless, the individuals enumerated in this entry each month are never very numerous and suggest that many months, only one or two men-of-war performed quarantine here, despite Malta's status as the seat of Britain's Mediterranean Fleet.

[26] Totals for both 1831 and 1835 derived from NLM (Valletta) LIBR 812/I.

[27] See Arthur Holroyd, *The Quarantine Laws: Their Abuses and Inconsistencies. A Letter Addressed to John Cam Hobhouse, Bart. M.P., President of the Board of Control &c.* (London: Simpkin, Marshall, 1839), 41.

[28] This approximate ratio of passengers in the lazaretto to crew members performing quarantine onboard ship is derived by comparing the summary of Bonavia's report in Holroyd's letter,

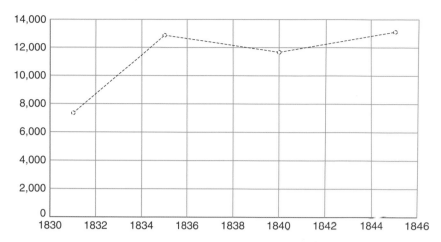

Figure 4.2 Graph of sailors and passengers arriving at Malta in quarantine, 1830–45 (line is an approximation). Calculations derived from National Library of Malta, Valletta, LIBR 810/I and 810/II.

numbers reported to Arthur Holroyd, who conducted an inquiry about Mediterranean quarantine practices in the 1840s, Signor Garcin, a Maltese quarantine official, estimated that the average number of individuals performing quarantine in the lazaretto during his years of service was roughly 800 to 1,000. After that point, according to Bonavia, there occurred a "very considerable increase."[29] Again, these numbers dwarf the typical passenger totals at Italian lazarettos and at Marseille (roughly 200–500 each year). Unlike Livorno, Malta was heavily used as a stopping point for ships en route from the East, and it saw less traffic from carrying routes along the Mediterranean coast of Europe (Figure 4.2).

In 1840, there were 653 ships performing quarantine at Malta, and 11,689 individuals. While the number of ships dropped after the dissipation of the first cholera epidemic in Southern Europe, the total number of individuals remained quite high – showing a growing average crew size. By this time, new kinds of ships, including steam ships, were routinely performing quarantine at Malta. In 1845, some 846 ships and 13,132 individuals performed quarantine there[30] – a high point of traffic, despite the fact that by this time, the British government had (for the first time) authorized a steam route to bypass quarantine altogether on its journey from

NLM 810/I (the lazaretto register), and NLM 812/I (the main register of ships arriving in quarantine) with respect to the mid-1830s.

[29] Holroyd, *Quarantine Laws*, 50–51. These numbers are consistent with Paul Cassar's estimate. See Cassar, *A Medical History of Malta* (London: Wellcome Institute, 1964), 296.

[30] Total derived from NLM LIBR 812/II.

Alexandria to Southampton. The 1845 total is significantly higher than Livorno and demonstrates how the British Mediterranean became central to quarantine operations over the course of the second quarter of the nineteenth century.

The data also give a sense of the changing social demographics of individuals in quarantine. In 1845, some 949 women performed quarantine at Malta (all of whom would have done so in the lazaretto) including some 364 Englishwomen.[31] This is an increase of more than 400 percent in the number of Englishwomen who performed quarantine in Malta in 1831. Most of these women would have been leisure travelers or wives of diplomats, colonial officials, and British merchants who had relocated to the Mediterranean – none, presumably, were the crew members, soldiers, or mercantile apprentices who had long formed the vast majority of the quarantined population. The increase suggests, then, a real change in the class of individuals performing quarantine. It finds an echo in Quarantine Superintendent Emanuele Bonavia's letter to Malta's Chief Secretary on assuming his office in 1837 that numerous repairs and additions were needed, as more and more people were arriving to perform quarantine, "many of them ladies and generally all persons of condition."[32]

Malta, Livorno, Marseille, and Genoa were the biggest lazarettos in the Mediterranean in terms of substantial traffic. While smaller, the lazarettos of Venice (Austrian control reduced Venice from its once "dominant" quarantining position in the seventeenth and eighteenth centuries), Ragusa, Naples, Cagliari, Port Mahon, Ancona, Messina, and Palermo also accommodated a significant number of ships. Additionally, there were scores of smaller lazarettos, coastal quarantine stations, and overland quarantine stations along the Austro-Ottoman frontier (Semlin and the Rothenthurm Pass were extremely busy terrestrial quarantine stations). By way of comparison, in Britain itself, roughly 720 ships were detained each year in the period that preceded moderate liberalization of quarantine rules in the late 1820s.[33] While such ships only rarely transported passengers, all their crew members add substantially to the annual population of those detained by quarantine. The picture one gets is that by 1830 – from Western European quarantine alone – in all likelihood well over 50,000 individuals experienced the system each year, sometimes vastly more. In the early 1830s, the French anticontagionist Nicolas Chervin

---

[31] The term is used in the Maltese records. The division is simply "Maltese," "English," and "Other"; it is unclear whether "Englishwomen" and "Englishmen" referred to individuals from all constituent countries of the UK.

[32] E. Bonavia to Hector Greig, November 8, 1837, NAM CUST/04/01. Greig, who had just been promoted to the role of Chief Secretary to the Government, had served as Superintendent of Quarantine until Bonavia's appointment and was well aware of the problem, having lobbied the government for the preceding decade to increase space available for quarantine accommodations.

[33] See Maclean, *Evils of Quarantine Laws*, 33.

estimated that just over 8 percent of all of France's ships were detained in quarantine at any given moment.[34] Quarantine harbors were often packed – an eerie spectacle of stationary ships, which no one boarded and from which no one disembarked. In Britain, limited space in the three major harbors reserved for ships with foul bills of health meant that ships often needed to wait for weeks for a spot to open up for them simply to *begin* serving quarantine.[35]

During the 1830s and 1840s – the decades just before universal quarantine's demise – the greatest number of passengers in history were caught up by it. Quarantine may have operated on the margins of Europe, but to hundreds of thousands of individuals, it was not a marginal concern, nor was it populated by a comparative handful of unrepresentative Levant traders. As the age of steam travel and Mediterranean imperialism dawned, quarantine evolved and expanded.

Varieties of Disinfection

On approach to a quarantine harbor, a ship would typically be met by a customs official and often a representative from the local board of health, who, from a distance, would ask an extensive set of questions. The answers to these would determine the scope and nature of quarantine. In British practice, largely adopted from procedure in the Mediterranean, more than fifty questions (divided into "preliminary questions" and "quarantine questions") would be put to each captain during this initial conversation. These focused on the state of health at his port of departure, a list of ports of call en route, specific details about all passengers on board, the health of the crew, and the nature and provenance of the cargo.[36] Across Western Europe, a ship liable to quarantine was bound to hoist the yellow flag and remain in isolation while the information from the captain's declaration was taken to the local board of health. In ports with a lazaretto, passengers and many goods would be disembarked to perform their quarantine there.

Quarantine lengths were mostly standardized in advance, though a ship with illness on board on arrival or a ship proceeding from a port where there were rumors of an epidemic would face additional detention. When ships were detained for longer than their set period (for example, the well-covered case of the HMS *Éclair* in Britain in 1845),[37] quarantine officials could face harsh criticism. Such cases were rare, but so was exceptional leniency. This did not

---

[34] "Periscope," *Medico-Chirurgical Review* 20 (1834): 234.

[35] On this problem, see V. Denis Vandervelde, "Quarantine at Milford Haven," *Pratique* 23, no. 1 (1998): 21.

[36] For a full list of Quarantine Questions, see Dyer Dew, *A Digest of Customs and Excise* (London: Richards and Co., 1818), 243–48.

[37] Harrison provides an exhaustive exploration of the *Éclair* episode in *Contagion*, chapter 4.

stop ship owners and trading companies from petitioning these bodies for an early release of their ships, crew, or merchandise. Such petitions for lenient treatment were duly noted and mostly ignored. For the bulk of this period, boards of health ruled without much regard to popularity.

On arrival, passengers lined up for inspection by a doctor, surrounded by fellow travelers with whom it was often impossible to communicate. Charles Terry, who performed a fourteen-day quarantine at Odessa in December 1846, noted that his party included "a Comte de V . . . . . ., his lady, their little son, and myself in the first class; a Russian officer, and a Greek in the second; and in the third class, a dozen or twenty of all sorts, including servants, Polish Jews, sailors, and a criminal, &c." This collection of individuals stood for some hours waiting to be examined, naked, by the doctor (or, for women, a "doctoress"), and assigned quarantine clothes while their own were expurgated with smoke. Terry was disgusted with his own costume: a pair of archaic trousers, enormous boots, and "a thick cotton pyramidal night cap."[38] Part of the confrontation of oneself as a foreign body thus involved a literal (as well as metaphorical) alienation from typical habits, standards, and appearances.

Sometimes, passengers themselves were fumigated (and not simply their clothes). This practice went out of vogue at most lazarettos around the turn of the nineteenth century, though the *spoglio* (as it was called) was still practiced at Malta into the 1820s.[39] During this process, passengers were often stripped and consigned to a room without ventilation. In the middle of this room, aromatic wood and herbs were burned until the individuals subjected to this cleansing came close to asphyxiation. Kept "coughing and sneezing all the evening," Claudius Shaw, a Briton who underwent the *spoglio* at Malta in 1810 insisted "I never wish to be disinfected again."[40]

Goods, more than passengers, were the central focus of fumigation procedures. Enumerated goods (those considered capable of harboring contagion) included major items of the Levant trade, and thus, much of the lazaretto's square footage was dedicated to storerooms for goods such as cotton, silk, wool, and fur. Like so much about quarantine, fumigation procedures were standardized in the course of the late eighteenth century; until about 1750, members of the Levant Company were simply instructed to fumigate their trade goods themselves before departure from Turkey. A few decades later, each item was synonymous with a particular fumigation technique. John Howard described the procedures at Venice in detail in the 1780s: when presented with cotton, expurgators "thrust their naked hands and arms into the bales . . . as far as the middle of the bag, for twenty days successively." Wool was "turned

---

[38] Charles Terry, *Scenes and Thoughts*, 247.
[39] Board of Health minutes for meeting no. 26, October 14, 1826, NLM LIBR 847.
[40] Quoted in Cassar, *Medical History of Malta*, 289.

and mixed"; cloth was hung on lines to be exposed to the air; beeswax and sponges were put in salt water; furs ("among the most dangerous articles") were "moved and shaken"; feathered animals were "purged by repeated sprinkling with vinegar"; and ostrich feathers – ambiguously and ominously – were "very diligently attended to."[41]

The rhythm of goods arriving at lazarettos was difficult to plan for. In Marseille, in 1821, some 133 ships hauling a commercial cargo arrived in quarantine from the Middle East, North Africa, or the Black Sea region.[42] While the average value of cargoes in that year was about 145,000 *francs*, the largest ships with the most expensive cargoes, including hundreds of bales of cotton and silk, and sometimes other items such as skins and dried fruit, carried goods worth up to 700,000 *francs* that year. These larger ships arrived throughout the year, and with the Marseille lazaretto serving as a frequent point of importation for ships from Sweden, Switzerland, and other European countries without a Mediterranean port, lazaretto authorities needed to retain a number of guardians and porters who were available for reassignment on fumigation duty at a moment's notice. Furthermore, while cotton and silk required fairly laborious fumigations, wheat (another common import, particularly from the Black Sea), did not. While cotton was by far the dominant import in 1821, wheat and oil (another commodity that was usually not fumigated) grew in importance in 1825 – again, this meant a recalibration of duties for lazaretto employees, who might have significant downtime depending on the rhythms of traffic.

While the fumigation of goods required substantial physical space and labor, the fumigation of letters (another crucial task of lazarettos) was faster. This was an area in which boards of health began to innovate, creating fumigation boxes to make the process faster, such as this example from a lazaretto in Venice (Figure 4.3). At most lazarettos, letters were often smoked with various chemicals and/or dipped in vinegar. In 1798, for example, French Foreign Minister Talleyrand wrote to the Marseille *Conservateurs* in a fit of pique that letters addressed to him from "the Levant and Barbary" had arrived stinking of vinegar and totally illegible. The *Conservateurs* rushed to assure him that this was a mistake and that they had instituted a dual-track procedure where ministerial letters were fumigated separately with the less-corrosive *parfum*.[43] Despite its name, that substance was unlikely to have smelled much better, composed as it was of a discordant mix of substances including sulfur, laudanum, cardamom, black pepper, and cumin.[44]

[41] Howard, *Account*, 21.
[42] Even though other ships were subjected to quarantine, the Marseille Agent of the Foreign Affairs Ministry tabulated these arrivals separately. All of the data that follow in this paragraph are derived from AN (Paris) AE/B/III/280.
[43] Conservateurs to Talleyrand, 14 Ventôse, An 6 (March 4, 1798), AN (Paris) AE/B/III 211.
[44] J. P. Papon, *De la peste, ou époques mémorables de ce fléau* (Paris: Lavillette and Company, 1800), 2:207.

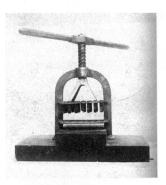

Figure 4.3 Mail fumigation device from Venice. Courtesy of the Wellcome Library. (CC BY license)

During the 1820s, the *Intendance* conducted a series of experiments and inquiries into the replacement of vinegar with chlorine for all fumigation purposes. Elsewhere, fumigators treated mail with such diverse substances as saltpeter, absinthe, and hot peppers.[45] Mail fumigation, it should be noted, was the fastest form of quarantine, and it could occur without the trappings of a full lazaretto. For example, although there were only a handful of lazarettos on the Habsburg-Ottoman frontier (with most travelers crossing at Semlin or the Rothenthurm Pass), there were dozens of smaller *rastels*, which were little more than huts, but were places where mail could be fumigated and some goods exchanged.

Lazaretto Life

Costs multiplied in quarantine. Many of these were born by trading houses and ship owners: fees for harborage, guardians sent onboard ships, fumigation of trade goods, and even the cost of sending the lazaretto surgeon to conduct a final examination and admit a ship to pratique.[46] For independent travelers arriving on passenger ships, or even poor parties of mobile peddlers and laborers, quarantine was also very expensive. At most lazarettos, these expenses included not only accommodation but also the salary of the guardian assigned to watch over the passenger's party, doctor's fees, and fees for food and furniture (for which certain tradespeople and the lazaretto restaurant often held effective monopolies).[47] For single travelers by the mid-1840s, guardian

---

[45] Karl Meyer, *Disinfected Mail* (Holton, KS: Gossip Printery, 1962), 22.

[46] See ASGe Sanità 1671.

[47] For a representative list of furniture prices provided by the Garçin brothers to passengers detained at the Lazaretto of Malta, see J. Quintana, *Guida dell'isola di Malta e sue dipendenze* (Valletta, [1845]), 209.

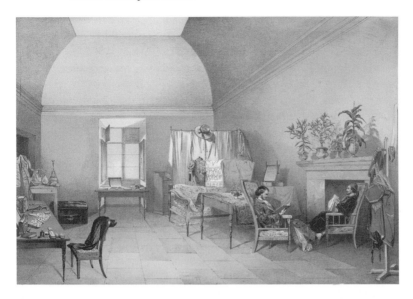

Figure 4.4 Two Hungarian aristocrats in their apartment in the Lazaretto of Malta. Lithograph of 1857 by Joseph Heicke after an 1842 painting by Iván Forray, one of the men in the image. © The British Library Board.

fees at Malta were 1s./3d. each day; if multiple travelers shared a guardian, he was paid double. Altogether, with good apartments, a standard menu of food ordered from the lazaretto restaurant, basic furniture rental, and the use of a servant and a washerwoman, the cost for a solo traveler in quarantine at Malta, estimated Sir John Gardiner Wilkinson, typically surpassed £11 ("without wine," as he is careful to note). Traveling as part of a large group and sharing the costs of the guardian could take this down, he estimated, to £6 or £7.[48] When one considers that the entire overland voyage between Bombay and London, at the time, cost £107 "for a gentleman," the substantial cost of quarantine as a proportion of a westward voyage becomes clear.[49]

Wilkinson's notation that his cost estimates are for "gentlemen" reveals the severe class demarcations that governed experiences at the large, Mediterranean lazarettos. Comfortable apartments came at a price (unsurprisingly, many rich travelers described their accommodation as surprisingly commodious) (Figure 4.4). And even here, commodiousness depended on

[48] Sir John Gardner Wilkinson, *A Handbook for Travelers in Egypt* (London: John Murray, 1847), xxiv.
[49] Ibid., xvi.

circumstances. At Genoa's Lazaretto della Foce (subsidiary to the more prominent lazaretto of Varignano that Genoa's *Magistrato* operated at La Spezia),
two passengers arrived on a ship from Odessa in late April 1828 and shared the
entire lazaretto with, at most, one other ship's passengers, but three months
earlier, another ship from Odessa disembarked eighteen passengers who, presumably, had a more limited choice of apartments (and, for unknown reasons,
a quarantine that was eight days longer).[50]

Official quarantine rhetoric often hid the variation in the way members of
different classes experienced quarantine; Francis Hervé was told "in a very high
manner" by the Health Bureau that "the Austrian government maintains the
lazaretto for the convenience of travelers, at its own expense, and takes no
money." But in reality, he wrote after he was discharged from quarantine at
Semlin, this would only be true if one camped outside; "but if you take your
quarters under any thing in the shape of a roof, you must pay for it, and that pretty
handsomely."[51] Camping outside was indeed a reality for many poor travelers.
However grim was Walsh's cottage at the Rothenthurm Pass Lazaretto, his own
accommodations in quarantine were far better than those of the bands of peasants
he observed. For the most part, Walsh notes, these groups would arrive and be
quarantined *en masse* in a small hut, with meat hooked around the exterior to serve
as provisions given that the food in the lazaretto restaurant was too expensive. Midway through his quarantine, however, a group of several hundred Wallachian
peasants arrived to find all such huts were full, and were forced to camp outside:

A body of two hundred, including women and children, had arrived, when there was no
place to shelter them. They were bivouacked of necessity, on the banks of the river; and
after suffering exceedingly from wet and cold, in very inclement weather, they were
suffered to proceed after ten days' detention, having had their clothes previously passed
through water.[52]

His chance observation leaves us with a sense of what could happen to such
large groups of groups of travelers, members of which, certainly, never wrote
travel narratives of their own.

In general, the smaller quarantine stations of Eastern Europe featured more
rudimentary accommodations and worse weather than the rooms designed for
large groups of poor travelers in Mediterranean lazarettos. But crowding could
make even the largest lazarettos unbearable; a letter from Malta's
Superintendent of Quarantine reveals that he had been obliged to consign
a party of sixty-one Maltese passengers to eight tiny rooms of twelve square
feet each.[53] That works out to about eight individuals forced to perform close to

---

[50] Data for February 1828–June 1828. See ASGe Sanità 1707.   [51] Hervé, *A Residence*, 2:335.
[52] Walsh, *Narrative of a Journey*, 263.
[53] Hector Greig to the Chief Secretary to the Government (hereafter CSG), February 14, 1837,
NAM CUST/04/1.

a month of quarantine in a space the size of a small closet. While better-off passengers were assigned buildings in the lazaretto itself, when Ottoman ships arrived at Malta with huge numbers of pilgrims returning from the *Hajj* (such ships carried about 300 passengers at once), these pilgrims were obliged to sleep as a group in the large plague hospital building adjacent to the Lazaretto proper.[54] An examination of the lazaretto death register of shows that such groups suffered the highest rates of mortality of all passengers in quarantine at Malta.[55]

Returning *Hajjis*, seasonal laborers, mobile peasants moving across the land borders of Eastern Europe, and soldiers returning to Western Europe from campaigns in Greece and North Africa were the major groups of poor travelers to experience quarantine in a European lazaretto. Captains and crew members (the latter of whom certainly could not have afforded quarantine fees) almost always remained on their ships, to which lazaretto guardians would be dispatched to superintend the work of fumigation, alongside a doctor if there were cases of illness on board.[56] The crowded shipboard conditions from this period are well known, and the infuriating experience of remaining in them at voyage's end (and in sight of the shore) can only be surmised. Sailors performing quarantine this way constituted the vast bulk of those who performed quarantine at all.

Though accounts written by individuals who performed quarantine onboard ship are rare, the hints we get demonstrate that the boredom of confinement created serious disciplinary problems. In Livorno, in 1830, for example, the guardians fumigating Captain Antoni Fattuta's brig related that having witnessed one sailor assault another the night before, the captain wanted permission to disembark the sailor into the stricter disciplinary space of the lazaretto, "not wanting to keep such a wild person on board."[57] Captains were always happy to send problematic sailors to the lazaretto – the Livorno letter books are filled with similar requests. This could be a boon for the sailors so disembarked – leaving the cramped quarters of a ship for the (usually) more spacious quarters of a lazaretto must have been a welcome change.

In addition to the expense of simply inhabiting a lazaretto, passengers frequently complained about the group of local merchants who made a specialty of being indispensable to quarantined individuals. They were also in a position to take advantage of their clients' need for provisions and their limited choice. Most passengers arrived in a quarantine port without knowing much of anything about the town behind the lazaretto walls and were often

---

[54] Register of ships in quarantine, September 1834, NLM (Valletta) LIBR 810/I.
[55] See NLM LIBR 822.
[56] In the 1820s, at Genoa, a doctor would be dispatched onboard a ship (there to remain, if necessary, for weeks), at the cost of 5 *lire* per day. See quarantine bills in ASGe Sanità 1671.
[57] Cantini to the Secretariat of the Sanità, October 8, 1830, ASLi Sanità 208.

assailed on arrival by traders offering anything from food, to mattresses, chairs, tables, writing materials, and books. Travelers often noted the conjunction of rapaciousness and fear of the plague that characterized such vendors. Observing a crowd of Maltese jewelry merchants outside the lazaretto, Terry was "greatly amused at the careful anxiety of all these little dealers in bijouterie lest we should touch any thing, and leave a plague-spot on it." This "careful anxiety" was a ritual and a performance, but it was also real. All money exchanged was immediately dipped in water "before it was considered fit for the possession of its new owners."[58] For those who needed to secure furniture quickly or make an arrangement about food provisions, the spectacle could be bewildering. Should one arrive at the lazaretto gates without having engaged a servant in advance, Wilkinson warned his elite traveling readers, many aspirants for the position typically waited in a mass "at the door of the lazaretto . . . with letters of recommendation from former masters, which may be read *but not touched*. When engaged, they come into quarantine and perform the same number of days as their master." Such servants were paid a daily rate of 1s/3d (the same salary as a guardian), with an extra 7 d. for living expenses (a salary that, over the course of a year, would likely far exceed the wages of an equivalent servant back in Britain).[59]

Quarantined travelers formed a captive audience for local merchants. Francis Hervé's traveling companion (Signor Castelli) had in his possession a letter of introduction to one "Signor Spirito," a Greek merchant in Semlin. Spirito advised the travelers about which officials to bribe and how best to make their onward journey from Semlin, though Hervé suspects much of this council was due to Spirito's wish to supply them with donkeys. In the end, Hervé complained that "the wily Greek merchant had a feeling in every transaction, which, by special favour, he undertook for us." Between paying off Spirito's commission and paying other "spungers [*sic*] on our purses," Hervé left the lazaretto furious about the "extortionate" cost of quarantine.[60] Many travelers had similar opinions. Edmund Spenser, who performed quarantine at Galatz (then on the Russian frontier of the River Danube), lamented that "the charges for refreshments would have been less at the London Hotel at Vienna, so famous for the excellence of its accommodations."[61] Others were luckier in their commercial interactions. Thomas Watkins, who performed quarantine at Ragusa in the 1780s, entered into an arrangement with a Muslim family who lived next to the lazaretto and was extremely pleased that the

---

[58] Terry, *Scenes and Thoughts*, 97.   [59] Wilkinson, *Handbook*, xix.
[60] Hervé, *A Residence*, 2:334–35.
[61] Quoted in V. Denis Vandervelde, "River Danube Quarantine," 44.

provisions they brought him daily enabled him to keep "a good table" at a moderate expense.[62]

In large lazarettos, like those at Malta or Marseille, the typical course of action was to order meals from the lazaretto restaurant. A look at the "menu" of the Marseille lazaretto shows this was expensive ("Table d'hôte" was given at 3 Fr/dinner or 2 Fr/lunch, though the à la carte menu could be much cheaper). Several entrées, ranging in expense from roast chicken or steak and potatoes down to macaroni or soup accommodated a variety of budgets, though the restaurant was far more expensive than others would have been outside the lazaretto gates.[63] Malta's set menu was slightly cheaper. It featured a meal of "soup, fish or beef ragout, . . . two kinds of fruit, and a bottle of Sicily wine," for 4 shillings.[64] Mrs. G. Darby Griffith called the food from Malta's lazaretto restaurant "excellent."[65] Robert Snow similarly approved of the food there and, in a quarantine defined by *ennui*, found dinner to be "the great event of the day."[66]

To ward off the common complaint of boredom, travelers practiced a similar set of activities. Many travel narratives record time in quarantine spent writing letters, reading, and attempting to use the solitude to complete work that had long been put off. Francis Hervé managed to pass hours each day touching up some of the paintings he had begun while in Anatolia. The French author and politician Alphonse de Lamartine wrote the entirety of his *Notes on Serbia* while in quarantine at Semlin,[67] and Benjamin Disraeli drafted the novels *Contarini Fleming* and *Alroy* in quarantine at Malta, crowing in a letter to his father about the "quantity I have planned and written."[68] (Disraeli also claimed quarantine enabled him finally to "understand politics" from reading old copies of *Galignani's Messenger* that were lying around the lazaretto.)[69] In its capacity as a clearing-house for news and for letters, the lazaretto could be a convenient stopping place during a long journey. It provided a stable address at which papers and mail could be received after weeks spent on the move.

---

[62] Thomas Watkins, *Travels through Switzerland, Italy, Sicily, the Greek Islands, to Constantinople; through Part of Greece, Ragusa, and the Dalmatian Isles; in a Series of Letters to Pennoyre Watkins* (London: T. Cadell, 1792), 2:335–36.

[63] See ADBR 200 E 877. Menu is undated but almost certainly from 1851 given its placement in the sequence of letters.

[64] E. Bonavia to H. Greig, April 15, 1838, NAM CUST/04/02. [65] Griffith, *A Journey*, 84.

[66] Robert Snow, *Journal of a Steam Voyage Down the Danube to Constantinople, and Thence by Way of Malta and Marseilles to England* (London: Moyes and Barclay, 1842), 77.

[67] Alphonse de Lamartine, *A Pilgrimage to the Holy Land; Comprising Recollections, Sketches, and Reflections Made during a Tour in the East* (New York: D. Appleton, 1848), 2:277–89.

[68] Quoted in Donald Sultana, *Benjamin Disraeli in Spain, Malta, and Albania: 1830–2* (London: Tamesis, 1976), 68.

[69] Ibid., 68.

"A Gate for the Whole Continent"

Sick and healthy, young and old, French, British, or Ottoman, quarantine produced unusual mixings, and despite different classes of apartments, some sort of social mixing was inevitable. The Lazaretto of Malta, concluded Cardinal Newman, was "a gate for the whole Continent."[70] Charles Terry, meanwhile, considered that "in every respect" quarantine "resembles a menagerie." Walking around the grounds of the lazaretto, he counted "twenty compartments . . . all double with high wooden gratings, and ticketed, as would be and is done in England to denote a hyena from Egypt, a lion from Barbary, or a bear from Russia."[71]

At many lazarettos, the diversity of quarantine's detainees was visible only at the *parlatorio*. This was a room (or a set of piers) where individuals in quarantine could speak to friends in pratique or to merchants from whom they wished to make purchases. In Malta, a special parlatorio was built in order to accommodate ships of war performing quarantine whose captains wished to communicate with other ships at different stages of quarantine or with officials on shore.[72] In either case, such places were under the careful watch of quarantine guardians and often featured a small channel of water or an iron grille creating a tangible demarcation between the sick and the well.

Despite this uncrossable barrier, the parlatorio was usually a jumble. "Peregrine," the anonymous traveler quoted above who experienced shipboard quarantine at Messina, compared the parlatorio to a cattle pen, replete with "guards ever and anon pushing their pikes between the rails, to keep you together, and making the most discordant noises: you may imagine a scene which would have well suited our inimitable Hogarth."[73] Perhaps the association with Hogarth's satirical imagery was a means of diffusing social awkwardness; for those who were well off, the parlatorio was the main opportunity to catch sight of the sailors, soldiers, or low-level traders that constituted the lazaretto majority.

While all lazarettos hosted detainees from many parts of the world, Malta's was particularly diverse – not simply because of its geographical position but also because of British dominance of Mediterranean shipping post-1815 and Malta's status as a (quasi) free port. As we have seen, British and Maltese

---

[70] Quoted in Paul Cassar, *A Medical History of Malta*, 303.

[71] Terry, *Scenes and Thoughts*, 254.

[72] The Coradino Parlatorio was built in the Grand Harbor. A guardian was dispatched from the Quarantine Department to be in constant attendance there, including sleeping in tiny accommodations next to the pier. A December 19, 1831 letter, Hector Greig to Chief Secretary of the Government (NAM CUST/04/01), states that the rooms appointed for the use of this guardian were so damp the unfortunate man had to be sent to the hospital twice due to aggravated rheumatism.

[73] Peregrine, "The Traveller: Letter IV," *The Kaleidoscope*, June 19, 1821, 401.

people were always a minority of those performing quarantine there. This situation was true, to a lesser degree, elsewhere. Records at Livorno show that Tuscan ships were always a minority of arrivals in quarantine in any given month throughout the 1820s and 1830s. By way of an example, there are medical reports for exactly one hundred ships performing quarantine at Livorno between January and June 1830. Of these, fourteen were Tuscan, twenty-six Austrian,[74] nineteen Sardinian, ten Neapolitan, eight Russian, eight American, five Greek, three British, three Dutch, and a single ship each from France, Spain, Sweden, and Denmark.[75] These percentages were not stable – as boards of health changed the rules for which countries were being subjected to quarantine, the percentage of ships under particular flags changed too. For example, when arrivals from Spain were being detained in the 1820s due to the yellow fever outbreaks there, Spanish ships constituted a far higher percentage of arrivals in quarantine at every Mediterranean port.

Quarantine's cosmopolitanism led to problems of communication. In December 1831, Hector Greig, Malta's Superintendent of Quarantine, complained that Greek vessels had been arriving with bills of health written in "modern Greek – a language that no one in this office understands" instead of the usual Italian. Greig proposed the retention of a translator with the cost to be borne by an additional charge to Greek Captains. "I do not think that Greek vessels can object to pay this charge . . . in order to render their bills intelligible," he continued, "as the modern Greek language cannot be considered one of the generally known languages of Europe."[76] At least in Marseille, the cost of translating Greek bills of health was a regular, and substantial, line item in the *Intendance Sanitaire*'s budget. In 1839, for example, it appears that more than 400 Greek bills needed to be translated, costing the considerable sum of 925 Francs.[77] If quarantine was a pan-European institution, it presupposed that quarantined individuals would be able to operate in a language seen to transcend national borders.

Travelers' opinions of what constituted a "generally known" language were idiosyncratic. On entering the Habsburg domains at the Rothenthurm Pass, Robert Walsh was outraged to find the lazaretto doctor capable only of speaking German: "I tried him in French, Italian, and finally in Latin, which I thought he

---

[74] Tuscany was an Austrian satellite state at the time, so it is unsurprising that Austrian ships constitute the single largest national group. Many among the crew of such ships were likely Tuscan.

[75] ASLi Sanità 208. These numbers are derived from medical report forms – the true number of ships in quarantine was higher because not every ship required this form, and not every form was preserved. Furthermore, these data reveal only the national flag the ship was flying; based on the incomplete manifests that are sometimes available, it is obvious that crew members and passengers on the same ship came from a variety of nations.

[76] Hector Greig to Acting Lt. Gov., December 23, 1831, NAM CUST/04/1.

[77] See ADBR 200 E 1064.

must know something of, but he could not comprehend or speak a word of it."[78] Italian (and to a lesser extent French) may have been a lingua franca for quarantine personnel in the Mediterranean, but this was clearly not the case in Central Europe. Despite his own incapacity in that language, Walsh was lucky to have a doctor capable of speaking German. Francis Hervé, for example, resigned himself to communicating in sign-language to his Serbian-speaking Guardian, "as he could not speak any language that was intelligible to us."[79]

Mutual incomprehension could sometimes force unexpected social encounters. Just so, Charles Terry and his aristocratic friends in quarantine at Odessa (who between them could muster French, Italian, German, and English) were forced to rely on a Greek man who understood some Russian, and could translate into French and English: "He is a dark, vulgar person with a blotched face, but he is civil, and we are indebted to him."[80] The exigencies of quarantine required this (grudging) social compromise.

The Suspicious Death of a Frenchman

In the lazaretto, every move mattered. Travelers who arrived on the same ship could commune with each other, but even an accidental brush against a traveler from another party could result in further quarantine. The traveler John Davy claimed to have known a man in pratique who was visiting a friend in an Austrian lazaretto and was summarily placed in quarantine with him when a guardian observed that "the tassel of the cap on his head touched a line on which some of the clothes were airing belonging to" his friend.[81] Robert Walsh, with typical acidity, mocked a guardian serving at the Rothenthurm Pass Lazaretto for fearing his touch:

Forgetting that I was supposed to have the plague, I approached this man; but he looked wild and staring, and rolled his eyes in the most extraordinary manner, and finally drew himself outside, and spoke to me through the door. Here, in a loud and solemn tone, he informed me in bad Italian, that I must not touch or even approach any person while I remained.[82]

Many travelers found the idea that they could be considered potentially pestiferous so insulting that it motivated a grudge against the quarantine system as a whole and also the vicious mocking of guardians. Frequently, elite British travelers made a sport out of the professional conscientiousness of lazaretto

---

[78] Walsh, *Narrative of a Journey*, 253.   [79] Hervé, *A Residence*, 2:326.
[80] Terry, *Scenes and Thoughts*, 249.
[81] John Davy, *Notes and Observations on the Ionian Islands and Malta with Some Remarks on Constantinople and Turkey and on the System of Quarantine as at Present Conducted* (London: Smith, Elder & Co. 1842), 2:338.
[82] Walsh, *Narrative of a Journey*, 253.

employees. For Walsh and Davy, since quarantine precautions mandated this presumption of guilt, it was convenient to decide that the precautions must be ridiculous. Mrs. Griffith, too, lampooned the procedures taken by guardians to maintain the segregation of the lazaretto: "It is quite laughable to see them lighting each other's cigar: for instance, this evening our guardian was smoking, when a friend in pratique entered; he brought out another cigar, and laid it upon the ground for the new comer to pick up."[83] One could laugh at these precautions, but it was necessary to take them seriously when the alternative was three weeks of detention turning into a six-week ordeal.

In these ways, for passengers, quarantine involved the close conjunction of minute precaution, boring routine, and high stakes for any false move. This often induced a range of lazaretto neuroses. Cardinal Newman became obsessed by the idea that mysterious sounds he heard at night indicated his room was haunted. Newman wrote to his sister that "you may say the noises came from some strange transmission of sound; or you may say that the quarantine island is hardly Christian ground. Anyhow, we cannot doubt that evil spirits in some way or other are always about us." This ghostly experience, he complained, had upset his sleep more than had sea-sickness and had also given him a cold.[84]

The psychic impact of quarantine could inspire serious hypochondria. In *Little Dorrit*, Mr. Meagles, while detained in Marseille's lazaretto, complains "I have had the plague continually, ever since I have been here. I am like a sane man shut up in a madhouse; I can't stand the suspicion of the thing ... I have been waking up, night after night, and saying, *now* I have got it, *now* it has developed itself, *now* I am in for it."[85] The constant need to adopt a neurotic avoidance of everyone and everything clearly unnerved many travelers. One David Lester Richardson remembered the "curious feeling" of thinking of himself and his party as "such marked and suspected people, and to know that strangers would be horrified at our touch. It was enough to convince a hypochondriac that plague was in his blood."[86]

More than simple hypochondria, Robert Walsh insisted that the fear quarantine inspired could actually predispose the body to infection. "Now if fear and alarm be depressing passions," he argued,

and so, according to the best medical opinions, be predisposing causes to the reception of contagion, a more effectual way could not be devised to cause the disease to develop itself, than by treating a man who had just come from where it was, as if he had the

[83] Griffith, *A Journey*, 2:95.
[84] Newman to (his sister) Jemima. See J. H. Newman, *Letters and Correspondence of John Henry Newman* (London: Longmans, Green, and Co., 1890), 1:294.
[85] Charles Dickens, *Little Dorrit* (Oxford: Oxford University Press, 1982), 13.
[86] David Lester Richardson, *The Anglo-Indian Passage; Homeward and Outward; or, A Card for the Overland Traveler*, 2nd ed. (London: James Madden, 1849), 84–85.

disease upon him, and shutting him up in a filthy, dismal room, the very look and atmosphere of which seemed contagious.[87]

Accommodations at Malta, for those who could pay, were more commodious than those Walsh described, yet no less an eminence than Lord Byron complained of the fever he suffered while in quarantine there.[88] Lazarettos had a reputation for insalubrity – a fact that was seized on by reformers. "I have often heard captains in the Levant trade say that the spirits of their passengers sink at the prospect of being confined in [a lazaretto]," recorded John Howard, "In those of them which I have visited, I have observed several pale and dejected persons, and many fresh graves."[89]

Mrs. Griffith witnessed the death of a French traveler (Remé or "Remy" Fondant) who had served nearly all of his quarantine in perfectly good health. A day before he was due to be granted pratique, he suddenly died. Happening to catch a glimpse of his coffin being taken to the lonely lazaretto burying ground, Griffith was horrified: "the melancholy scene . . . made so deep an impression on my mind that I could not shake it off. I cannot think of anything more horrible than to breathe one's last in a lazaretto."[90] In sympathy, perhaps, she began to feel unwell herself, and on requesting quinine, incurred the deep suspicion of the lazaretto doctor. The vague worry that one might be getting ill was a freighted one; consulting the lazaretto doctor or revealing symptoms too overtly could easily result in an extension of quarantine.

Griffith assumed that, lamentable and disturbing though it was to her, such deaths were more or less common in quarantine. What she could not have known was that, in fact, the Maltese treated the death of Fondant as anything but ordinary. A letter from Charles Delfy, the French consul at Malta, to the *Intendance Sanitaire* of Marseille, noted that the deceased man was carefully examined by the lazaretto doctor, who was greatly alarmed by the presence of mysterious tumors and a large lump on Fondant's groin. The Maltese Quarantine Department immediately convened an extraordinary council. Considering the "origin of the illness and the speed of death," the Council decided the plague could not be ruled out and doubled the quarantine duration of all those who had shared apartments with Fondant.[91] Emanuele Bonavia, then Superintendent of Quarantine, provided a series of updates to all Mediterranean boards of health on the uneventful quarantine of these passengers.[92] In the end, the Frenchman's illness was never satisfactorily defined, and the lazaretto burial register describes the cause of death simply as "vague suspicion of the plague."[93]

[87] Walsh, *Narrative of a Journey*, 253–54.   [88] Lord Byron, "A Farewell to Malta," ll. 11–12.

[89] Howard, *Account of the Principal Lazarettos*, 23.   [90] Griffith, *A Journey*, 2:92.

[91] Charles Delfy to the Intendants Sanitaire, undated (August, 1842), ADBR 200 E 463.

[92] See ADBR 200 E 970.   [93] "Sospetto remoto di peste" [*sic*], NLM LIBR 822.

Fondant's demise is one of the few instances in which an observation by a quarantined individual matches a visible archival record of the vast machinery of quarantine diplomacy. The death struck Griffith as a horrifying element of lazaretto life. "I never thought of the plague till now," she had written regarding her arrival in Malta. Subsequently, events in quarantine made her "almost terrified of it."[94] Death seemed close in the lazaretto. Its employees, on the other hand, had different concerns. A case of suspicious illness necessitated the tedious obligation of writing constant updates to interlocutors in other ports. Once the quarantine on Fondant's fellow passengers expired without event, the issue was successfully concluded as far as Mediterranean boards of health were concerned. For Griffith, the psychic effects of the episode made a boring stay in the lazaretto terrifying. This disjunction between the official mind of quarantine and the experience passengers had of it shows how the system could appear so regular, routine, and ordinary in its archival remains and yet stimulating, unusual, and extraordinary in the writings of travelers.

While cases of plague sometimes occurred in Mediterranean lazarettos (almost always following the arrival of a plague ship), no full-scale epidemics broke out inside their walls. And yet, death itself was common. The reformer John Howard was inspired to perform his survey of European quarantine institutions in the 1780s because a campaign against their reputed lack of hygiene seemed a logical follow-up to his prison reform efforts. Decades later, deaths of passengers or sailors confined in close quarters continued apace. Ambiguous fevers, apoplexy, and inflammation appear most commonly in lazaretto records as the causes of death. Though cases of plague were rare, there are numerous records of death from yellow fever and cholera, diseases that were equally concerning to boards of health.

Fondant was one of 338 individuals to die in quarantine and be buried in Malta's lazaretto cemetery between 1832 and 1842.[95] In the preceding decade (between 1823 and 1832), more than 600 people died in quarantine at Marseille, although these numbers are particularly inflated because of the French campaigns in Algeria from 1830.[96] Still more lethal, the quarantine harbors and four lazarettos superintended by the Genoa *Magistrato* saw about thirty deaths each month throughout the late 1820s and early 1830s.[97] Dedicated to decontamination it may have been, but the lazaretto itself was not a healthy environment.

---

[94] Griffith, *A Journey*, 2:78.   [95] NLM LIBR 822.   [96] ADBR 200 E 1004.
[97] ASGe Sanità 1114.

Sanitary Infractions and Sanitary Disasters

The strictures and the rituals of quarantine were so precise that it remains a surprise that so few passengers were arrested for violating the rules. Certainly, the archives of boards of health are full of anecdotes of individuals attempting to communicate with other ships waiting in the quarantine harbor, but outright attempts to flee to shore and abrogate the quarantine laws were exceedingly rare. Exceptions were more common along land-based quarantine frontiers, especially temporary ones. In 1828, for example, when the *Magistrato di Sanità* of Nice constructed a temporary cordon against Marseille during a smallpox epidemic there, several travelers were actually shot while trying to cross the border.[98] By contrast, passengers detained inside a lazaretto were constantly under the eye of lazaretto employees. Boards of health recognized that adherence to the quarantine laws depended on the rigorous rule-keeping of these guardians and set salaries high. The records of quarantine administration suggest that the vast majority of lazaretto employees believed in the merits of their work.

But temptations there were, and occasionally the zeal of lazaretto employees was not enough to preempt sanitary sinning. At the most serious end, soon after the quarantine of foul bill ships was permitted off the Kentish Coast at Stangate Creek, members of the Levant Company began to complain that silk and cotton were going missing from their ships during quarantine. A series of urgent letters between the Levant Company and the Privy Council shows that, in 1804 and 1805, rumors were flying that (ostensibly smuggled) Levantine cotton and silk were being openly sold on the streets of Rochester at cut-rate prices. A "confidential Person" sent to Rochester by the Company to conduct enquiries turned up nothing much "owing to the unwillingness of people in general to incur the odium attaching to informers," but nevertheless found evidence of wrongdoing at Stangate Creek.[99] The Company could make a persuasive argument that to admit the necessity of quarantine legislation was to acknowledge the extreme danger of such a practice,[100] and finally, the government was pushed to action when they ordered an inquiry by the Customs Service (published in April 1805).[101] This inquiry seems to have put an effective stop to the practice, but the damage to Levant Company coffers was substantial.[102]

Even at the ostensibly stricter Mediterranean lazarettos (where, in many cases, the death penalty remained on the books for sanitary infractions), there

---

[98] See Bon, "Cholera Epidemics," 49.
[99] J. Green to Sir Lucas Pepys, January 26 and February 12, 1805, TNA SP 105/122.
[100] Samuel Bosanquet to Lord Hawkesbury, October 20 and 26, 1804, TNA SP 105/122.
[101] See Bosanquet to Stephen Cottrell (PC Clerk), April 22, 1805, TNA SP 105/122.
[102] See Russell, *Later History*, 321–23.

were occasional reports of abuse. The meticulous notes of various "*procès verbaux*" conducted by the Marseille *Intendance* reveal cases like that of François Germaine, an unfortunate porter who had been caught red-handed with a bale of quarantined coffee concealed "under his arm" while walking in a lazaretto courtyard.[103] Other smuggling attempts were much more elaborate. Another inquiry from Marseille shows the captain and crew of a French ship proceeding from New Orleans in 1818 attempted to conceal (without success) a large quantity of cloth, several sets of clothing, a barrel of molasses, and four sixteen-kilogram cartons of tobacco.[104] Because the collection of customs tariffs was often accomplished by way of a declaration by lazaretto officials of goods received in quarantine, the desire to evade the gaze of customs officials often *also* involved the committing of a sanitary crime. Fixed quarantine duties paled beneath customs charges and fees such as the (roughly two percent) commission owed to the Levant Company (in Britain) or the Marseille Chamber of Commerce (in France). Sanitary crimes, then, though clearly rare, were far more common than they would have been if there had been no coordination between quarantine employees and customs officials.

While the archives of Marseille's Board of Health make sanitary crimes particularly visible, it is clear that smuggling and other violations by quarantine personnel occurred at other lazarettos as well. In Malta, a guardian was actually sentenced to death for an ambiguous quarantine breach in 1814 (at the conclusion of the 1813–14 plague). Fortunately for the life of this guardian (one Felix Camilleri), though a gallows was constructed and the execution organized, he was pardoned (and a plaque visibly displayed) to demonstrate the generosity of British imperial justice. Elsewhere, too, the death penalty remained more theoretical than real. At Marseille, in 1798, a captain who was convicted of failing to provide an accurate manifest of his cargo to quarantine and customs officials was given the rather light sentence of augmented quarantine fees and a mandatory 100 *franc* donation to a local hospice.[105]

Evidently, even the gallows erected at Malta failed to instill employees of the Quarantine Department with much fear if they were determined to break the law. In 1831, after years of accusations and vigorous defenses of his honor by Superintendent of Quarantine Hector Greig, Captain Pulis of Malta's lazaretto was suspended from his duties after irrefragable proof was presented that he had smuggled grain out of the lazaretto to hide it from customs inspectors. Apparently the £200/year salary granted to the Captain of the Lazaretto was not sufficient to guard against temptation. Nevertheless, perhaps as a sign of Pulis's

---

[103] Legal proceedings of François Germaine, porter, May 19, 1819, ADBR 200 E 1014.
[104] Note by Captain Dalmais, July 10, 1818, ADBR 200 E 1014.
[105] *Procès*, 27 Frimaire, An 6 (May 16, 1798), AN (Paris) AE/B/III/211.

belief in the reality of the concerns quarantine addressed, he apparently only began to smuggle out the grain in question on the last day of its quarantine.[106]

Some quarantine employees did break the law, as the above examples show. But just as Captain Pulis apparently attempted to mitigate the consequences of his criminality for public health, most lazaretto employees seem to have taken their work very seriously; the annals of quarantine justice make clear that rule-breaking was relatively rare. A further inducement to good behavior was the dependability of the work and the high salary. Many quarantine guardians kept working until they were quite elderly (the problem of immobile or hearing-impaired guardians recurs frequently in the letters of lazaretto captains and boards of health). The lucrative careers one could expect in a lazaretto encouraged a belief in the norms and rituals of quarantine practice – exactly what boards of health intended. Indeed, it should not surprise us that a career spent "performing sanitation" should make one a believer in "performative sanitation."

Many emerged from quarantine convinced that it was, as the antiquarantinist doctor Charles Maclean put it, a "forty-days farce."[107] But whether willing, resentful, or resigned, travelers and crew members in quarantine, alongside lazaretto employees, gave shape and meaning to a sanitary border that was the subject of continual negotiation. As we turn, in the next chapter, to the arena of international sanitary diplomacy, we should be conscious of how many thousands of people were affected by every change in quarantine lengths, fumigation procedures, or bill of health documentation. Later in this book, as we consider medical arguments about quarantine, it is important to remember how many of the doctors who participated in debates surrounding bubonic plague had experienced Mediterranean quarantine themselves.

---

[106] Hector Greig to Frederick Hankey, December 19, 1831, NAM CUST/04/01.

[107] Charles Maclean, *A Dissertation on the Source of Epidemic and Pestilential Diseases* (Philadelphia: William Young, 1797), 227–28.

5   A European System

Like the xenophobic Mr. Podsnap, in Charles Dickens's *Our Mutual Friend*, many Victorians considered other countries to be "a mistake." Bernard Porter has persuasively delineated this "Little Englander" mentality in suggesting that for many in the nineteenth century, the European continent seemed to be oriented between poles of "bureau and barrack"[1] (excessive officialdom and the overt presence of the military). This idea surfaces again and again among those who complained about the quarantine system – with its forms of bureaucracy and impositions on liberty, the lazaretto seemed to many to be both bureau *and* barrack. Charles Meryon, the young doctor and companion of the eminent traveler Lady Hester Stanhope, termed the lazaretto "a legalized panoptikon," suggesting that Jeremy Bentham's hypothetical prison was the epitome of illiberal planning. "Quarantine ought never to exist in a civilized country," Meryon wrote, "neither ought passports."[2]

But just as Britain would follow the trend of introducing passport requirements in the early twentieth century,[3] the British government simultaneously considered itself to be both an administration that believed in "liberty" *and* one that engaged in quarantine administration. The most zealous opponents of quarantine in Parliament conceded that commercial and strategic relationships with European allies made independent action impossible. The Radical MP Joseph Hume called the quarantine laws "a family compact" between European states specifically geared against epidemic disease in "the states of Barbary and the other Turkish states,"[4] while a French reformer considered it to be an implicit "contract," which bound its implied signatory nation-states in a shared mission of "protecting the public health of Europe."[5] Even for the system's opponents, it was clearly a common opinion that to be European *was*

---

[1] Bernard Porter, "'Bureau and Barrack': Early Victorian Attitudes towards the Continent," *Victorian Studies* 27, no. 4 (1984): 407–33.

[2] Charles Meryon, *Travels of Lady Hester Stanhope* (London: Henry Colburn, 1845), 1:358–59.

[3] On this trend, see John Torpey, *The Invention of the Passport* (Cambridge: Cambridge University Press, 2000), chapter 4.

[4] Hansard, House of Commons Debate, July 10, 1823, Vol. 9, c. 1526.

[5] Louis Aubert-Roche, "Des quarantaines: nécessité de les réformer en France par suite de leur abolition en Angleterre et en Autriche," *Revue de l'Orient* 1, no. 1 (1843): 69.

to quarantine. John Bowring, another Radical MP, was quarantine's most formidable parliamentary foe, but conceded in the 1830s that "our own sanatory [*sic*] legislation could scarcely be changed unless the governments of Europe were willing to concur in some general modification."[6] The same critics (like Bowring and Hume) who considered quarantine practice to be barbaric also recognized it to be the necessary price of participation in a freer form of trade with Europe.

This concession was relatively new. As we have already seen, it remained possible into the middle of the eighteenth century to imagine a world in which quarantine was not universal and in which changes to the rules did not need to be coordinated with European allies. What caused the move toward a coordinated system? In an era before telephones and telegraphs, and amid much discord among European states, how did independent boards of health in different port cities coordinate quarantine practice across the Continent? What place did Britain have in a quarantine regime largely based in the Mediterranean? This chapter's central argument is that Mediterranean quarantine came to demarcate a kind of transnational "biopolity"[7] in the course of the late eighteenth and early nineteenth centuries, and that Britain and its colonies came to recognize themselves as members of this evolving, transnational association. The system was forged by corresponding quarantine administrations (boards of health) in different Mediterranean ports; it had many quasi-independent authorities for whom independent action was gradually circumscribed by common norms and assumptions.

Mild deviations, crisis points, and violations of rules had the effect of making the system more robust by forcing its advocates to make their assumptions more explicit. In 1799, on an occasion when two Scandinavian consuls issued clean bills of health in Tunis despite the presence of the plague, the members of the Marseille Board of Health enumerated for the Foreign Minister Talleyrand the importance of obtaining reliable sanitary information from French consuls: "Here, *Citoyen Ministre*, are the rules for the general health of Europe, and the nations which live in it, forming among themselves a common union [*union commune*] against the curse of the plague."[8] Regular, cross-Mediterranean

---

[6] John Bowring, *Observations on the Oriental Plague and on Quarantines as a Means of Arresting Its Progress. An Address Given to the British Association of Science, August 15, 1838, at Newcastle* (Edinburgh: William Tait, 1838), 35.

[7] Foucault's conception of "biopolitics" refers to a new priority in the administration of the modern state (at the turn of the nineteenth century) to regulate health on the level of the entire population. In using the term *biopolity*, I wish to emphasize that population health as a subject of concern was growing across Western Europe at this time. Here *biopolity* indicates an association of states in agreement that the health of their populations was linked together and that the presence of even one plague-ridden body outside the lazaretto gates in any single European state could compromise the sanitary integrity of the whole Continent.

[8] Conservateurs to Talleyrand, 1 Germinal, An 7 (March 21, 1799), AN (Paris) AE/B/III/220.

communication enabled the formation of a border regime that spanned many different states. The sharing of epidemiological information was the salient feature of the European biopolity for these *Conservateurs de Santé*, and so it became more generally. From the late eighteenth century onward, I argue, networks of exchange among boards of health and consuls allowed procedures to be harmonized and threats to be recognized before disasters loomed. Reciprocal correspondence among such actors achieved paramount importance. This practice focused on the Mediterranean, and as an increasingly important Mediterranean imperial power in the nineteenth century, Britain played an integral role. Boards of health were the hubs of sanitary information exchange. From Marseille to Gibraltar, from Malta to Venice, they facilitated European sanitary integration from the ground up. As I demonstrated in Chapter 3, they were local authorities with a national (even international) remit.

After 1815, Western Europe (Britain included) emerged from a convulsive set of wars as a single biopolity, in which border control was effectively shared and in which unilateral sanitary action was impossible without controversy. The idea of any kind of single "polity" for Europe at this time might seem surprising – the nineteenth century, after all, is so often seen as the golden age of the European nation-state. Quarantine, however, created the sense of a shared border and gave a coherence to the epidemically secure interior. Subscribing to what French reformer Pierre Ségur-Dupeyron called "*le droit sanitaire de l'Europe*" meant a circumscription of independent national action on sanitary matters.[9] The system suggested clear boundaries between a vulnerable "us" and a contagious "them." Given the extent to which quarantine impinged on other areas of legislation – from public health reform to trade policy – it is right to recognize the way it bound Europe together politically as well as conceptually. This biopolity circumscribed independence only in certain areas, but it required much more regular transnational coordination than the contemporaneous high diplomacy that followed the Congress of Vienna.

The system forced compliance from would-be innovators. This is well demonstrated by the Continental reaction to Britain's passage of a reformist Quarantine Act in 1825. The final portion of this chapter addresses this episode, in which the British government was quickly persuaded to retreat from far-reaching reforms and promise fidelity to the strictures of Mediterranean quarantine. I argue that the entire controversy shows a Britain eager to innovate *and* deeply committed to remaining a member in good standing of the European biopolity. To some reformers, quarantine could appear to be a corps of the coerced rather than a coalition of the willing. The fact remains, however, that

---

[9] See Pierre Ségur-Dupeyron, *Des quarantaines et des pertes qu'elles occasionnent au commerce* (Paris: Madame Huzard, 1833), 23.

Britain could not "go it alone" when it came to revising the quarantine laws in 1825. As Mediterranean boards of health saw it, if one part of Europe reduced its precautions, there was no guaranteeing the security of the whole.

Though many have noted that the late nineteenth-century International Sanitary Conferences, which dismantled the quarantine system from the 1850s onward, were a predecessor of such institutions as the World Health Organization (WHO),[10] I argue that earlier transnational arrangements for quarantine set the pattern for future sanitary cooperation and European bureaucratic integration. Many Europeans inveighed against quarantine for its indiscriminate mandates and its inefficiencies, but it was, in the end, a European system, and in many ways, it suited the European powers and was shaped by their interests – Britain included. While British quarantine critics often painted their island nation as the dupe of Continental bureaucrats, their government managed to swing the machinery of quarantine in its direction rather often, and other powers were forced to take note.

While the international cooperation among the low-level bureaucrats who composed boards of health was unique, it was rendered more likely by the incentives built into the system and a preexisting consensus that quarantine was the appropriate response to the plague. The dynamic in which retaliatory quarantines stifled deviation and reciprocal information sharing generated complementary favors resembles the "tit-for-tat" strategy that the political scientist Robert Axelrod found to be the most successful path to cooperation (as derived from prisoner's-dilemma-style games).[11] That said, board members engaged in the behavior that they did for historically specific reasons. Explanations include the growing transnational circulation of newspapers toward the end of eighteenth century, the expansion of European diplomatic corps in the Middle East, and the Napoleonic public health crisis that endowed the fight against epidemic disease with a reenergized intensity. As Chapter 1 made clear, that last factor is particularly important. The mechanisms of sanitary cooperation explored here show that the imagined geography of a shared frontier against a common threat inspired an intuitive inclination toward comprehensiveness. Performative sanitation, as we saw in the last chapter, consisted of an accumulation of rituals that converted a risky body

---

[10] See Mark Harrison, "Disease, Diplomacy, and International Commerce," *Journal of Global History* 1, no. 2 (2006): 197. Also Valeska Huber, "The Unification of the Globe by Disease? The International Sanitary Conferences on Cholera, 1851–1894," *Historical Journal* 49 (2006): 458–59, and Marcel Chahrour, "A Civilizing Mission? Austrian Medicine and the Reform of Medical Structures in the Ottoman Empire, 1838–1850," *Studies in History and Philosophy of Biological and Biomedical Sciences* 38 (2007): 702. Finally and most canonically, see Norman Howard-Jones, *The Scientific Background of the International Sanitary Conferences, 1851–1938* (Geneva: WHO, 1975).

[11] Robert Axelrod, *The Evolution of Cooperation* (New York: Basic Books, 1984), esp. chapters 2 and 9.

into a safe one. In this chapter, I show how sanitary diplomacy was *itself* performative; an exercise that fostered a sense that comprehensive protection had been achieved. Universal quarantine depended on its transnational application, and in ensuring (and frequently testifying to) reciprocity, members of boards of health sought to give universality meaning. In this way, the idea of contagion and its seductive, transhistorical corollary impulse of "stamping out"[12] disease impelled scalar expansion and incentivized cooperation. In the diplomatic history of Mediterranean quarantine, "tit-for-tat" emerged instinctively.

The durability and success of sanitary cooperation among so many different poles of authority is extraordinary. But perhaps its very multipolarity made this system *more* rather than less likely to succeed. It was easier for board of health members to oppose changes demanded by politicians in their own countries once they pointed to the multitude of other authorities who had to agree to any change. Consciously or unconsciously, then, health board members committed to the maintenance and security of quarantine were predisposed to seek reciprocal links across the Mediterranean.

Reciprocity and Reputation

Reciprocal correspondence itself had existed since the seventeenth century.[13] Yet, even eighteenth-century correspondence between boards was highly variable. While correspondence was at a peak during episodes such as the plague of Marseille and Provence in the early 1720s, its volume declined as urgency waned. As Daniel Panzac has shown, of the roughly one hundred letters sent between boards of health at Marseille and Cadiz in the eighteenth century, about two-thirds were written between 1749 and 1755, during a North African plague epidemic.[14] In addition, the horizons of communication were limited in the eighteenth century. Circulars written by Venice's *Provveditori alla Sanità*, for example, were mainly sent to other Italian health administrations – the only non-Italian authorities ever addressed on such letters were the boards of health of Geneva, Zurich, Bern, and Marseille.[15]

---

[12] Tom Crook aptly characterizes this as a central ambition of the modern public health regime. See Crook, *Governing Systems*, chapter 6.

[13] See Takeda, *Between Crown and Commerce*, 115–16. Also Panzac, *Quarantaines et Lazarets*, 91–92.

[14] Panzac, *Quarantaines et Lazarets*, 91.

[15] See ASVe Provv. Sanità 160. Also Comitato alla Sanità di Venezia to "Magistrati Esteri di Sanità," May 20, 1797, ASVe Provv. Sanità 793. This latter source is the letter that announced the demise of the old Venetian Board of Health and the founding of a "Comitato alla Sanità" under the new, Napoleonic regime. As such, it was one of the most important circulars sent in the entire eighteenth century. Of the twenty-nine foreign boards to receive it, twenty-five were in modern Italy, three were in Switzerland, and one was in France.

By contrast, from the late eighteenth century and early nineteenth onward, better communication, new epidemic pressures, and the experience of the Napoleonic Wars ensured that contacts became more regular and more diverse. The boards of health of Trieste, Ancona, Cagliari, and Palermo became regular participants in information exchange, as did Malta's quarantine officials, and other British sanitary bureaucrats in the Ionian Islands. Greek, Turkish, and Egyptian interlocutors began to correspond with their Western counterparts in the 1830s. Correspondence among boards of health became a regular, transnational phenomenon during the period covered by this study. In general, in the nineteenth-century Mediterranean world, these expanding circuits of exchange increased the sense of a Western European sanitary alliance. The biopolity was forged, in many ways, through the mail.

From the late eighteenth century onward, no single type of correspondence was more common than tables of standard quarantine lengths for different countries and parts of the world. Such quarantine tables gave a specific number of days an average ship would be quarantined depending on its port of departure and the types of items onboard. Boards of health constantly sought to reassure each other of the strictness of their procedures. Hence the elaborate preamble to the Portuguese rules forwarded to the Genoese in 1816. Given that the assumptions about "infected ports" were widespread, for example, Genoa's *Magistrati* surely did not need to read that "The ports currently considered to be contagious with Oriental Plague include the ports of Egypt ..., Constantinople, Rhodes, Smyrna, Cephalonia, Salonika, and Macedonia"[16] for their own edification. They were no doubt pleased, however, to hear that Portugal operated under that assumption. In 1825, a member of Genoa's *Magistrato* made a careful translation and annotation of Britain's Quarantine Act of that year.[17] This was common procedure for major changes to legislation, but the archives of all major boards of health show that hundreds of copies of standard quarantine lengths and descriptions of operating procedure were sent back and forth among quarantine ports. The logic of quarantine meant that it was always better to be forthcoming about local procedures. Constant communication meant ports cohered around a shared understanding of a minimum level of severity.

The British colony of Malta presents a telling case study of this phenomenon. After its disastrous plague of 1813–14, the island colony's ships were denied free pratique in Continental ports for more than ten years. This was a major source of concern for Malta's merchant community and its British governors, given that the vast majority of the local economy depended on small-scale

---

[16] Portuguese Quarantine Rules, composed by Luigi Antonio Rebella da Silva, 1816, ASGe Sanità 1365.
[17] See ASGe Sanità 1921.

commercial exchange with Sicily, Marseille, and ports on the Italian coast. Sustained pressure from Maltese merchants (including a rare, direct petition to the British Parliament) led to intermittent protests from British officials, but serious action to achieve free pratique was only undertaken in the mid-1820s. The effort reached all the way up to the Earl of Bathurst at the Colonial Office and George Canning at the Foreign Office. Canning sent a directive to all British consuls in the Mediterranean to conduct inquiries about the quarantine regulations operating in their ports of station. Simultaneously, diplomatic pressure was applied to the highest levels of the French foreign ministry in Paris. Frederick Hankey, a high-ranking colonial official in Malta, was sent on a tour of inquiry to the lazarettos of Marseille, Naples, and Palermo.[18]

Augustus Foster, the British consul in Turin, having received Canning's circular, undertook inquiries of his own. Malta (and Gibraltar, which had long experienced fifteen-day quarantine imposed against fears of yellow fever), he determined, suffered from a reputation problem. Despite the presence of an enormous lazaretto and an experienced staff, there was the sense that Malta, having committed the unthinkable crime of admitting the plague, was no longer a safe holder of the *droit sanitaire*. In a letter to Canning, Foster recounted a conversation he had with Count de la Tour, an influential member of the Sardinian Court. The Count, he reported,

owned to me that a prejudice did, pretty generally, exist in the Mediterranean Ports in regard to the sanatory [*sic*] establishments of that Island [i.e., Malta], which took its rise during the war when it was believed that great relaxations of the health laws, had occasionally taken place ... which had left an unfavorable impression upon the boards of health of the neighbouring countries, where the utmost strictness is observed.[19]

De la Tour was optimistic that with gentle diplomatic pressure, Maltese shipping would once more obtain free pratique in European ports. Not so for Gibraltar. "I am sorry to say," wrote Foster, "that the prejudice against Gibraltar seems to be still stronger than that against Malta." He was informed by the Count de la Tour, in fact, that Malta itself had recently instituted a heightened quarantine against Gibraltar in consequence of a rumor of a plague outbreak in nearby Morocco.[20] Sharing a colonial power, clearly, did not inspire the Maltese with a sufficient sense of affinity to allow Gibraltarian shipping into their ports without quarantine.

As de la Tour's response suggests, the campaign to achieve free pratique for Malta was eventually successful.[21] Both in setting up a new board of

---

[18] Joseph Planta to Robert Hay, July 31, 1826, TNA CO 158/52.
[19] Augustus Foster to George Canning, May 11, 1826, TNA CO 158/52.   [20] Ibid.
[21] That said, in the course of the late 1820s and 1830s, due to perceived sanitary violations, Maltese merchants would find themselves in and out of quarantine in European ports. These were, however, brief episodes, and the norm after 1826 was that Malta would remain in free pratique with Continental ports.

health (again, in the past, a superintendent was the sole official in charge of Maltese quarantine) and in formulating new rules, Maltese quarantine officials emphasized their conformity to shared norms. "Having assimilated, by the above measures, the Sanitary Laws of this island with those of the Continental Lazarettos," board members wrote, as they concluded an introductory circular letter to the other Mediterranean health boards, "we can entertain no doubt that all vessels arriving from this island will henceforth be admitted into immediate pratique at your Ports."[22] Sometimes, the process of standardization actually meant a *diminution* of sanitary rigor. At one of the first meetings of Malta's Board of Health, it was decided that the colony should end its anachronistic requirement that passengers should be fumigated as well as goods.[23] "The board of health," recorded its secretary, "with the constant view of assimilating the regulations of the Continental Lazarettoes [*sic*], has been pleased to order that from this day henceforth, the *spoglie* of passengers and other persons be abolished."[24] The final change, which the French Foreign Minister conceded was the most crucial in persuading Continental boards of health to grant Maltese ships free pratique, involved lengthening the quarantine imposed on British warships – a move that had long been resisted by the military establishment on the island.[25] It is all the more telling, then, that the pressure to standardize quarantine procedures overrode such a strong interest. In the end, these changes in Malta made the decisive difference – Maltese shipping was granted free pratique at Marseille in the late fall of 1826.

Malta's success in persuading Marseille's *Intendance* to end its quarantine fed on itself; other boards followed suit, again in the name of standardized procedure. In his letter to the *Intendants* on first being informed of Malta's new Board of Health and its policies, the President of Genoa's *Magistrato* noted that it was his aim to act toward the Maltese in concert with the Marseillaise, given "the reciprocal harmony, which always governs the important decisions, between my *Magistrato* and your eminent *Intendance*."[26] This emphasis on "reciprocal harmony" recurs throughout the archives of boards of health. In operating thus, health board members accepted that major questions about the operation of quarantine in their ports were often decided abroad. Quarantine was a subject of local regulation and national law, but also supranational expectation.

---

[22] Hector Greig to the Intendants Sanitaire de Marseille, April 6, 1826, NAM CSG 03–71.1.

[23] Such a decision was, no doubt, heartily welcomed by thousands of travelers. At the same time, as will become clear in the next chapter, the *spoglio* mimicked the disinfection procedures employed on a daily basis by Western Europeans in the Middle East.

[24] Minutes of the Board of Health meeting of October 14, 1826, NLM LIBR 847.

[25] Baron Damas to Viscount Granville, May 30, 1826, TNA CO 158/52.

[26] Pallavicini to the Intendants de Santé of Marseille, April 29, 1826, ADBR 200 E 423.

The system had hiccups, but these fashioned greater congruity. In 1836, for example, Maltese ships were quarantined once again in France and Italy because of information that two frigates from Corfu were granted pratique in Malta after only ten days quarantine. A formal letter to the Genoese signed by all the members of Malta's Board of Health vigorously defended the action. It asserted that the diminished ten-day quarantine for ships with clean bills coming from Greece was thoroughly appropriate given that this was "exactly how ships originating in Greece are treated at Livorno."[27] In reality, Malta's Board was trying to pass off an attempt at reform as if it were an effort to assimilate procedure. Threatened with a retaliatory quarantine, board members conceded the point. A month after having claimed a ten-day quarantine was eminently reasonable, Malta restored the original length of eighteen days. As they attempted to pressure the Maltese to restore their more severe quarantine, Marseille's *Intendants* and Genoa's *Magistrati* coordinated their responses.[28] The whole episode reveals not only how correspondence among boards of health forced the assimilation of quarantine procedure, but also how the invoking of precedent in another port (Malta's references to Livorno's procedures) could serve as justification. In the end, it was impossible to reduce quarantine lengths substantially without simultaneous agreement by a majority of boards of health. Marseille's *Intendants*, for example, were able to convince Parisian ministers about the need to maintain a quarantine on France's new colony of Algeria for more than a decade after French colonization thanks to the threat of retaliatory quarantine on French ships in Italy if Algerian ships were admitted in free pratique.[29]

Reciprocal correspondence generated reciprocal procedures. Even when a change of procedure was not being contemplated, however, board members were aware that a main task of this correspondence was to build up confidence in foreign ports about quarantine enforcement at home. In October 1825, for example, G. Falconcini of Livorno's *Consiglio di Sanità* sent a letter to the President of Genoa's *Magistrato* informing him of the severe and extraordinary measures he took against a ship which was then in perfect health but was known to have disembarked a passenger with plague in Alexandria. In the conclusion to the letter, Falconcini noted that this information (even though it might make the Genoese suspicious) was offered up "as a proof of loyal participation in reciprocal correspondence".[30]

---

[27] Board of Health of Malta to the Magistrati di Sanità of Genoa, December 27, 1836, ASGe Sanità 1184.

[28] Maltese Board of Health circular letter to foreign boards, December 14, 1836. Also Intendants de Santé de Marseille to the Marchesa di Pallavicini, November 30, 1836, ASGe Sanità 1184.

[29] See correspondence between Laurent Cunin-Gridaine and Marseille's Intendants, ADBR 200 E 208.

[30] G. Falconcini to the Marchesa di Pallavicini, October 21, 1825, ASGe Sanità 1178.

A central perk of being seen as a willing participant in this exchange of information was that, in return, members of a board of health could expect to receive additional medical intelligence. Thus, in 1830, Sir Hector Greig, Superintendent of Quarantine at Malta, learned of plagues at Kolah and Usciak on the Anatolian coast from sanitary correspondence with boards of health in Venice and Livorno. This enabled him to suggest that the Naval Commander-in-Chief should instruct Royal Navy captains operating in the Mediterranean to refrain from taking a cargo onboard in any part of the Levant, as the presence of cargo during a plague epidemic could drastically augment quarantine on the warships' return to Western Europe.[31] From Greig's perspective, accurate information from abroad could make life easier for captains, consuls, and quarantine officials across the British Mediterranean.

Some boards were known to have better information than others. In the late eighteenth century, Venice was typically the most *au courant* with sanitary news about Dalmatia and the rest of the Balkan Peninsula – Marseille's *Intendance*, for example, established a routine of giving Venice's *Provveditori* information about North Africa in return for bulletins about plagues on the Dalmatian coast in the 1790s. On the whole, however, the *Intendants* were usually ahead of all competitors when it came to achieving an accurate sanitary picture of the entire globe. Almost once each week, they prepared a *Note Sanitaire*, which summarized the latest sanitary intelligence for every region of the world (based on information received from captains arriving at Marseille, from foreign boards of health, and from French consuls in correspondence with the *Intendance*). Foreign consuls who managed to get their hands on one of these "sanitary notes" regularly sent them along to boards of health in their home countries.[32]

Diplomacy and Sanitary Information

A cog is missing in this network of exchange as I have painted it thus far – the role played in sanitary information exchange by consuls. Consuls have appeared obliquely until this point – watching ships come in at the quarantine harbor, interceding if a board of health put their home country's shipping in quarantine. Their role, however, was crucial in the information exchange that enabled quarantine to function.[33] First, consuls stationed in the "East" routinely forwarded prominent boards of health in their respective countries sanitary information about the Ottoman Empire and North Africa. Second, consuls in

---

[31] Hector Greig to Sir Frederick Hankey, January 5, 1830, NAM CUST 04/01.

[32] See, for example, Sardinian Consul-General Pagano to the Marchesa di Pallavicini, July 2, 1825, ASGe Sanità 1178.

[33] On the general importance of consuls in relation to sanitary regulation in the late eighteenth and early nineteenth centuries, see Arner, "Making Commerce Global."

other quarantine ports or European capitals reported on quarantine affairs abroad. This allowed boards of health back home to enforce the threat of retaliation. Thus, in many cases, consuls – corresponding directly with boards of health – acted as medical intelligence agents on foreign shores.

Consuls posted in port cities often operated from buildings situated directly on the harbor (Figure 5.1). Among other reasons, this was because their presence was often necessary there – to oversee the arrival of their country's ships or to receive prominent nationals in their offices soon after their arrival. But another, and crucial, reason that necessitated a consul's frequent attendance at a port was his duty of issuing and signing a bill of health. Across the Mediterranean, boards of health accepted any consul's bill of health as legitimate. Though it was normal for a ship flying the British flag to receive a bill from the British consul if possible, the fact that patents issued by all consuls were accepted at all ports makes the bill of health analogous to a passport – after all, its receipt was a required part of receiving pratique. This makes it a unique document for its time; a more or less standardized international form that was essential to achieving admission to any given nation. The importance of these bills is a further proof of the way in which consuls formed a central cog in the

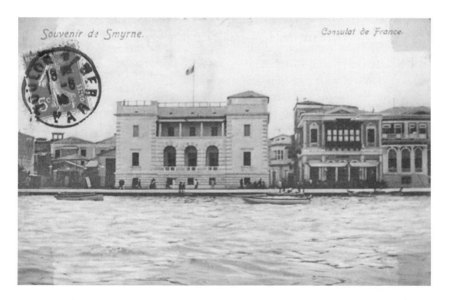

Figure 5.1 Postcard showing French Consulate along Smyrna's waterfront from around the turn of the twentieth century. Many other powers (including Britain and Austria) had consulates on Smyrna's harbor. Courtesy of the Levantine Heritage Foundation.

sanitary network and also an indication of the way in which quarantine fostered greater intra-European coordination.

In each Ottoman port city, there are indications that the European consuls closely coordinated the issuing of bills of health. It was up to each consul individually to decide whether local conditions merited a "clean," "suspected," or "foul" bill, but where one consul went, there was pressure to follow. In the 1840s, when a profusion of local quarantines came into being *within* the Ottoman Empire, the pressure became even more acute. Mrs. G. L. Dawson Damer, a British traveler through the Ottoman Empire and Egypt in 1840, describes an anxious moment she experienced in Smyrna while waiting for her ship to depart for Syria:

Mr. Brant, our consul, came on board, and after a little interchange of civilities, he proceeded to tell us, as an agreeable communication, that a case of the plague had occurred at Smyrna, or rather, as he added, a strong suspicion; and that, in consequence, he, the French and Austrian consuls, had issued *des patentes noires* [foul bills of health] and that a quarantine of twenty-one days would ensue at Alexandria, or at whatever port we touched, and this would be independent of the ultimate quarantine at Malta, and no *pratique* likely to be afforded at either Beyrouth or Jaffa.[34]

And yet, Damer's party was saved this excessive quarantine through the "delightful" intervention of the Dutch consul, who insisted on continuing to issue clean bills of health as the plague case had not yet been substantiated.[35] Consuls were pressured to operate in concert, lest they subject their own country's ships to comparatively long delays or, conversely, betray too much laxity in issuing clean bills when other consuls issued foul ones.[36] For the most part, consuls seem to have taken seriously their charge to remain aware of potential plague cases and issue patents accordingly.

The cooperative atmosphere between European ambassadors in Constantinople became urgent in 1818 when a serious sanitary crime threatened the integrity of the process of issuing bills of health. In a letter from October of that year, the French ambassador to the Porte (the Marquis de Rivières) wrote the *Intendants* of Marseille to warn that "*un inconnu* presented himself . . . at the printer's room in the British Embassy of this city and asked there that they print for him 50 copies of the enclosed blank form of one of your bills of health." On being informed by the printer, the British ambassador (Sir Robert Liston) immediately ordered the blank bill of health to be seized and

---

[34] The Hon. Mrs. G. L. Dawson Damer, *Diary of a Tour in Greece, Turkey, Egypt, and the Holy Land* (London: Henry Colburn, 1841), 1:240–41.

[35] Ibid., 242.

[36] Note, for example, the condemnation in France of the Swedish and Danish consuls in Tunis for apparently issuing clean bills of health after reports of plague deaths in North Africa in March of 1798. Conservateurs to Talleyrand, 1 Germinal An 7 (March 21, 1799), AN (Paris) AE B/ III/220.

alerted Rivières. Noting that this plan could have resulted in false bills being issued by someone other than a French diplomat, Rivières urged the *Intendance* to take measures to prevent the counterfeiting of bills of health.[37] The *Intendants* immediately obtained the authority to affix a stamp to the bills they forwarded to consuls,[38] and there are no further examples of comparable crimes.

Enforcement, in such a case, depended on the French and British ambassadors' belief that insuring the integrity of quarantine across Europe was a matter of mutual concern. Furthermore, the form of correspondence generated by this incident is suggestive of broader patterns of sanitary information exchange. Rivières's immediate action of writing to the *Intendance* rather than the responsible Paris Minister (who was only kept in the loop by the *Intendance* itself) helps demonstrate a pattern of direct communication between diplomats and boards of health. This was essential to the proper functioning of quarantine.

Such correspondence involved a variety of issues. Just as in Rivières's letter asking for lenient quarantine for the Ottoman Ambassador to France, consuls often wrote to boards of health when eminent individuals were known to be departing for Europe and included requests for lenient quarantine on their arrival. Should the government of a consul or ambassador's station be considering sanitary legislation, boards of health were always kept in the loop. Sometimes, in fact, they helped shape laws themselves. Marcel Chahrour, for example, has shown how integral the Austrian *Internuncio* at the Ottoman Porte was during the development of the initial Ottoman quarantine system in the 1830s and 1840s.[39] The declaration eventually negotiated by the Internuncio and Rifaat Bey, an Ottoman vizier, stipulated that three individuals in the employ of the Lazaretto of Semlin would be sent to Constantinople to give their advice on implementing new quarantine procedures.[40]

Diplomats, then, took an active role in crafting quarantine rules. Many knew more about typical Mediterranean procedures than occasionally more parochial members of boards of health. For example, no single individual was more responsible for the strict observance of Maltese quarantine procedure in the early 1830s than Dominique Miège, the French consul in Valletta. In constant correspondence with the Marseille *Intendance*, Miège persuaded the Maltese to

---

[37] Rivières to the Intendants of Marseille, October 10, 1818, ADBR 200 E 460.

[38] Intendants of Marseille to the Minister of the Interior, November 18, 1818, AN (Pierrefitte) F/8/29, Dossier XI.

[39] See Chahrour, "A Civilizing Mission?" As Teodora Sechel has shown, Habsburg thinking about epidemics had long been influenced by the cross-border studies of provincial Austrian doctors. See Sechel, "Contagion Theories in the Habsburg Monarchy (1770–1830)," in *Medicine within and between the Habsburg and Ottoman Empires, 18th–19th Centuries*, ed. Teodora Sechel (Bochum: Winkler, 2011), 55–78.

[40] Declaration by Rifaat Bey and Baron d'Ottenfels, Istanbul, May 21, 1838, Haus, Hof, und Staatsarchiv, Vienna (henceforth HHStA) MdÄ AR F50-2.

further tighten their scrutiny of warships, to construct better parlatorios, and to create a stricter regime for arrivals from locales suspected of cholera.[41] Miège saw his role as pushing for Maltese severity in order to establish "confidence between you [Marseille's *Intendants*] and the *Comité Maltais*."[42] Indeed, Marseille's *Intendants* sent Miège precise questions about Maltese procedure, urging him, for example, to determine the number of days for which the Maltese typically quarantined Black Sea wheat.[43] On occasion, Miège's zeal to encourage greater Maltese severity seems to have exceeded that of Marseille's *Intendants*. In October 1831, for example, the indignant consul expressed his "astonishment," that the *Intendance* had failed to respond to his four most recent reports of Maltese laxity by establishing a temporary quarantine on Malta (though they did a month later).[44]

Needless to say, this intervention by the French consul was extremely irritating to Maltese authorities. On the occasion of the 1831 quarantine Marseille slapped on Malta due to supposed laxity in the face of cholera, Frederick Hankey (the Chief Secretary of the Government) was outraged to hear from the British consul in Marseille that the *Intendance*'s decision had been made entirely based on material received from Miège and summoned that zealous consul to the Government Office to explain himself.[45] But, due to the nature of Mediterranean diplomacy, it was impossible to ban this form of intelligence sharing. The retaliatory quarantining that happened so often among Mediterranean ports in the 1820s and 1830s was almost entirely based on information transmitted to boards of health by consuls – ambiguous diseases in the hinterland, suspiciously short quarantines, and unacceptable fumigation procedures were all duly noted by Miège and his ilk. As a result, boards of health across the Mediterranean were pushed into greater standardization of procedures and greater reluctance to grant exceptions when it came to quarantine traffic. The advent of Mediterranean steam ships and more reliable mail service meant quarantine ran more efficiently, but also that in many ports it was harsher than it would have been without such efficient forms of communication.

While boards could improve their reputation for conscientiousness by relaying any information about deviations in a particular quarantine port to other boards, tattling was less common than the more good-spirited method of gaining foreign approbation by sharing sanitary information. Epidemic news

---

41 Dominique Miège to the Intendants of Marseille, March 6, 1830 (warships), July 2, 1831 (parlatorios), and August 28, 1831 (cholera), ADBR 200 E 463.
42 Miège to the Intendants of Marseille, November 8, 1831, ADBR 200 E 463.
43 Miège to the Intendants of Marseille, August 10, 1830, ADBR 200 E 463. The answer, it turned out, was thirty days of quarantine. Marseille's Intendants seems to have been satisfied with this.
44 Miège to the Intendants of Marseille, October 18, 1831, ADBR 200 E 463.
45 Sir Frederick Hankey to Dominique Miège, November 7, 1831, ADBR 200 E 463.

became a kind of currency, which boards could leverage to their advantage. In the mid-1820s, when Malta's Superintendent of Quarantine, Hector Greig, was making a broader push to achieve permanent free pratique status for Malta in Continental ports (described above), he attempted to dangle the possibility (to foreign boards) that good relations with Malta would enable them to access valuable sanitary information obtained from Britain's arsenal of consuls. "Being in perfect knowledge how useful it is to the common institutions [of quarantine] to hold frequent reciprocal relations between boards of health ... relative to the state of health of ports in the Levant and Barbary," Greig wrote in a circular to foreign boards, "I intend to adopt a constant system of sending off such correspondence at least once a month."[46]

Here, Greig was clearly envisioning a Maltese equivalent to Marseille's "*Note Sanitaire*" as a ticket to Malta's inclusion within the "in-crowd" of Mediterranean lazarettos. The intelligence he provided in this initial letter, however, was hardly likely to impress the other Mediterranean boards, being a set of general comments to the effect that the plague was present in all of the Levant, but that Greece and North Africa were enjoying good health. Though his future communications were by no means regular, in 1829, for example, Greig sent a circular to "the Sanitary administrations of the Continent" containing a detailed description of a plague epidemic menacing Odessa and Varna.[47] On the whole, his efforts seem to have been largely sincere, even when British consuls did not hold up their end of the bargain and send up-to-date sanitary information to Malta. In 1830, after an episode where he was only informed of a troubling plague epidemic in Anatolia by the Livorno Board, Greig complained to the Maltese government that he received "few or no sanitary advices ... from HM Consuls in the Levant."[48] Greig was frustrated that he was not able to put potential British contacts in the East to good use in the game of building up credibility with other boards of health.

Still, slowly but surely, ascendant British Mediterranean power made itself felt in older sanitary networks. Even prior to achieving free pratique with the Continental ports, British officials in Malta knew it was wise, in corresponding with foreign boards of health, to sing the praises of the huge value of "loyal, faithful, and reciprocal correspondence" between sanitary bureaucrats.[49] And even if Malta's Quarantine Superintendents did not receive as many sanitary notices as they would have liked, they put the information they did receive to good use. Dominique Miège, that great skeptic of British-run quarantine in

---

[46] Hector Greig to the Magistrati di Sanità of Genova, October 4, 1825, ASGe Sanità 1178.

[47] Circular Letter from Hector Greig to foreign boards of health, October 19, 1829, ADBR 200 E 463.

[48] Greig to Sir Frederick Hankey, January 5, 1830, NAM CUST/04/01.

[49] Robert Grieves to the Superintendent of Quarantine at Palermo, November 11, 1818, NLM LIBR 843.

Malta, nevertheless routinely forwarded sanitary intelligence he received from interacting with the British. In 1837, for example, in an effort to convince him they were taking the threat of plague-importation from Libya seriously, Maltese officials forwarded Miège a dispatch from Hanmer Warrington, British consul in Tripoli, about the course of plague in that city. Miège dutifully translated Warrington's letter into French and forwarded it to Marseille's *Intendants*.[50] Far more frequently, Miège alludes to epidemic intelligence he received from speaking with captains arriving at Malta, and sent advice so derived to Marseille. In this way, the fact that ascendant British Mediterranean power and a liberal trade policy was gradually turning Malta into an *entrepôt* for intelligence from all sides of the Mediterranean placed it closer to the center of networks of sanitary information. Finally, the proximity of the Ionian Islands to the Greek mainland meant that dispatches referencing diseases there, written by British officials on Corfu, were voraciously consumed by French and Italian boards of health.[51] In sum, Britain's growing Mediterranean Empire, its dominant Mediterranean Fleet, and its ever-greater population of merchants and consuls inhabiting Ottoman and North African cities meant that its citizens increasingly conveyed sanitary news that was consumed by boards of health across the French, Italian, and Austrian coasts.

By contrast, countries that could not boast such extensive Mediterranean networks fell behind in the pursuit of sanitary information. At various occasions when epidemic disease in the Mediterranean excited alarm in the 1820s, the Danish consul at Genoa, Anton Morellet, wrote letters pleading with Genoa's *Magistrato* to give him some news he could share with his information-starved government. On the occasion of the 1820 plague of Mallorca, for example, Morellet wrote to the *Magistrati* "needing, as I do, to share some information with my Government on the contagious malady which is infesting the island of Mallorca, and not being able to rely with certainty on the stories in the newspapers ... which, often for commercial reasons, exaggerate the true state of things, I am driven to [ask you to] share with me some positive information known by your Illustrious Magistracy."[52] Morellet appears to have been successful in his request, because he asked the same from the Genoese during the Spanish yellow fever epidemics of the mid-1820s. Given their contacts with foreign boards of health, with consuls serving abroad, and their information obtained from arriving captains, Mediterranean boards could be counted on to possess current sanitary information that would be especially valuable to governments (like Denmark's) that did not have an extensive network of consuls in the Middle East. Their place at the center of networks

---

[50] See ADBR 200 E 463.
[51] See, for example, the circular letter from A. Broadfoot, Inspector of Health in Corfu, to the boards of health of the Mediterranean, August 5, 1825, ASLi Sanità 37.
[52] A. Morellet to the Magistrati di Sanità of Genoa, July 13, 1820, ASGe Sanità 1365.

of sanitary information gave immense prestige to Mediterranean boards of health and undergirded, strengthened, and regulated the quarantine system as a whole.

The Power of Rumor

In December 1824, the Sardinian consul in Tunis wrote to the Genoa *Magistrato*, alluding to an event that demonstrates the problems boards of health had in obtaining an accurate picture of health in the Mediterranean. Noting that his November letter had suggested "that there were many dead in the city of Tunis from the bubonic plague," this diplomat wrote that he had since determined that this information had been spread by "some spiteful individual." "Many of the foreign Consuls," he reported, "as well as the Faculty of Medicine" had since determined that "this city, as well as its environs, maintained and continues to maintain the most perfect health."[53] As further proof of this encouraging news, he included a supplementary letter signed by numerous French and Italian doctors residing in Tunis, which stated that its sanitary affairs were in good order.[54]

On receipt of these letters, the apprehensions of Genoa's *Magistrato* were quelled and the quarantine on Tunis was returned to its more moderate clean bill regimen. But the episode demonstrates that it was necessary to formulate quarantine rules (the length of detention, thc type of fumigation to be ordered) based on reports whose validity was an open question. One individual (for example, a merchant whose goods would not be shipped for another several months and wished to delay the trade of his competitors) could spread rumors of disease that could have far-reaching effects across the Mediterranean. Still, the system had mechanisms built within it – the slower, but coordinated action of investigating consuls in any given port – which could counteract false reports.

Even when extraordinary quarantines were shown to be based on faulty information, however, a rumor could involve the unnecessary detention of dozens of ships and serious financial losses by merchants whose trade goods were so detained. Before Britain's 1800 Quarantine Act allowed ships with foul bills of health perform quarantine at home, a report by PC clerk William Fawkener suggested that the Dutch, Greeks, and Italians habitually conspired to delay British commerce by spreading plague rumors that forced foul bills to be issued.[55] Other rumors were not intentionally spread, but developed due to the necessarily patchy nature of sanitary intelligence.

---

[53] Enrico to Magistrati di Sanità of Genoa, December 24, 1824, ASGe Sanità 1267.
[54] "The Doctors of the City of Tunis" to the Magistrati di Sanità of Genoa, November 27, 1824, ASGe Sanità 1267.
[55] See Fawkener, "Enclosed Report," in Lord Hawkesbury's "Note on Levant Ships," June 1, 1796, BL Add. Ms. 38354.

In part, this sprung from the lengthy time it took for European communities of major Middle Eastern cities to get news of the presence of a plague. A death outside the European quarter would only be immediately known to Western diplomats and merchants if it was attended by a European physician. Constantinople, Smyrna, Aleppo, Cairo, Alexandria, and Tunis all had substantial communities of French, Italian, British, and Austrian doctors by the early nineteenth century, though such physicians were thin on the ground in the poor or outlying districts in which epidemics often began. Reports picked up steam as the number of victims grew. The often random set of local contacts a European doctor, consul, or merchant interacted with might share the news of plague reports, but most often Greek physicians (who were much more integrated into Ottoman society and who staffed the major plague hospital of Constantinople) would serve as intermediaries for the spread of epidemic rumors to their more isolated Western European colleagues.

Consuls might receive word of suspicious deaths at any time – from a day or two after a potential plague victim had died to several weeks later. As Mrs. Damer's experience shows, consuls might decide to postpone announcing reports of plague until concrete information was received from multiple sources. Still, they often alerted boards of health before more detailed information was received – hence reports of dubious validity. Board members were then forced to judge whether the information they had been sent was enough to merit a change in the quarantine rules for the given locality. Given their understandable reluctance to be blamed for ignoring intelligence of an epidemic (should it be imported), board members often acted on the receipt of very vague information even as they pressed consuls for updated reports.

All epidemics in Constantinople, suggested the French traveler A. Brayer, were preceded by "premature plague rumors."[56] Plague's status as a favored subject of gossip can be seen in Mrs. Damer's description of the British consul telling her there were reports of the disease "as an agreeable communication." Boards of health, being in receipt of so much intelligence from consuls, boat captains, and merchants, were part of this network of gossip and often got reports of epidemics long before they had been substantiated. In 1808, for example, Florimond de la Tour-Maubourg, in his capacity as secretary of the French embassy at the Porte (he would later become ambassador), wrote the *Intendants* at Marseille simply to inform them that "the state of health of this capital of the *échelles* of the Levant is highly satisfactory. The rumors which suggested the plague had manifested itself at Smyrna are entirely without foundation."[57] Presumably, de la Tour-Maubourg had previously sent along the rumors himself.

---

[56] A. Brayer, *Neuf Années a Constantinople* (Paris: Bellizard, Barthès, Dufour, et Lowell, 1831), 2:68.

[57] Florimond de la Tour-Maubourg to the Intendants of Marseille, October 7, 1808, ADBR 200 E 460.

Given that the quarantine lengths meted out to ships with *clean* bills were still quite long if the ship had proceeded from the Middle East, among the most significant rumors were those that cast doubt on the health of another European port city, arrivals from which were more numerous and usually received in free pratique. It should be clear from the numerous epidemics to hit European cities and the tales of reciprocal quarantines imposed for diplomatic reasons, that even among European ports, free pratique was only a provisional guarantee. Thanks to the yellow fever epidemics (in Spain and Italy) from 1799 until the 1820s, cholera after 1831, and harsh responses to news of a plague ship in a given quarantine harbor, such intra-European quarantines were common.

Rumor-induced intra-European quarantine was particularly common on the continent's periphery, where proving or disproving a tale of epidemic disease took more effort. In 1824, for example, Britain's Board of Trade was outraged at the news that the Kingdom of the Two Sicilies had placed all ships arriving from Limerick and the County of Muenster under a long quarantine at the ports of Palermo, Naples, and Messina. Having made inquiries, the Board of Trade could find no evidence of any kind of disease outbreak in Ireland at all, still less one that could justify "a measure so unusual and so vexatious to the commerce from this country to Sicily."[58] The Kingdom of the Two Sicilies appears to have been notorious for its frequent excessive reactions to rumors of suspicious diseases: an important exception to the principle that boards of health generally cohered around similar quarantine standards. Summarizing the state of quarantine against Malta to Admiral Penrose (the Commander of the Mediterranean Fleet), a Quarantine Superintendent of Malta complained that the Sicilians "keep this island in a constant quarantine of seven days, doubling that period on every idle rumor propagated." He concluded that he could name many more examples of "of the vacillating absurdity of the people of Sicily in their conduct toward this Island under the denomination of Health security," but that he would spare the Admiral further details.[59] It is clear, however, that though Malta was in quarantine across the Mediterranean in this period (arrivals from Sicily, it should be noted, were also given a quarantine of observation at Marseille at this time), the quarantine at Palermo and Messina was particularly damaging given the vital commercial links between Malta and these Sicilian ports.

Malta itself occasionally imposed premature quarantines. In spring 1830, Malta revoked the free pratique granted to ships arriving from northern Italy based on reports suggesting a suspicious "contagion" had broken out there. This was eventually revoked based on definite information received from

[58] "Quarantine Note" from the minutes of the December 30, 1824, meeting of the Board of Trade, TNA BT 5/33, ff. 262–64.
[59] Robert Grieves to Admiral Charles Penrose, undated, but clearly late winter 1819, NLM LIBR 843.

British consuls in the area.[60] It should be noted that particularly malignant outbreaks of typhus, smallpox, or "fever" could be treated as grounds for quarantine alongside more exotic diseases, making the frequency and consequences of rumors even greater. Given this, as the episodes I have brought forward show, it was essential for boards of health to present to each other the appearance of sanitary respectability. Some of Malta's reactiveness to rumors received from abroad, then, should be considered from this perspective – the Maltese quarantine official who decided to act on a potentially premature rumor was a wiser official than one who did nothing until after *Le Chevalier* Miège had heard the same rumor.

Clearly aware of the cost of rumor-induced quarantines, boards vigorously defended their sanitary impeccability when they sensed they themselves were the subject of sanitary gossip. Marseille's Revolutionary-Era *Conservateurs*, for example, were aware in 1796 that the integrity of their quarantine procedures had been called into question by rumors circulating among Italian boards of health that the quarantine on two plague ships recently arrived from Algiers had not been strict enough. Not waiting for news that French ships had been quarantined, the *Conservateurs* wrote the Venetian *Provveditori* to preemptively rebut any intelligence they might hear: "*Messieurs*, we must write to you to stop the false rumors which might spread *chez vous* about the state of health of our lazaretto." Presenting a lengthy description of the ideal position of their lazaretto and quarantine harbor and emphasizing the severity of their procedures, the *Conservateurs* said they were writing "to calm all the fears which vague and ever-exaggerated rumors might give you about public health."[61] The *Conservateurs* hoped that reciprocal correspondence and exhaustive sharing of "case histories" of quarantine events (plague ships, unusual episodes, etc.) would militate against the pernicious power of vague rumors.

Given that rumors often had a kernel of truth – a small outbreak of disease that was reputed to be a large one, a plague ship in the harbor that was mischaracterized as plague running wild in the city – their existence encouraged the kind of information sharing that I have demonstrated was so prevalent in this period. Their ubiquity also expands our sense of how sanitary news might spread. Vague reports made by captains were taken very seriously, and boards of health frequently relied on items in newspapers or shipping gazettes that suggested anomalies had occurred in foreign ports. Meanwhile, consuls trawled the harbor docks for sanitary information they could send to boards of health back home. Bartolomeo Cornet (the Venetian consul at Marseille for more than forty years in the late eighteenth century) gave a hint of that latter

---

[60] Sir Frederick Hankey to Dominique Miège, February 4, 1830, ADBR 200 E 463.
[61] Conservateurs de Santé of Marseille to the Provveditori alla Sanità at Venice, August 20, 1796, ASVe Provv. Sanità 551.

phenomenon when hunting for information about the sanitary state of a convoy of seventy French ships recently arrived from Ottoman ports: "In fact, it was whispered in my ear by one person that three men had died, but [my informant] did not know enough to tell me whether this had happened in one boat of the fleet or in many, although the officials and *Intendants* deny everything."[62] The complex web of sanitary communication in the modern Mediterranean meant quarantine actions were never undertaken in private, and dubious events could not be hushed up; it was usually better to air one's dirty laundry publicly.

Testing Reciprocity: Britain's Quarantine Act of 1825

As the European biopolity took shape from coordinated action, the standardization of procedures, and the sharing of information, the paradox of national quarantine legislation seemed ever more apparent. Reciprocal correspondence among Mediterranean sanitary authorities had resulted in common practices of disinfection, but at any time, national legislation could override the confidence built up among boards of health. Any legislative change was watched closely in foreign ports. A sudden lurch toward reform, or even the suspicion of such a change, was not possible without retaliation. The drama surrounding Britain's mildly reformist 1825 Quarantine Act presents just such an instance in which the ambiguities of quarantine's status were brought to the fore. Was quarantine based on a set of national rules? Or was it an early example of international law? All of the aspects of quarantine in the Mediterranean addressed in earlier sections of this chapter were crucial to the development of this episode: communication among boards of health, the importance of sanitary information networks, and the invidious power of rumor. The event emphasizes how difficult it was to legislate on matters of quarantine (by the early nineteenth century) as a national power within an international system. It also demonstrates the extent to which Britain was implicated in Mediterranean sanitary networks and its need for resourceful diplomacy in order to resolve the debacle the law introduced.

We have already broached the topic of this law in Chapter 2. Again, the dramatic uptick in Britain's trade with the Ottoman Empire and George Canning's consequent decision to revoke the charter of the Levant Company coincided with a decision to revise the quarantine laws. The complaints of captains about exorbitant quarantine charges, fears that quarantine in Britain was unusually strict, and efforts by the anticontagionist doctor Charles Maclean to persuade Parliament to adjudicate the question of the plague's contagiousness all contributed further toward a reformist climate. Parliamentary select

---

[62] Bartolomeo Cornet to the Provveditori alla Sanità at Venice, August 11, 1781, ASVe Provv. Sanità 378.

committees in 1819 and 1824 had considered the validity of the doctrine of contagion and the links between the quarantine system and the Levant trade. By 1825, in concert with the formal end of the Levant Company and in the midst of high hopes for further trading success, MPs felt ready to revise the Quarantine Act of 1800.

Changes proposed included a more rigorous effort to integrate Irish ports into the British quarantine system and a clause that mandated that all goods considered liable to infection (so-called enumerated goods) be accompanied by a written declaration that they were not the produce of the Ottoman Empire or North Africa. The most controversial aspect of the law, however, was Section 22, which allowed the Privy Council to exempt from quarantine on their arrival in Britain all ships with clean bills of health *including those from the Middle East*.[63] Still, although this was considered reformist, the change put British quarantine procedure on roughly the same footing as in the Mediterranean, where, theoretically, a board of health could radically change the quarantine length mandated for any individual ship. Even if the Privy Council *did* intend to exempt a ship from quarantine, there would still be a delay of several days as the captain's report was taken to London and ruled on before word could be sent back to the coast. In the end, this power was not used to excuse ships from detention until the 1840s.

For most ship owners, by far the most important change included in the 1825 Act was the government's assumption of the responsibility for paying many of the quarantine fees they had had to bear in the past. The 1824 Quarantine Committee found that the method used to calculate duties in Britain resulted in fees at Stangate Creek that were between twenty and fifty times greater than the corresponding costs in Marseille and Trieste. It was precisely, the report lamented, thirty-seven times cheaper for British ships to perform quarantine in Holland than it was in Kent (low quarantine fees and short quarantine durations in Holland were a frequent source of British commercial angst).[64] The primary motivation behind the reform seems to have been a desire to mitigate iniquities like these rather than to strike at the heart of the quarantine laws, though the records of the debate in the House of Commons show that many members did indeed take the occasion to put their weight behind more fundamental changes.

There is reason to believe that based on its text alone, the 1825 Quarantine Act would have been carefully read in Mediterranean ports, but that it would not have been seen as a radical break with past procedure. Unfortunately for Britain, the debate on the bill coincided with a serious breach of the quarantine laws in Liverpool. In the winter of 1825, a ten-ship convoy hauling cotton from

---

[63] For a summary of the various clauses of this Act, see Booker, *Maritime Quarantine*, 401–3.
[64] 1824 Select Committee Report, 7.

Alexandria arrived at Liverpool's quarantine harbor only to find it full. After much vacillation by port officials, more than ten thousand bales of cotton were permitted to be disembarked without any quarantine, not least because the ships all had clean bills of health. Cotton, though the chief import from Egypt to Britain, was one of the classic "enumerated goods" and was usually extensively fumigated. As usual, the arrival of this fleet and the disembarkation of its cargo was announced in the *Liverpool Gazette*. It was presumably this paper that caught the eyes of the Board of Health of Trieste and caused a serious crisis of quarantine diplomacy.[65]

Immediately on reading that this breach had occurred, the President of Trieste's Board sent letters to every major Mediterranean board of health. These indicated that the full facts of the case still needed to be confirmed but that, if this event had occurred as it seemed from the papers, ships arriving from Britain would need to be quarantined across the Mediterranean. This was a breach of the quarantine laws on an apparently nationwide scale by a major European power. The receipt of this intelligence set the transnational sanitary information network alight with indignation.

G. Falconcini, of the Livorno *Consiglio di Sanità*, informed the Marseillaise in May that Livorno was now formally quarantining ships arriving from Britain because of "the new maxims and the new systems, now followed in Britain, which allow for ships from the Ottoman Levant and from Barbary to be admitted to free pratique." This behavior, he noted, was "in opposition to the sanitary principles generally adopted by all the civilized nations of Europe."[66] By the late spring, Trieste, Genoa, Naples, Messina, Ancona, Marseille, Toulon, and other boards of health placed British ships under an equivalent fifteen-day quarantine. Sounding a similar note to the Livorno *Consiglio*, Genoa's Marchesa di Pallavicini wrote that "such a grave irregularity undertaken by a civilized government" was hardly credible, especially as it would suggest that Britain was not chastened by "the experience of what the consequences had been when sanitary discipline was ignored in its possessions of Malta and Corfu."[67] This was a reminder that Britain had allowed the plague to invade two of its new Mediterranean colonies (in 1813–14 and 1816, respectively), and should be the last power to contemplate abandoning quarantine.

From the late eighteenth century onward, as I have emphasized, quarantine was transformed from a set of idiosyncratic local practices into a standardized European system – a collection of reciprocal procedures that enforced a common biopolitical border. It took the sudden threat of a gaping hole in

---

[65] Costanzi of the Trieste Sanità to the Intendants de Santé of Marseille, April 8, 1825, ADBR 200 E 427.

[66] G. Falconcini of the Livorno Sanità to the Intendants de Santé of Marseille, May 5, 1825, ADBR 200 E 427.

[67] Marchesa di Pallavicini to the Governor of Livorno, April 20, 1825, ASLi. Sanità 240.

that border for this idea to be acknowledged explicitly. As spring 1825 wore on, Genoa's Pallavicini lamented the "irregularity that has taken place in the British ports, in opposition to the Sanitary System of Europe" ("*sistema sanitario Europeo*").[68] The response was even more damning from P. Mangelli of the Ancona Sanità. Referencing reports that anticontagionist doctors in Britain were responsible for the new policy, Mangelli slammed the "new maxims embraced in Britain," which, he said, were "fatal to the meticulous reciprocal institutions of public health." Mangelli announced an indefinite imposition of "the most rigorous measures" on all ships arriving from Britain and noted his intention of inquiring whether "it will be necessary to augment the quarantine already in operation against ships arriving from the Ionian Islands, Gibraltar, and Malta (all subject to the influence of the British Government), in case an equally pernicious system is now operating there."[69]

Mangelli's letter is a reminder that, in Mediterranean diplomacy, Britain no longer operated as an outside power. As British trade expanded, and as the Ionian Islands and Malta joined Gibraltar as British colonies in the area, a sense that Britain was renouncing its sanitary commitments had wider implications than it would have had in the eighteenth century. Having received word of this new anti-British skepticism at exactly the same time that they were pushing to achieve free pratique with the Continent, British administrators in Malta scrambled to reassert the island's sanitary reputation. Sir Frederick Hankey wrote a circular to all British consuls in the Mediterranean urging them to inform the boards of health at their respective stations that Maltese procedures would not change whatever the British government decided:

It appearing ... that a supposition prevails, that this Government intends some relaxation of the existing Quarantine restrictions to which invariably are subject all Vessels, Persons, and Goods arriving at Malta, from Egypt, the Coast of Barbary, or any other place liable to suspicion, I am directed to request that you will immediately notify the *Sanità* Department at your Port, that no relaxation of the existing quarantine will be allowed at Malta, on any pretence whatever; and that the *Sanità* regulations as at present established will continue to be maintained with the utmost rigor.[70]

This strong response was largely successful. Malta, not yet in free pratique with the Continent, does not seem to have suffered substantial augmentation of the quarantine imposed on ships from its ports elsewhere in Europe as a result of the 1825 controversy. Yet for British quarantine officials there, who were seeking desperately to prove their sanitary competency, the sense of ineptitude emanating from the metropole was distinctly unhelpful.

---

[68] Marchesa di Pallavicini to the Consiglio di Sanità of Livorno, June 15, 1825, ASGe Sanità 1056.

[69] P. Mangelli of the Magistrato Centrale di Sanità per la Costa Pontificia dell'Adriatico to the Livorno Consiglio di Sanità, May 13, 1825, ASLi Sanità 240.

[70] Circular, Sir Frederick Hankey to "British Consuls or Vice Consuls at the Principal Ports of the Mediterranean," June 28, 1825, NAM CSG 07/1.

Meanwhile, by May 1825, the situation seemed to be spiraling out of control. Naples's Board of Health had dedicated an entire meeting to debating Britain's new health regime and applied a fourteen-day quarantine to all ships arriving from British ports.[71] Meanwhile, Marseille's *Intendants* took the opportunity to inform the Italian boards that the Low Countries were adopting similar quarantine procedures to Britain; arrivals from Holland, consequently, were placed under a similar quarantine regime in France and the Italian states.[72] To Mediterranean boards, in the late spring of 1825, it must have appeared that Northern European governments were losing their senses. Britain's quarantine bill, winding its way through Parliament in the late spring, only came up as a subject of notice well into this maelstrom. It was taken in the Mediterranean as a codification of the "new maxims" that rejected the contagiousness of the plague. When Genoa's *Magistrato* sent inquiries to the Count d'Aglié, the Sardinian Ambassador to Britain (Genoa being the central port of the Kingdom of Piedmont-Sardinia), Aglié sent back a copy of the bill as well as the *1824 Select Committee Report*. This only seems to have further provoked the Genoese. In a letter to Marseille's *Intendance* announcing that the *Magistrato* had translated the bill into Italian and was now able to read it, Pallavicini zeroed in on Section 22, noting that codified quarantine would be restricted to foul bill ships and that the Privy Council could newly exempt ships with clean bills from detention.[73] To the members of Mediterranean boards of health, it seemed clear that Parliament was planning on upending centuries of quarantine practice.

Aglié himself evidently thought that the Mediterranean health boards were overreacting. He noted that Mediterranean protection could hardly completely isolate Britain, as its ships still arrived in free pratique at northern French ports like Calais.[74] Far from taking this as a signal to back down, the Genoa *Magistrato* immediately sent a letter to Marseille's *Intendance* lamenting continued French admittance of British ships at its northern ports. "Such chaos [in French policy]," Pallavicini warned the *Intendants*, "renders the cautions we have adopted somewhat illusory, and makes the *Magistrato* anxious."[75] This was both a threat to put all ships from anywhere in France under quarantine and a tacit admission that, within Europe, frontiers were difficult to regulate. Once the transnational compact began to fracture, board members' instincts were to go it alone. To prevent the system from falling apart entirely, the *Intendants* petitioned the Interior Ministry to address the problem by instituting anti-British precautions at all French ports, Calais included.

---

[71] Minutes from the May 11, 1825, meeting of the Magistrato di Salute of Naples, ASN Mag. Salute 505.

[72] See Corsini to Livorno Consiglio di Sanità, May 26, 1825, ASLi Sanità 37.

[73] Pallavicini to the Intendants de Santé of Marseille, June 16, 1825, ADBR 200 E 423.

[74] Comte d'Aglié to the Magistrati di Sanità of Genoa, May 22, 1825, ASGe Sanità 1267.

[75] Pallavicini to the Intendants de Santé of Marseille, June 16, 1825, ADBR 200 E 423.

Boisbertrand, their correspondent at the Ministry, tended in most situations to be skeptical about the *Intendants'* inflexible severity. On this occasion, however, he promised to watch the bill as it made its way through Parliament. In the meantime, Boisbertrand promised to instruct officials at all of France's northern ports to "be vigilant" about British ships and to detain all cotton which might have arrived in Britain from the Middle East.[76] By the end of June 1825, then, the sanitary organization of Europe appeared to be in disarray. British and Dutch ships were placed under a minimum fourteen-day quarantine at all major Mediterranean ports. Malta was under pressure to quarantine the ships of its colonial power, while France was contemplating the unthinkable policy of denying free pratique to the thousands of British ships that docked each year at Calais and Dunkirk.

But far from proving Britain's nature as a Continental outlier, the episode's eventual resolution shows how tightly bound Britain had become to the *sistema sanitario Europeo*. By early May 1825, the Board of Trade became aware of the foreign quarantines levied against Britain. Foreign Secretary George Canning correctly intuited that the skepticism about pestilential contagion expressed by various elements of Parliament and the British press was encouraging the action taken by foreign boards of health and urged, in a June 3 debate on the quarantine bill, that MPs "keep such opinions a little more to themselves."[77] The British government, Canning noted, had no intention of overturning or questioning the doctrine of contagion. British consuls were given instructions to emphasize in European ports that the bill's main intention was to reform quarantine fees, not to admit ships from the Middle East and North Africa in free pratique. The authority of the king and PC to set quarantine lengths was a codification of a presumption that had existed before, British consuls stressed in letters to Mediterranean boards of health.[78]

Concurrently, correspondence at Genoa and Marseille shows that William Huskisson (the President of the Board of Trade) met with Sardinia's Aglié and the French Ambassador. Huskisson persuaded both men that the Liverpool cotton affair was an aberration and that the Quarantine Act would change nothing. They were provided with a full report of the episode by an official from Liverpool's port. Concurrently with the bill's final passage, the government ordered the official publication of a dispatch from Sir Thomas Maitland, Governor of Malta during the plague, which emphatically proclaimed the contagiousness of that disease. By the end of this apparent lobbying campaign, Aglié was singing

---

[76] Boisbertrand to the Intendants de Santé of Marseille, July 2, 1825, ADBR 200 E 298.

[77] Hansard, House of Commons Debate, June 3, 1825, Vol. 13, cc. 1036–39.

[78] See, for example, J. Harting (British Consul at Genoa) to the Magistrati di Sanità of Genoa, June 19, 1825, ASGe Sanità 1365.

the praises of British officials' commitment to the quarantine system to Pallavicini and Genoa's *Magistrati*.[79] Before long, the Mediterranean boards were mollified. By the end of July, Livorno, Genoa, and Marseille had all (in close coordination) ended their extraordinary quarantine on Britain,[80] with Naples following on August 3.[81]

An Order in Council was issued by the Privy Council in mid-July, which set out the terms of British quarantine under the new regime. It showed little change from the previous system. This caused some in the Mediterranean to assume that their diplomatic pressure had impelled the British to reverse course. But that view accompanied a conviction that the original British plan had been to declare an end to all quarantine and admit all arrivals from the Levant and North Africa in free pratique (a misreading of the Liverpool cotton affair).[82] In fact, it was not the Order in Council that changed Mediterranean hearts and minds. By mid-June, correspondence between Marseille and Genoa shows that the tide had already turned based on materials received from national ambassadors in London.[83] Furthermore, economic damage alone can hardly explain the PC's conservative order. Only ten ships from Britain were quarantined in Livorno during this episode,[84] for example, and only three at Marseille.[85]

Britain and the European Biopolity

Although the economic ramifications of this quarantine were limited, the threat to Britain's reputation as a respected nation within the European sanitary system was serious. The society doctor Augustus Bozzi Granville wrote an anguished public letter to the President of the Board of Trade at the height of the controversy:

Sir my prediction is fulfilled! England is declared to be an infected country; she is put on a footing with Turkey at some of the principal ports of the Mediterranean, ... in consequence of the reported relaxation in the sanatory [*sic*] laws said to have been recommended by this government to the legislature, and still more in consequence of the singular doctrines proclaimed in Parliament.[86]

---

[79] Aglié to Magistrati, June 24, 1825, and July (day missing), 1825, ASGe Sanità 1267.

[80] Falconcini to Intendants de Santé of Marseille, July 28, 1825, ADBR 200 E 427.

[81] Summary of Magistrato di Salute meeting on August 3, 1825, ASN Mag. Salute 505.

[82] See, for example, Venturi to the Intendants de Santé of Marseille, June 15, 1825, ADBR 200 E 427.

[83] See June 1825 correspondence between Marseille's Intendance and Genoa's Magistrato, ADBR 200 E 423.

[84] See ASLi Sanità 716.   [85] ADBR 200 E 780.

[86] Augustus Bozzi Granville, *A Letter to the Right Honble. W. Huskisson. M.P., President of the Board of Trade, on the Quarantine Bill* (London: J. Davy, 1825), 1.

What rankled Granville most was the sense that Britain's policy makers had rendered British ships as suspicious as those coming from the Ottoman Empire. The whole episode threatened to put Britain on the wrong side of the *cordon sanitaire*, a classification that connoted much more than medical status. As the situation makes clear, the idea that Britain was willing to abandon prophylaxis against the "East" implied that it was cutting itself off from "civilized" government.

As the French quarantine reformer Ségur-Dupeyron put it, it was not enough to be a "habitually healthy country" but also necessary that ministers follow "usages generally adopted." Ségur approvingly noted that the British government acted "sagely" in recanting its seemingly radical measures, which he noted were particularly problematic for Malta.[87] On the one hand, this simply restates the logic of the British government itself. But, by emphasizing that enjoying national health was less important than capably managing quarantine, Ségur's work undergirds the sense that the fight against contagion occurred, at least partially, on the level of symbolism and reputation.

One could analyze episodes like this and find evidence, as Peter Baldwin, Erwin Ackerknecht, and John Booker have done, that Britain was always equivocal about its adherence to European sanitary norms.[88] On the other hand, I have shown that tit-for-tat quarantines to enforce sanitary standards were hardly unusual. Although it was Trieste's Board of Health that first brought the British reforms to the attention of other Mediterranean boards, ships from the city of Trieste were themselves in quarantine throughout the Mediterranean during spring 1825 because that city's Board had admitted Lord Strangford (the British ambassador to the Porte) without the appropriate quarantine on his arrival from Constantinople.[89] Consequently, one could take the Trieste Board's revelation about British infractions as an effort to regain sanitary credibility.

For Britain itself, any sense of a major disjunction with Mediterranean practice was based on a series of misunderstandings. British administrators were obviously taken aback at the swift reaction to a proposed reduction in quarantine, but they were also very willing to reverse course. In the event, British quarantine policy did not change significantly in the wake of 1825. This episode is telling not because it reveals an embarrassing reversal by British cabinet ministers bamboozled by conservative Mediterranean bureaucrats, but because it shows that Britain had learned to play the game of Mediterranean

---

[87] Ségur-Dupeyron, *Des Quarantaines*, 7.

[88] Peter Baldwin, "The Victorian State in Comparative Perspective," in *Liberty and Authority in Victorian Britain*, ed. Peter Mandler (Oxford: Oxford University Press, 2006), 54–55. Also Baldwin, *Contagion and the State*, chapter 1; Booker, *Maritime Quarantine*; Ackerknecht, "Anticontagionism."

[89] Roisbertrand to the Intendants de Santé of Marseille, May 4, 1825, ADBR 200 E 298.

sanitary diplomacy rather well. British ministers may have been eager to reform the system, but they also knew how to be patient. They took Britain's membership within the "*sistema sanitario Europeo*" very seriously indeed.

In this vein, it is instructive to consider the case of Britain in relation to the case of Spain. Under Spain's post-1823 restored monarchial regime, its quarantine laws were rigorous and were not subjected to any reformist legislation prior to the later nineteenth century. Yet, because of successive epidemics of yellow fever, boards of health across Mediterranean Europe subjected ships proceeding from Spanish ports to quarantine for most of the 1820s. Indeed, ships from Spain saw far more quarantine in that decade than did ships from Britain. British authorities during the 1830s appear to have continued to view Spanish quarantine practice with some suspicion, especially given their long-held desire to improve Gibraltar's reputation as a quarantine port. In 1839, there was significant disquiet in Gibraltar about a ship (recently arrived from Cuba) that had a certificate showing it had performed quarantine in the port city of Vigo, on Spain's northern coast. While the Spanish government did indeed institute a foul bill quarantine station at Vigo soon after,[90] this was not yet in operation, and British officials were bewildered by the deviation from typical procedures.[91] The decision of authorities in the Spanish port of Algeciras to admit this ship (the *Concepcion*) on an authority not acknowledged and regularized by long-held practice led to a serious diplomatic incident. Alexander Woodford, Governor of Gibraltar, noted his "uneasiness on the score of public health, the communication between Algeciras and this fortress being so immediate" and noted that the event was so serious as to almost necessitate "putting all Spain in quarantine" at Gibraltar.[92]

Despite being assured by the Governor of Algeciras that the officials at Vigo acted in accordance with their understanding of Spain's quarantine laws,[93] Woodford wrote to the British government about his anxieties surrounding the incident, drawing the attention of Lord Palmerston, and, later Lord Aberdeen (successive foreign secretaries). Further inquiries indicated that in anticipation of new rules, the provincial health boards of Spain's north coast were admitting ships from America during yellow fever season in a manner inconsistent with the presumed policy of Spain's central government in

[90] On the disposition of quarantine ports in mid-and late nineteenth-century Spain, see Quim Bonastra, "Quarantine and Territory in Spain during the Second Half of the Nineteenth Century," in Chircop and Martínez, *Mediterranean Quarantines*, 17–46.
[91] See Woodford to the Marquis of Normanby, August 21, 1839. Contained in *Correspondence Relative to the Contagion of the Plague and the Quarantine Regulations of Foreign Countries* (London: T. R. Harrison, 1843), 210.
[92] Woodford to Southern, August 17, 1839. *Correspondence Relative to the Contagion of the Plague*, 212.
[93] See Fernando de Butron to Woodford, August 15, 1839. *Correspondence Relative to the Contagion of the Plague*, 211.

Madrid. This knowledge prompted Palmerston to urge the British mission at Madrid to impress upon the Spanish government the importance of a "uniform and intelligible system of proceeding in matters of quarantine."[94]

All told, the episode demonstrates that during a decade when we typically assume Britain's participation in quarantine was simply down to Continental enforcement, depending on the context, British diplomats themselves could be the enforcers. During this same period, the British government was in negotiations with France and Austria to convene a reformist quarantine summit; Spain did not participate in these efforts, and can generally be considered to be one of the more conservative powers in Europe with regard to quarantine practice, at least in the first half of the nineteenth century.[95] Indeed, the letters surrounding this episode show that from the perspective of Spanish authorities, nothing unusual had occurred; they noted that allowing secondary quarantine ports on Spain's Atlantic coast to receive ships from the Americas without disease on board was analogous to France's practice of allowing such ships to perform quarantine at ports such as Bordeaux, Bayonne, and Havre de Grace.[96] British officials continued to press the issue, both because of their apparent belief in the protocol that suggested a state needed formally to publicize its quarantine rules and because of genuine fears in Gibraltar that suspected negligence on Spain's north coast could lead to the reintroduction of yellow fever (Gibraltar itself having been particularly hard-hit in an epidemic in 1828).

In conclusion, numerous incentives and impulses drew states to participate in the European biopolity. While this biopolity may have had a limited legislative reach, it encompassed legislation pertaining to trade, naval administration, and public health. It also had staying power undergirded by the evolving Mediterranean context. As we know from Chapter 2, British engagement with the quarantine system is inextricable from broader military, political, and diplomatic trajectories. And as we have seen here with the 1825 Quarantine Act, the development of British sanitary legislation depended on links between Britain and Continental powers. Even well after the cholera epidemics and transformations of opinion in favor of anticontagionism during the 1830s, as we see in this final example regarding Gibraltar and Spain, British diplomats could find themselves in the position of urging sanitary severity. In the 1840s, when Britain made its first tentative steps toward ending quarantine for some steamship routes between Alexandria and Southampton, they were operating

[94] Palmerston to Southern, September 26, 1839. *Correspondence Relative to the Contagion of the Plague*, 217.

[95] A French defender of quarantine in the 1860s called the Spanish "the last defenders of public health" in contrast to French, British, and Italian willingness to loosen quarantine rules in the preceding decade. Quoted in Arrizabalaga and García-Reyes, "Case of Nicasio Landa," 179.

[96] Perez de Castro to G. W. Jerningham, November 18, 1839. *Correspondence Relative to the Contagion of the Plague*, 219.

with the full understanding of French and Austrian ministers. Acting otherwise would have rendered a huge sector of the British export trade open to severe delays – that this sector was larger than Britain's trade with the Ottoman Empire is a crucial reason quarantine lasted so long. British economic vitality, diplomatic credibility, and political prestige required free pratique with the Continent.

Over the period from 1780 to 1840, coordination among sanitary authorities across the Mediterranean contributed to a quarantine system that was increasingly seen as a unitary barrier protecting a coherent European biopolity (Britain firmly included). This polity's members were sometimes at odds, and approaches to health and disease varied among nation-states. But that low-level sanitary bureaucrats began to generate a shared border is a clear demonstration of the lingering power of Mediterranean rhythms to generate convergence among different kinds of states. By setting Europe on the path of sanitary congruity, by providing it with a shared border, and by fostering trust among officials at all levels as they confronted epidemic disease, quarantine facilitated European integration. The Mediterranean Sea was the fundamental border of a biopolity. The English Channel was not.

Part III

Imagining the Plague

6   Plague and "Civilization"

A study of how Europeans and Ottomans negotiated plague epidemics in the Middle East, and an analysis of the way the plague shaped understandings of civilizational difference, could do no better than to join one of the most popular travel writers in history, Alexander Kinglake, as he stood on the terrace of the Lazaretto of Semlin in 1838. Six years in the future, Kinglake would go on to write a bestselling narrative of his travels: *Eothen; Or, Traces of Eastern Travel* (1844). It begins here, at the lazaretto, as Kinglake paused at the border between and the Habsburg and the Ottoman domains and prepared to journey, via a Turkish boat, down the river to Constantinople. In the course of his travels he would visit Syria, Egypt, and the Holy Land.

But that lay in the future; at the beginning of his journey, the East appeared to Kinglake as a piquant suggestion behind an imposing barrier. The lazaretto, Kinglake noted, marked the "end of this wheel-going Europe." Behind him lay the familiar vistas and routine experiences of life in the West; across the River Save lay "the splendour and havoc of the East." Kinglake observed Ottoman Belgrade "austere and darkly impending" just across the river. Habsburg Austria and the Ottoman Empire – the lazaretto terrace and the fortifications of Belgrade – were "less than a canon-shot distant," but Habsburg and Ottoman subjects held "no communion" with each other (Figure 6.1).[1]

This border was made implacable by quarantine: "It is the plague, and the dread of the plague, that divide the one people from the other. All coming and going stands forbidden by the terrors of the yellow flag."[2] Crossing over to the potentially infected zone meant making one's body a possible locus of Eastern contagion. It was a moment heavy with gravity. Given that any return from Austria after contact with a single Ottoman subject meant a mandatory fourteen-day quarantine in the "odious lazaretto" of Semlin, Kinglake and his fellow travelers anticipated their departure "with nearly as much solemnity as if we had been departing this life." The final passage was mediated by "the compromised officer" – an Austrian soldier who passed his term of service in exile from his

---

[1] Kinglake, *Eothen*, 1.   [2] Ibid., 1.

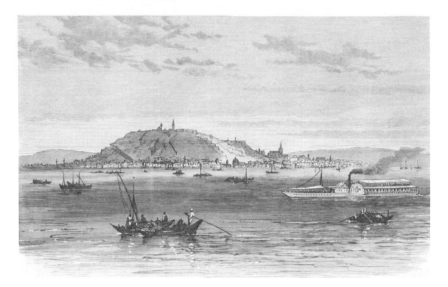

Figure 6.1 The harbor of Semlin, with a view toward the fortifications of Belgrade. From *The Illustrated London News*, 1876.

compatriots because of his status as a conductor of travelers to the Ottoman domains. At the final moment of departure,

> We shook hands with our Semlin friends, who immediately retreated for three or four paces, so as to leave us in the centre of a space between them and the "compromised" officer. The latter then advanced, and asking once more if we had done with the civilised world, held forth his hand. I met it with mine, and there was an end to Christendom.[3]

Once past this dramatic encounter, Kinglake found that the "Easterness" of the scene that awaited him on the other side was dramatically accentuated. "I have since ridden through the land of the Osmanlees, from the Servian Border to the Golden Horn – from the gulph of Satalieh to the tomb of Achilles; but never have I seen such ultra-Turkish looking fellows as those who received me on the banks of the Save."[4] The presence of quarantine thus intensified Kinglake's perception of cultural difference, and the plague serves as a dramatic marker throughout his narrative. The symbolism of a West identified with "fear of the plague" and an East identified with the disease itself would be a recurring trope. Just so, once he reached Constantinople, Kinglake noted that:

[3] Ibid., 2–3.   [4] Ibid., 3–4.

All the while that I stayed at Constantinople the plague was prevailing, but not with any degree of violence. Its presence, however, lent a mysterious and exciting, though not very pleasant, interest to my first knowledge of a great Oriental city; it gave tone and color to all I saw, and all I felt – a tone, and a color sombre enough, but true, and well befitting the dreary monuments of past power and splendor. With all that is most truly oriental in character, the Plague is associated.[5]

What precisely did Kinglake mean by this? What was it about plague that lent itself to an essentialized vision of the Middle East? In addressing these questions, this chapter aims to explore how plague informed Western stereotypes, preconceptions, and fears about the lands outside the *cordon sanitaire*. I argue that plague prevention formed a crucial part of the self-perception of Western Europeans as a distinct and cohesive community when visiting Ottoman cities. At the same time, I emphasize how some of the very travel narratives expressing that view simultaneously reveal how extensively Christian and Muslim responses to plague in those cities resembled each other. Such narratives, like Kinglake's, form the focus of this chapter – these works shaped the contours of sanitation and civilization for the British reading public.

In the past three chapters, we have explored the ways in which quarantine impelled Britons and Continental Europeans toward a sense that sanitation and civilization went together. In Chapter 5, we saw how quarantine itself fostered a European sanitary system, where entry at one port implied at least a medical right to enter the entire Continent. It should not surprise us that Mrs. Griffith felt herself "comparatively at home" on reaching Malta's lazaretto.[6] The country might have been Catholic and the architecture foreign, but the lazaretto marked a border that lent a sense of sanitary harmony to the lands inside it: from Malta to Manchester, from Ancona to Aberdeen.

By the nineteenth century, however, the same structures that promoted a sense of shared sanitary integrity at home also gave a sense of coherence to the threatening Orient outside. It was a world of contagion, of unrestrained microbes that correlated easily with an orientalist stereotype that the East was the home of unrestrained passions. To Western observers, it figured as a land in decline, in which apparent civilizational descent corresponded with the lingering power of premodern epidemics.[7] Finally,

---

[5] Ibid., 29. On Kinglake's role in a longer intellectual trajectory of establishing the plague as an "Oriental" disease, see Nükhet Varlık, "'Oriental Plague' or Epidemiological Orientalism," *Plague and Contagion in the Islamic Mediterranean*, ed. Nükhet Varlık (Kalamazoo, MI: Arc Humanities Press, 2017), 57–58.

[6] Griffith, *A Journey*, 2:77.

[7] See Nigel Leask, *Curiosity and the Aesthetics of Travel Writing: 1770–1840* (Oxford: Oxford University Press, 2002). David Arnold explores the conjunction between new styles of travel writing and the construction of "medical topographies" in *The Tropics and the Traveling Gaze* (Seattle: University of Washington Press, 2006).

it was in the Orient that despotism supposedly had its seat,[8] and the implacable power of the plague mapped easily onto the ostensibly terrible justice of sultans, viziers, and beys. To travel to the East was to flirt, by necessity, with transgression. Kinglake's analogy between venturing past the lazaretto gates and "departing from this life" found literal expression in the fact that life insurance policies, which travelers may well have taken out, frequently restricted travel to areas considered medically secure. The life insurance policy of the Church of England, for example, retained a clause until the 1850s limiting residence abroad to "any place in Europe not subject to the Quarantine Laws or affected by Epidemic or Endemic Disease."[9] In this official language, to venture outside the limits of the *cordon sanitaire* was literally to flirt with death.

In these ways, there was a fundamental interpenetration of Western conceptions of "plague" and of "the East." So too, in a practical sense, the disease mediated relations between Westerners and Muslims. Prevailing traditions (inspired by quarantine) about techniques to ensure immunity from the plague induced the extensive communities of Western expatriates in Ottoman cities to develop specific procedures designed to curtail contact with locals during periods when disease prevailed. The social and economic life of Western traders, diplomats, and missionaries resident in the Ottoman Empire moved, in many ways, according to epidemic currents.

In his 1864 *Bible de L'Humanité*, the historian Jules Michelet characterized the "miraculous Orient" by its "dreamy torpor." Nevertheless, he wrote, "it advances, invincible, fatal to the Gods of the light, by the charm of its dream, by the magic of its chiaroscuro."[10] However much a fear of an Oriental "invasion" is a Western fantasy, the presence of plague unnerved many travelers, and formed a recurrent point of interest. To detect this fear, it is necessary to read beneath the nonchalance many travel writers retrospectively claimed to have maintained in the face of the plague. Most British travelers made a point of ridiculing the extensive self-quarantines and disinfection precautions undertaken by other Europeans residing in Ottoman cities. A feigned unconcern with the disease comes across as an unconvincing retrospective attempt to impose

[8] For a genealogy of the idea of "Oriental Despotism," see Lucette Valensi, *The Birth of the Despot: Venice and the Sublime Porte*, trans. Arthur Denner (Ithaca, NY: Cornell University Press, 1993). Also see Ann Thomson, *Barbary and Enlightenment: European Attitudes to the Maghreb in the 18th Century* (Leiden: Brill, 1987), 54–55.

[9] Church of England Fire and Life Assurance Society Board Minutes. London Metropolitan Archives (formerly Guildhall) MS 12160D, vol. 3. I am grateful to Timothy Alborn for drawing this source to my attention.

[10] Jules Michelet, *Bible de L'Humanité* (Paris: F. Chamerot, 1864), 277. Edward Said quotes a condensed version of this statement in *Orientalism*, though he questions its representative character. See Said, *Orientalism* (New York: Vintage Books, 1978), 73. Epidemic disease, however, is one area where Michelet's fear would appear to be representative.

a spirit of *sang-froid* to an Eastern sojourn. Perhaps from the vantage point of London, surveying a trip concluded without any plague, the disinfection procedures looked ridiculous. And yet, most Britons in the East appear to have adopted them without question. Conscious of the potential dubiousness behind the prophylactic power of many techniques, most still reached for anything that might stop the march of the most terrifying disease they knew. Once on the far side of the *cordon sanitaire*, quarantine's geography inspired a persistent consciousness of the omnipresence of plague.

Evaluating the "Sick Man of Europe"

Though Kinglake was intrigued by the exotic distinctions he saw on crossing into the Ottoman Empire, it did not take the self-satisfied barrister long to make himself at home. In Jerusalem, Kinglake emphasized his complete comfort and assured fellow elite travelers that they would find the city eminently familiar, even English: "Your club is the great Church of the Holy Sepulchre, where everybody meets everybody every day ... Your Bond Street is the Via Dolorosa."[11] Contributing to Kinglake's sense of familiarity was surely the increasing number of Britons making similar journeys. Across Western Europe as a whole, as Yehoshua Ben-Arieh has shown, the 2,000 travel narratives published about journeys to the Holy Land between 1800 and 1850 exceed the 1,500 published at any time before 1800.[12] Narratives about travel to Egypt and Anatolia were even more ubiquitous, and it is a mark of this that many such works begin with an extensive "apology" for adding to the growing number. The proliferation of these accounts encouraged a transformation already under way in the Romantic period from a form of travel narrative centered on straightforward description to one grounded in introspection and affect. This new mode of writing privileged emotion, imagination, and reverie.[13] Too often, such production is limited to the realm of literary analysis and cultural history without a serious consideration of travel literature as a political source. Imaginative reveries, for example, form an especially potent device through which Western European observers expressed political evaluations of the Ottoman Empire and mixed them with perceptions of Ottoman plagues.

For many European travelers, the presence of plague in the Ottoman Empire and its absence in Europe was more of a political dilemma than an

---

[11] Kinglake, *Eothen*, 159.
[12] See Yehoshua Ben-Arieh, "Jerusalem Travel Literature as Historical Source and Cultural Phenomenon," in *Jerusalem in the Mind of the Western World: 1800–1948*, ed. Yehoshua Ben-Arieh (Westport, CT: Praeger, 1997), 2.
[13] On the increasing importance of reverie in nineteenth-century travel narratives, see Barbara Stafford, *Voyage into Substance* (Cambridge, MA: MIT Press, 1984), 400.

epidemiological one. It seemed to pose a question of the capability of the Ottoman state. While the idea of Ottoman "decline" as a general historical phenomenon has been fatally undermined by generations of historians,[14] it was certainly a concept that preoccupied diplomats in Western European capitals in the nineteenth century, and a piece of debatable conventional wisdom that many nineteenth-century Europeans thought they knew. While conceding that importation of the plague to the West was theoretically possible, an anonymous author in the *Quarterly Review* concluded that "progress in the arts of civilization and improvements in polity have disarmed epidemics of a considerable portion of their power."[15] J. P. Papon reminded his readers that "In other times, the same foyer of corruption which fosters the plague in Egypt and Ethiopia was in France and Italy: enlightened thinkers destroyed it." Such a thing, Papon insisted was possible in the East too: "I would like to believe that Cairo and Constantinople might become one day just as healthy as Paris and London."[16] In Mary Shelley's *The Last Man*, one character expresses the hope that an epidemic disease could be beaten by an extension of British civilization: "The favoured countries of the South will throw off the iron yoke of servitude; poverty will quit us, and with that, sickness."[17] For Shelley, the hope is meant to appear as a vain one; the idea that progress offered a bulwark against contagion appears as a delusion in the novel. To many of Shelley's readers, however, it would have seemed like common sense.

The use of plague as a metric for reading civilizational capacity shows us how high political discussions of the Eastern Question often filtered down into casual discourse. During Lord Palmerston's first stint as a turcophilic Foreign Secretary in the 1830s, for example, numerous travelers seem to have been aware that the official line was optimism about signs of progress. Some remained dubious, and here we see again how often domestic political divisions translated into evaluations of Ottoman prospects. The wife of the Tory MP George Dawson Damer refused to buy the official line, despite having received a bracing dose of turcophilia in a discussion with Lord Ponsonby (then British ambassador at Constantinople). There was no rousing the Ottoman Empire, Damer claimed, from "its present state of decrepitude." Furthermore, "the

[14] For a succinct summary of the problems with "declinist" narratives of Ottoman history, see Suraiya Faroqhi, *Approaching Ottoman History: An Introduction to the Sources* (Cambridge: Cambridge University Press, 2000), chapter 7. On the distinctions between early modern and nineteenth-century versions of "decline," see Şevket Pamuk, *The Ottoman Empire and European Capitalism, 1820–1913* (Cambridge: Cambridge University Press, 1987), 6–8. For a persuasive case that significant aspects of the Empire remained resilient into the nineteenth century, see Donald Quataert, "Overview of the Nineteenth Century," in *An Economic and Social History*, 761–76.
[15] "Contagion and Quarantine," *Quarterly Review* 27, no. 54 (1822): 553.
[16] Jean-Pierre Papon, *De la Peste*, ix.
[17] Mary Shelley, *The Last Man* (Lincoln: University of Nebraska Press, 1993), 159.

doctrine of fatality" was not "as much lessened among the Mussulmen as it is generally reported to be."[18] Ottoman subjects, she was suggesting, were content to let foreign civilizations pass them by. Travelers like Mrs. Damer made such decisions based on a few interactions and quick observations. But the fact that many travelers interested themselves in these debates shows how readily the concepts of the "Eastern Question" came to the minds of travelers.

As travelers questioned the possibilities for regeneration and investigated the potential for greater mercantile engagement, the recurrent plagues to which the Ottoman Empire was continually subjected appeared to be a potent sign that such progress remained far off. In travel accounts, stereotypical condemnations of supposed Ottoman despotism, stasis, and backwardness were linked to the persistence of the plague. On the other hand, turcophiles often tried to downplay the disease and to suggest aspects of the medical state of Ottoman society that appeared relatively healthy. Travelers used the plague as a metric to consider the question of Ottoman decline and the potential of Ottoman reform.

"The insalubrious state of a country and the impurity of the atmosphere seem best to account for the existence, or introduction, of the plague: but in inhabited countries, these physical evils are induced chiefly from moral causes."[19] So noted Thomas Thornton, a Levant Company consul and merchant, whose *The Present State of Turkey* (1807) presents a particularly favorable account of the Ottoman Empire. Despite the positive tone of his book, however, Thornton suggested the Ottoman government was directly responsible for the plague: "If the sin of David brought pestilence upon the innocent house of Israel; how much more must the despotism of the Turkish government, a system at which nature revolts, excite the anger of heaven, and provoke the infliction of augmented evil."[20] Thornton, inspired by the Book of Samuel, saw misgovernment and contagion to be emphatically linked.[21]

Sometimes, travelers drew on this association between misgovernment and pestilence because of concrete links between state policy (or lack thereof) and the existence of disease. Thomas Watkins, for example, found the lack of urban planning in Smyrna to be largely responsible for plague epidemics there.[22] William Eton, a future Superintendent of Quarantine at Malta and a savage critic of the Ottoman government, suggested that the Empire's travails were largely due to a vicious cycle of agricultural problems and economic decline brought about by depopulation. This problem derived in part from frequent

---

[18] Damer, *Diary of a Tour*, 1:163 and 1:172.
[19] Thomas Thornton, *The Present State of Turkey* (London: Joseph Mawman, 1809), 2:218.
[20] Ibid., 218.
[21] David's "sin," to which Thornton refers, was simply ordering a census – something that Thornton may well have seen as *good* government by the Ottoman sultan rather than the reverse.
[22] Watkins, *Travels through Switzerland*, 2:274.

plague epidemics, but it also predisposed the Empire to face more epidemics in the future.[23]

Needless to say, Eton took a grim view of the Ottoman future and held that its problems made almost inevitable "the expulsion of the Turks from Europe."[24] Only three years after his *Present State of Turkey* was first published, Eton established a set of draconian quarantine regulations at Malta. It is clear that in his mind, disease remained the last and most potent way a decaying power could threaten the West. Indeed, to some observers, the very nature of Ottoman government seemed to suit its reputation as a center of epidemic disease. Despotism – in the view of eighteenth- and nineteenth-century European observers – was a predisposing cause. Thus, the French plague authority Alexandre Raimond suggested that "general health is inconsistent with extreme servitude."[25]

Some believed that improvement from this state of affairs was impossible. The American traveler Edward Morris, for example, possibly influenced by Montesquieu's arguments about governments in hot climates, considered despotism an inevitable state of affairs: "It is a strange fact, that the oriental governments, from the earliest times, have always been despotisms. It would certainly be a hopeless task to essay to introduce self-government among the ignorant and enslaved populations of the East."[26] Such deterministic arguments aligned with a fairly widespread view, influenced by the growing popularity of anticontagionism and enduring theory of miasmas, that the Middle East was condemned to suffer from the plague forever, by dint of its geography and climate. Clot Bey, a French medical advisor to Mohammed Ali and a devoted opponent of quarantine, argued that despite those who located its origins more precisely, the plague was endemic to the entire Levant, thanks to "circumstances that were probably meteorological."[27] Another school of thought proposed historical and civilizational reasons for the ubiquity of plague in the East. As the Napoleonic *savant* F. C. Pouqueville noted, Herodotus found no plague in Egypt. Subsequently, however,

when it passed under the feeble power of the eastern emperors, its physical no less than its moral nature underwent a dreadful change; and the cradle of the arts, a spot once so celebrated, once so splendid, ornamented with such magnificent towns and buildings, – this spot became what? – the seat of the plague.[28]

---

[23] William Eton, *A Survey of the Turkish Empire* (London: T. Cadell, 1798), 254–55.
[24] Ibid., viii.   [25] Quoted in Thornton, *Present State of Turkey*, 2:218.
[26] Edward Morris, *Notes of a Tour through Turkey, Greece, Egypt, Etc.* (Aberdeen: George Clark, 1847), 34.
[27] A. B. Clot "Bey," *De la peste observée en Égypte* (Paris: Fortin, Masson, et CIE, 1840), 232–33.
[28] F. C. Pouqueville, *Travels in the Morea, Albania, and Other Parts of the Ottoman Empire*, trans. Anne Plumptre (London: Henry Colburn, 1813), 190–91.

In this way, social factors and climatological ones seemed to reinforce each other. Another French doctor, Étienne Pariset, wrote in the 1820s that Egypt had gone from "primitive salubrity" to a country that, "if it is not the only foyer of plague in the world, is certainly the principal one, as Montesquieu wrote."[29] Though Pariset cites Nile flooding and humidity as reasons the plague found Egypt such a congenial home, his citation of Montesquieu reveals the influence of socio-political reasoning; hot weather, despotism, and plague appeared to run together. Writing almost two decades later, the British doctor Gavin Milroy made cultural explanations for Egyptian plagues even more explicit: "Egypt was once a remarkably healthy country," he wrote in 1846, "subsequently to this period, the ignorance and fanaticism of the Mussulmen have brought it to [a] frightful state of moral degradation and physical wretchedness."[30] Milroy offered no theories on how the Egyptians might reverse this transformation but predicted Britain could be confident the disease could be avoided even without quarantine, given its integral association with despotism and Islam.

Plague appeared to endow the East with a parasitical grandeur. At first, Alexander Kinglake warned his British audience, "you go out from your queenly London – the centre of the greatest and strongest among all earthly dominions – you go out thence, and travel on to the capital of an Eastern Prince, you find but a waning power, and a faded splendour." A Briton's first reaction to the declining Orient would be "to laugh and mock." But, continued Kinglake,

Let the infernal Angel of Plague be at hand, and he, more mighty than armies, more terrible than Suleyman in his glory, can restore such pomp and majesty to the weakness of the Imperial city, that if, *when HE is there*, you must still go prying amongst the shades of the dead empire, at least you will tread the path with seemly reverence and awe.[31]

In this way, the association between despotism and plague not only linked the Sultan's government to the disease, but found disease to be inherent in his polity's power.

If a despotic regime marked out a diseased polity, disease itself was also described like a despot. John Bowring, like Milroy, a committed believer in the idea that plague could not exist in Britain, insisted that it was "in the East" that "the plague takes up its natural abode and reigns in its most despotic power."[32] Britons during the 1830s and 1840s referred to "King" Cholera. More evocatively, the late-century colonial administrator Walter Miéville cast cholera as a mythical, almost magical oppressor: "those who have never been in a cholera-stricken city can scarcely realise the awesome sensation as of an unseen messenger flitting through the streets, who willfully and without reason signs

[29] Étienne Pariset, "Note sur la peste," 1828, Wellcome Ms. 3767.
[30] Milroy, *Quarantine and the Plague*, 26.   [31] Kinglake, *Eothen*, 29.
[32] Bowring, *Speech Given to Parliament*, 7.

to the Angel of Death to strike down this one or that one or a whole household."[33] The randomness of epidemics accentuated their association with despotic government. If Ottoman despotism signified a state, as one traveller put it, "where the laws are regulated at the will and caprice of one man,"[34] epidemic disease itself was often described in strikingly similar terms. As an Anglo-Indian plague doctor described it later in the century, "caprice" was something that united cholera and plague into an epidemic type.[35]

Despotism had a distinctly premodern aura. The idea that plague followed naturally from the descent into despotism was related to a link between the plague and a "backward" East, steeped in the remains of antiquity and abstracted from the rhythms of the present. Mrs. Damer found the Ottoman Empire falling behind on the "march of civilization."[36] The idea of being left behind and a sense that the Middle East was defined by changelessness went hand in hand. Eliot Warburton opens his immensely popular travel narrative *The Crescent and the Cross* with a declaration that "immutability is the most striking characteristic of the East."[37] This was a popular idea; the French historian Alfred Assolant called residents of the Orient "people who, in the most fundamental way, cannot move with history."[38]

It was a short leap from being "stuck in the past" to being "stuck with the plague." We should recall Alexander Kinglake's sense that the "tone and color" with which plague imbued the Ottoman capital was "well befitting the dreary monuments of past power and splendour" he saw throughout Ottoman domains. After a night of glorious decline, epidemic disease figures as the hangover. It is on entering Constantinople on the occasion of the city's military capitulation that the main characters of Mary Shelley's *The Last Man* encounter the first evidence of the plague. Similarly, Thomas Thornton associated political collapse with the plague by noting that in Europe's own past, plague belonged to "the period in history ... most fertile in calamities, ... the age when disorder and distress had attained their greatest height." The disease began to vanish when "governments began to re-assume their vigour."[39] As the *English Cyclopaedia* succinctly put it, "wherever civilization has advanced, there plague has receded."[40] Europe's path had led it from barbarism and chaos to order and civilization; critics saw the inverse path under way in the Ottoman

---

[33] Walter Miéville, *Under Queen and Khedive: The Autobiography of an Anglo-Egyptian Official* (London: William Heinemann, 1899), 120.

[34] Griffith, *A Journey*, 1:65.

[35] See C. R. Francis, "Endemic Plague in India," *Transactions of the Epidemiological Society of London* 4 (1881): 401.

[36] Damer, *Diary of a Tour*, 1:164.

[37] Eliot Warburton, *The Crescent and the Cross* (London: Henry Colburn, 1845), 1:v.

[38] Quoted in Darcy Grigsby, "Out of the Earth," in *Edges of Empire: Orientalism and Visual Culture*, ed. Jocelyn Hackforth-Jones and Mary Roberts (London: Blackwell, 2005), 46.

[39] Thornton, *Present State of Turkey*, 2:220.   [40] Knight, *English Cyclopaedia*, 436.

Empire. To European observers, its capacity to alter its course depended on the extent to which it could throw off the despotism, superstition, and fatalism they criticized as so prevalent within it. It should go almost without saying that these denunciations actually *suited* the exotic associations European writers sought to evoke by referencing the Ottoman state. If half the thrill of visiting Crusader sites and Biblical landscapes was to see a landscape ostensibly abstracted from history, it is unsurprising (and not a little hypocritical) that the same observers deemed the Ottoman state itself to be falling behind on the march of history.

Despite the imaginative incentive to perceive decline, some European observers were more optimistic. Thomas Thornton is a good example: writing explicitly in opposition to William Eton, he found much to admire in Turkish civilization. He argued that "veneration for the law" was at the core of Eastern society, favorably compared the Persian poet Hafez to Shakespeare, and contested numerous anecdotes about barbarism and cruelty in Eton's narrative.[41] Coincident with this effort, his narrative is full of attempts to minimize the extent of the plague. Noting that many Europeans "ascribed the frequent appearance of the plague to a neglect of cleanliness," Thornton protested that the Turks paid "the greatest attention" to cleaning their homes and themselves.[42] In contrast to Europeans, whose "vain terrors and pusillanimous apprehensions" during epidemics left them more vulnerable to the plague, Thornton argued that "the Turks, from temperance, from consequent robustness of constitution, and from firmness of mind, frequently escape after infection."[43] Indeed, Thornton emphasized, excepting the plague, "Constantinople is not exposed to local disorders," and in any case, "in nine instances out of ten," reputed cases of the plague were some other disease entirely.[44] Thornton was not alone in stressing the positive sanitary aspects of Turkish society. Citing him, the medical writer Joseph Adam argued that "excepting the poor" of the Ottoman Empire, "few ... suffer by the plague" and reminded his readers that the now thoroughly respectable doctrine of inoculation derived from the Turks.[45] Finally, a nineteenth-century edition of the travels of James Porter, espousing a generally pro-Turkish line, suggested that at least "the climate in European Turkey [was] generally very healthy and mild" and that in general, the plague had been in retreat as habits improved.[46]

No matter one's view of the Ottoman Empire, the plague was a powerful lens through which to judge progress and regress, reform and stasis. Quarantine was crucial to this understanding of the plague; it provided a sense that the disease was not simply a divine scourge, but a concrete problem that governments could choose whether or not to address. Even among those skeptics who disputed

[41] Thornton, *Present State of Turkey*, 1:2, 1:52–53, and 1:24–26.   [42] Ibid., 2:213–14.
[43] Ibid., 2:211.   [44] Ibid., 2:208–9.   [45] Adam, *An Inquiry*, 44.
[46] George Larpent and Sir James Porter, *Turkey; Its History and Progress* (London: Hurst and Blackett, 1854), 1:28.

quarantine's efficacy, few took the view that there was nothing that governments could do to fight the plague; anticontagionists tended to stress sanitation, poverty reduction, and moral improvement rather than insisting on the futility of all action against epidemic disease. Plague blended so easily into evaluations of the Ottoman Empire because it provided a clear, catastrophic event, in the face of which, the tradition of quarantine suggested, government action was necessary.

Was it within the capacity of the Sultan's government to deliver such a response? Here, the question of the plague, and explanations for its continuing presence, bled into one of the major ideas of Orientalism – alleged Eastern "fatalism." This ascribed characteristic held that Islamic belief in predestination precluded intervention against anything which could be considered "the will of God," plague being a prime example. Louis Macleane went so far as to use "predestinarianism" as the central dividing line between zones of plague and zones of security: "the countries most liable to this dreadful calamity are in a manner destitute of Physical Knowledge, and to a man predestinarians."[47] The Franco-Hungarian Baron de Tott (an eighteenth-century reformer of the Ottoman military and the author of a weighty set of memoirs on his observations of the Turks) characterized belief in predestination and consequent "fatalism" as a central theme of the Ottoman state.[48] Well into the nineteenth century, "Turkish fatalism" had become a truism that was often repeated, frequently without reference to the Ottoman Empire at all.[49] It was advanced as a casual explanation for the endurance of the plague in the works of numerous authors. Some, like Thornton, disputed the idea that the Turks were fatalistic at all,[50] and with regard to the question of plague prevention, it is clear that there was evidence available whatever one's view. Although Birsen Bulmuş has shown that conservative elements of the *ulama* did oppose certain sanitary reforms in the early nineteenth century, she demonstrates a long-standing diversity of Ottoman thought and practice regarding the prevention of epidemic disease.[51] The idea that Turks were natural anticontagionists, she demonstrates,

[47] Louis Macleane, "Thoughts on the Plague, Lazarettos, and Quarantine with an Estimate of Expense," handwritten report contained in TNA PRO 30/29/3/2/16.
[48] Baron de Tott, *Memoirs of the Baron de Tott: Containing the State of the Turkish Empire, Translated from the French* (London: G. G. J. and J. Robinson, 1786), 2:74–78.
[49] Yaron Ayalon points out that medical historians stressing fatalism and resistance to flight and isolation have relied too much on plague treatises based on theoretical ideas or even conservative Muslim scholars who wished paint a picture of Muslim behavior during plague epidemics that was "consonant with the faith." He highlights stray comments in other sources showing that Turkish responses resembled European ones (namely, those with means fleeing epidemics of plague and poor people largely staying put). See Ayalon, "Religion and Ottoman Society's Responses to Epidemics in the Seventeenth and Eighteenth Centuries," in Varlık, *Plague and Contagion in the Islamic Mediterranean*, 179–97.
[50] Thornton, *Present State of Turkey*, 36.
[51] Birsen Bulmuş, *Plagues, Quarantines and Geopolitics in the Ottoman Empire* (Edinburgh: Edinburgh University Press, 2012), chapters 2–5.

was in large part a construct of European authors like Charles Maclean, who saw the point as useful for their own polemical writing.[52] Indeed, as Nükhet Varlık has recently demonstrated, during premodern Ottoman epidemics, reactions varied as dramatically as they did in western Europe.[53]

Travelers, too, recognized this diversity by noting that more well-to-do Muslim Ottoman subjects tended (like Western Europeans, and many Greeks, Jews, and Armenians) to isolate themselves during plague epidemics.[54] And just as the anecdotal evidence from travelers paints a picture of Ottoman sanitary practice that was not so different from Western European traditions, a state-level analysis shows a similar perspective. Not only did Ottoman governors in North Africa routinely impose maritime quarantines long before such initiatives were linked to diplomacy with Western Europe,[55] but, as Andrew Robarts has recently demonstrated, Ottoman administrators in the Black Sea region considered the management of plague epidemics a chief priority of the state. Throughout an era of Russo-Turkish wars, skirmishes, and refugee crises, the attempt to control mobile populations in the area was inextricable from concerns about the transmission of plague.[56] Ottoman leaders clearly considered the disease to be a source of disorder, an economic threat, and a humanitarian disaster in ways that intersected with the views of sanitary authorities in Western Europe. It was the simple presence of plague and the Orientalist tradition, far more than any interaction with Ottoman medical experts or administrators that convinced Western observers of the ubiquity of "fatalism."

The Exoticism of Epidemics

In travelers' mental schemas of the Ottoman Empire, plague constituted more than a measure of Ottoman capability. The disease was implicated in an admixture of Orientalist exoticism that incorporated other elements – excess, indulgence, and a lack of restraint. This helped reinforce the exoticized reputation the disease possessed in the nineteenth century, and, as we will see in the next chapter regarding cholera, shaped the perception of other diseases as well. A nebulous concept of "pestilence," freighted with the imaginative paraphernalia of cultural and moral corruption along all these lines, formed a convenient

---

[52] Ibid., 117.
[53] See Nükhet Varlık, *Plague and Empire in the Early Modern Mediterranean World: The Ottoman Experience, 1367–1600* (Cambridge: Cambridge University Press, 2016).
[54] See, for example, Andrew White, *A Treatise on the Plague* (London: John Churchill, 1846), 77.
[55] See Nancy Gallagher, *Medicine and Power in Tunisia, 1780–1900* (Cambridge: Cambridge University Press, 2002). See also Salvatore Speziale, "Epidemics and Quarantine in Mediterranean Africa from the Eighteenth to the Mid-Nineteenth Century," *Journal of Mediterranean Studies* 16 (2006): 249–58.
[56] Andrew Robarts, *Migration and Disease in the Black Sea Region* (London: Bloomsbury, 2017).

foil for famous Victorian sanitary reformers such as Edwin Chadwick and Thomas Southwood Smith. For now, it is important to examine how the links among fatalism, luxury, and illness fostered the discursive development of exotic contrasts in which epidemic disease was often cast as the counterpoint to ostensible Eastern indulgence.[57] The protean metaphor of the plague enabled that disease to stand in as a conveniently adaptable symbol of ultimate punishment. As such, it became an exceptionally versatile foil for the exotic extremes of luxury that travelers sought and described.

Often, this tendency appeared at moments when a traveler was wary of being lulled into a false sense of security. Charles Colville Frankland enthuses at great length over the beauties of the gardens outside the city walls of Damascus, but that precise enthusiasm recalls him to the sense of the plague:

The groves and gardens which surround the city are indeed beautiful; here, by the side of purling streams and bubbling fountain, the Turks sit in groups, and pass away their days in contemplation, smoking the finest tobacco through amber and jessamine and drinking the best sherbets and Moka coffee, out of cups of the clearest porcelain. But lovely as are such spots, they teem with danger; for here the pestilence shoots her arrows in silence and rapidity.[58]

In this description, the plague functions as a kind of *memento mori*, a tangible reminder that even (especially?) in an Eastern arcadia, epidemics were always smoldering.

But a deeper conceptual link bound basic images of Orientalist exoticism to the plague simply by virtue of their extremity. In Mary Shelley's *The Last Man*, the plague is initially confined to the Middle East, prompting the narrator to exhort the reader to:

Weep for our brethren, though we can never experience their reverse. Let us lament and assist the children of the garden of the earth. Late we envied their abodes, their spicy groves, fertile plains, and abundant loveliness. But in this mortal life extremes are always matched: the thorn grows with the rose, the poison tree and the cinnamon mingle their boughs.[59]

Heterodox and indulgent, Eastern luxury, by its very nature, appeared to demand an equally extreme consequence. Plague, says the narrator, is "of old

---

[57] Nükhet Varlık shows how considerations of supposed Turkish "fatalism" regarding epidemic disease shaped the historiography of plague as well as evaluations by Orientalist observers. Although before the eighteenth century, the Eastern and Western Mediterranean shared a common medical position vis-à-vis the plague and also a common tradition of medical scholarship, histories of early modern plague have often assumed an essential difference between Ottoman and Western experiences of plague without a clear basis. See Varlık, *Plague and Empire*, 73–74.

[58] Charles Frankland, *Travels to and from Constantinople, in the Years 1827 and 1828* (London: Henry Colburn, 1829), 2:101.

[59] Shelley, *The Last Man*, 169.

a native of the East, sister of the tornado, the earthquake, and the simoon. Child of the sun and nursling of the tropics, it would expire in [European] climes."[60] In the novel, such an assessment represents the deluded prediction of a Briton, but in writing it, Shelley was undoubtedly familiar with a common British tendency to view Northern European "cold" as a sufficient protection against epidemic diseases. Thus, while the British narrator's hope is soon shown to be a vain one, Shelley nevertheless makes explicit a widespread association in her society between extreme luxury and extreme mortality. A core assertion of nineteenth-century Orientalist exoticism could be expressed by the idea that in the East, life was more intense and death more catastrophic. One plague-minded British traveler, for example, noted his ambivalence about confronting the exotic wares at a Constantinople market in the midst of a plague epidemic – "I tremble, as I admire."[61]

If plague was positioned as the conceptual counterpoint of "Eastern" excess and opulence, the disease itself was rendered more glamorous by the connection. Alexander Kinglake, for example, found that the disease lent a "mysterious and exciting interest" to his experience of Constantinople.[62] Elsewhere, he describes joking about catching the plague as a kind of intimate flirtation with local women.[63] As Allan Christensen points out, the transmission of the plague takes on a similar sexual connotation in *The Last Man*, when its first visitation appears to be summoned up as a kind of erotic revenge by Evadne, a discarded lover of the Byronic hero.[64] The very extremity of the disease, and the unspecified but horrific symptoms it promised to inflict on the body corresponded to an extreme "Eastern" sensuality. After all, if the contagionist line was that touch alone spread epidemic disease, intimate touch could appear to spread it most devastatingly.

David Arnold notes a powerful undercurrent in nineteenth-century imperial medicine, which held that individuals, like plants, gradually but inevitably declined when they spent too long outside their native country.[65] Constantinople, argued the traveler E. D. Clarke, might be an interesting city to visit but it "is by no means a healthy place of residence."[66] He advocated specific diets for travelers who wished to remain healthy in the East, while Griffith found health impossible among the "plagues of Egypt" (to her, heat and insects).[67] This sense of sanitary siege had literal meanings: there were obvious

[60] Ibid., 169.   [61] Watkins, *Travels through Switzerland*, 237.   [62] Kinglake, *Eothen*, 29.
[63] Ibid., 33.
[64] See Allan Christensen, *Nineteenth-Century Narratives of Contagion: "Our Feverish Contact"* (London: Routledge, 2005), 156.
[65] Arnold, *Colonizing the Body*, 39. The idea of certain constitutions being best suited to certain climates can, of course, be traced back to the Hippocratic tradition.
[66] E.D. Clarke, *Travels in Various Countries of Europe, Asia, and Africa* (London: T. Cadell and W. Davies, 1818), 8:135.
[67] Griffith, *A Journey*, 1:119.

dangers to Europeans not simply from the plague, but also from malaria, ophthalmia, and dysentery. But the anxiety that the East might somehow desta- bilize a European, constitution also centered on the fear of a suspension of rationality in favor of hallucination and fantasy. For such a besieged European, the East could appear to be contagious; it threatened those who came into contact with it with an infectious agent that could attack both body and mind.

"A man coming freshly from Europe," wrote Alexander Kinglake, "is at first proof[ed] against the nonsense with which he is assailed, but often it happens that after a little while the social atmosphere of Asia will begin to infect him . . . he will yield himself at last to the faith of those around him."[68] To Kinglake, this kind of effect was half the appeal of Eastern travel. In a more negative sense, however, the same language was used in medical texts. "The inhabitants of ague countries," suggested Joseph Adam, in an 1809 work of epidemiology, "may be in a certain degree familiarized to the air, even in bad seasons; but to those who arrive fresh, the effect will be sudden, as the cause is new and more powerful."[69] In a literal sense, then, novelty itself was conceptually linked to contagion. Experiencing the exotic could destabilize the constitution. Just so, Florence Nightingale, upon visiting a mosque and being caught up in the prayers of the Egyptians surrounding her, "began to be uncertain whether I *was* a Christian woman."[70] Quarantine not only set the boundaries of a world in which to travel was to flirt with violent sickness and death but it also imposed a logic in which to communicate too closely or to experience too deeply was to risk contamination.

An "Anti-Social Malady"

Between 1800 and its final major plague outbreak (before the third pandemic) in 1841, Constantinople experienced plague epidemics in twenty-six different years. Egypt, which experienced its final plague epidemic in 1844, had featured twenty-eight "plague years" since 1800.[71] In many areas, then, Ottoman sub- jects faced plague with terrifying regularity. Though Western Europeans often assumed the universal attitude toward the plague among Muslims to be "fatal- istic" acceptance, it is clear that among all segments of the Ottoman populace there existed a diversity of practice. Western attitudes to the plague also varied. Given that many Western European travelers to the Ottoman Empire visited both Constantinople and Egypt (and that almost all traveled in one place or the other), plague epidemics appear regularly in travel narratives and induced a similar range of reactions. Europeans called it their own "Frankish" custom

---

[68] Kinglake, *Eothen*, 102.   [69] Adam, *An Inquiry*, 48.
[70] Quoted in Michael Calabria, *Florence Nightingale in Italy and Greece: Her Diary and "Visions"* (Albany: SUNY Press, 1996), 26.
[71] These statistics are derived from Panzac, *Peste*, 198 and 626.

to observe a draconian self-imposed quarantine during plague epidemics –
a custom sufficiently well known to be a reference point for governments and
medical writers back in Europe. Again, however, this custom may have been
observed by the "Frankish" quarter, but it was also observed by numerous rich
Muslims. To the extent that Europeans saw locals continuing to go out in public
during plague epidemics, we have no evidence that this showed fatalistic
nonconcern rather than the simple economic impossibility of total retirement
for a period of months.

Touch, as I have shown, became highly problematic during an epidemic.
This made extreme vigilance necessary during even mundane daily tasks. As
Thomas Watkins saw it, simply passing through a crowded part of a city could
be a life-threatening activity:

It is not, as some thing, caught from the *exhalation* of pestiferous bodies, but by *contact*:
therefore you may suppose I am particularly careful among the crowds of
Constantinople. I am even suspicious of every body, since I have heard that a menial
servant of the ambassador was on Friday last taken sick of it to the hospital.[72]

Drop your guard for an instant, many advised, and you could get the plague.
Alexander Kinglake mocked the tendency of Europeans during plague epidemics to "carefully avoid the touch of every human being whom they pass."[73]
Francis Hervé suffered frequent rebuffs in the street when he tried to shake
hands with acquaintances, causing him to write "it certainly is a most anti-
social malady."[74] Older accounts, like the American traveler John Antes's
description of his travels to Egypt during the plagues of the late 1770s, contain
more dramatic encounters. While Hervé tried to avoid shaking hands, Antes
apparently dodged corpses on Cairo's streets: "I have even myself been walking in the street, where people dropped down dead, before I locked myself up in
the house, and I only took good care not to touch any body."[75] The eighteenth-
century spelling of "anybody" has eerie resonance in a scenario where Antes
was literally dodging people who "dropped down dead" in the street.

The practice of self-imposed seclusion during an epidemic was known as
"shutting up." This involved observing a rigid and almost total quarantine by
remaining in a house during the entire period of a major epidemic, receiving no
visitors, and admitting supplies only via a basket and pulley or through small
slots in the door. Shut-up merchants, in Aleppo at least, typically received

---

[72] Watkins, *Travels through Switzerland*, 237.   [73] Kinglake, *Eothen*, 30.
[74] Hervé, *A Residence*, 2:181.
[75] John Antes, *Observations on the Manners and Customs of the Egyptians, the Overflowing of the
Nile and Its Effects; with Remarks on the Plague and Other Subjects* (London: John Stockdale,
1800), 35–36. F. C. Pouqueville, however, argues that the frequent stories of spontaneous death
by plague were fabricated. "It is not true that the plague comes on with such rapidity, as that
people fall dead in the streets, struck with it as by a stroke of thunder." Plague corpses in the
streets, he insists, were the bodies of the homeless. See Pouqueville, *Travels in the Morea*, 191.

letters with a pair of iron tongs and fumigated them with vinegar and sulfuric smoke before opening.[76] Antes describes the custom adopted by European merchants in Egypt of dousing all goods received, including foods, with water or vinegar before use.[77] Patrick Russell noted that "shutting up" was already a long-standing practice in the 1750s, and suggested that it was invented in the fifteenth century by Venetian traders who took their cue from early quarantine efforts.[78] His half-brother Alexander, who had preceded him as a Levant Company doctor in Aleppo between 1748 and 1760, noted a whole range of social rituals surrounding the "shutting up" process. He relates that most merchants divided themselves into small groups, chose the individual with the largest house, and shut themselves up together therein. Given that even this attempt to ward off boredom became irksome after a while, Alexander Russell notes that some people called on other parties via roof terraces. But others warned against this laxity: "yet, when the plague rages much, it is reckoned safest not to trust to any one, lest they should be guilty of irregularities."[79]

This absolutist approach to prophylaxis often left more recent "Frankish" arrivals disoriented. The medical traveler R. R. Madden lamented that his arrival in Alexandria coincided with the beginning of a plague outbreak and thus "every Frank was in quarantine, the hotel was declared infected, and a lodging was nowhere to be found." Forced to return to his ship, Madden was eventually given hospitality from an English merchant who "had the kindness to break through his quarantine, and received me into his house." In the midst of an epidemic, Madden noted that the conversation often centered upon folk wisdom about avoiding disease:

The laws of infection were handled by young ladies in the drawing-room: "a cat could communicate the plague, but a dog was less dangerous; an ass was a pestiferous animal, but a horse was non-contagious ..." If you complained of a headach [sic], there was a general flight; if you went abroad with a sallow cheek, the people fled in all directions ... and if you talked of McLean, your intellect was suspected to be impaired. Heaven preserve you from a quarantine in Egypt! It is not the death of one's neighbours which is so overcoming ... but it is the horror of eternally hearing of plague; it is the terror of contagion, which is depicted in every face; it is the presentation of pestilential apparitions and discourses to the eye and to the ear, morning, noon, and night.[80]

Despite his disdain for what he saw as paranoia, Madden appeared to echo the local dread of the plague hospital (ubiquitous among Muslims and Christians alike). Noting the case of a Dr. Giordano who died of the plague in disgusting circumstances, abandoned by his friends, Madden rhetorically asked his reader,

---

[76] Alexander Russell, *The Natural History of Aleppo, and Parts Adjacent* (London: A. Millar, 1756), 256–57.
[77] See Antes, *Observations*, 34–35.   [78] Russell, *Treatise of the Plague*, 316.
[79] Russell, *Natural History of Aleppo*, 254.   [80] Madden, *Travels*, 251–53.

"Do you imagine that a medical man can visit a case of plague in Alexandria, without having the offensive corpse of poor Giordano before his eyes[?]"[81] In this way, even among those who affected nonchalance (especially in travel narratives written once back home), it is difficult to imagine that anyone in the midst of an epidemic truly felt secure.

Self-quarantines severely disrupted the social and economic life of major Middle Eastern cities. Russell suggested that Ottoman merchants so feared the loss of European business during plague epidemics that they would try to conceal reports of disease to forestall the complete withdrawal of a rich clientele.[82] "Shutting up" thus had an impact on businesses run by locals as well as "Franks." The period of detention considered necessary could be much longer than quarantine on a journey to Western Europe. For a hypothetical trader who traveled back and forth between Europe and the Levant, between time "shut up" in an Ottoman city and time in a lazaretto, one might pass six months in a year in quarantine.

The strict adherence to this custom among Levant Company traders and other merchants stationed permanently in the East was well known. The 1805 Board of Health quoted the Russells extensively on how "shutting up" functioned and praised the system as responsible for preserving the "Frankish" communities of Aleppo and Constantinople from the plague.[83] And yet, "irregularities" did occur. John Antes relates a story of a man, having shut himself up in a house at Alexandria, who arranged to break his self-quarantine in order to receive a shave. This he did by sticking only his head out of a small door and allowing a barber to trim his face. "However," warns Antes, "he paid dear for his folly, and died a few days after."[84]

If shutting up was the norm throughout the eighteenth century and into the nineteenth, its strictures appear to have broken down during the 1820s and 1830s – at least during relatively mild epidemics. During the 1830s, Kinglake and Hervé certainly ventured outside while the plague raged. Still, Hervé was subjected to onerous prophylactic procedures deemed necessary by his fellow guests at a European-run boarding house:

At one period [the plague] was very virulent at Pera, to my extreme annoyance, as I was compelled, every time I returned home, to undergo the operation of perfuming, or rather fumigating. For this purpose you enter a sort of sentry-box, where you stand on an iron grating under which herbs are burnt; and there you remain, putting your head out of a hole, as if in the pillory, till it is considered that you are sufficiently purified.[85]

Despite his professed nonchalance, Hervé considered information about plague behavior to be "a topic of vital importance to those who may chance to visit the

---

[81] Ibid., 274.   [82] Russell, *Natural History of Aleppo*, 253.
[83] *First Report of the Board of Health*, 3.   [84] Antes, *Observations*, 35.
[85] Hervé, *A Residence*, 2:178.

East."[86] Hervé noted a divergence of opinion between Western doctors (who, he says, increasingly adhered to anticontagionism) and the bulk of Western European expatriates who continued to view contact with potentially infected people and goods as anathema. Certainly in the 1830s, then, "shutting up," was not the result of compulsion by medical authorities, and yet from custom and from fear, it remained common practice.

In the absence of direction from doctors, the "Franks" appear to have relied on other sources for knowledge about the plague. Hervé mentions a Jewish man who had caught, and then recovered from, the plague, and who was thus considered "one of the best judges in doubtful cases."[87] He paints a picture of expanding awareness among the Muslim community that the plague was something to be actively avoided. Should the Ottoman government get wind of a plague victim, Hervé wrote, the unfortunate sufferer could be hauled off to the pest house – a fate essentially tantamount to death.[88] Though this may have prompted some to conceal the disease, Captain Frankland, who traveled in Anatolia and Syria in the late 1820s, noted that individuals from "infected areas" were marked out by yellow sticks (indicating they "were either infected themselves or were of infected houses").[89] The practices of separation and demarcation, when it came to responding to the plague, were clearly adopted by Ottomans and Western Europeans alike. From the color of yellow being used to signify isolation, to the reliance on isolation hospitals during epidemics, to the eventual institution of maritime quarantine rules in 1839, Ottoman and Western European practices regarding the plague clearly resembled each other during the first half of the nineteenth century.

Europeans in the Middle East liked to tell themselves that proper procedures made their communities immune. This was transparently not the case – though, obviously, all the travel narratives that survive were written by individuals who lived long enough to return home and publish. During the devastating 1835 plague at Cairo some 515 "Franks" perished.[90] In the midst of an 1825 plague outbreak at Alexandria, the Tuscan consul Cavaco informed the Livorno *Consiglio di Sanità* that the excellent segregation procedures undertaken by the captains of Tuscan and Austrian ships waiting in the harbor had preserved those fleets from the disease. But, he notes, "among the fleets of other [European] nations, more than one boat has suffered the lethal consequences of failing to maintain the same level of attention."[91] Given the numerous rituals

---

[86] Ibid., 189.   [87] Ibid., 184.
[88] Ibid., 182–83. The Greek Hospital in Istanbul, which received numerous plague victims, certainly had a reputation for abysmal care, and most treated the first sign of plague as a sign that one way or another, death would soon follow. See Charles Maclean to Lord Grenville, February 14, 1816, BL Add. Ms. 59265, f. 94. See also Thornton, *Present State of Turkey*, 2:212.
[89] Frankland, *Travels to and from Constantinople*, 102.
[90] Bowring, *Speech Delivered to Parliament*, 8.
[91] Cavaco to Governor Venturi of Livorno, June 21, 1825, ASLi Sanità 240.

and procedures that marked out a strict "level of attention" to the plague, it was always possible to find fault with an unlucky individual's (or community's) sanitary habits as a means of explaining the fact that they caught the plague.

Perhaps it comforted Europeans residing in the Middle East to assume that even in a city stricken by the plague, practices they assumed to be exclusive would preserve them. Sometimes, the death from plague of a single European was the subject of community-wide concern. In 1827, for example, two British travelers (Fox Strangeways and Henry Anson) claimed they had been assaulted and enslaved by an Ottoman official in Aleppo. Mathieu de Lesseps, the French consul there, gave shelter to the two travelers as they attempted to recover from their injuries.[92] It soon became clear that Anson was in fact suffering from the plague and subsequently died from it, after which Strangeways and the entire de Lesseps family performed a lengthy decontamination process with chlorine.[93] De Lesseps and a British diplomat memorialized the then Foreign Secretary and Prime Minister, George Canning, writing, "We think it proper to represent to you as Consul-General of France and representative of the English nation in this city, a breach on which the security of all Franks equally depends."[94]

The death from the plague of a young English nobleman (Anson was a younger son of a viscount) seemed to result in the European community in a major Middle Eastern city drawing ranks. And yet, as an obituary noted in passing, the doctor employed by de Lesseps to treat Anson was "a Turkish physician, celebrated for his practice in the treatment of that terrible malady."[95] Despite its rhetoric of sanitary separation and disengagement, then, the "Frankish" community evidently shared medical practitioners with wealthy Turks. Not only, in fact, did Europeans patronize Turkish doctors, as with the Anson/Strangeways incident, but Muslim Turks and Arabs also consulted Western European doctors. Mrs. Damer praised one "Dr. McG–" (who attended her husband) by noting that he had "a hugely expansive practice" and "has been enabled to attain a knowledge of Turkish manners and customs, such as, I should think, no other European possesses; for which, indeed, he has great advantages, as he has constantly attended the principal harems, and was physician to the late and present sultans."[96] This "Dr. McG–" is presumably

---

[92] Mathieu de Lesseps, a longtime French diplomat, was the father of Ferdinand de Lesseps, the developer of the Suez Canal.

[93] The *Gentleman's Magazine* translated a record of the incident in the *Journal des Débats*, which noted that "M. Strangeways . . . is indebted solely for the extraordinary good fortune of escaping contagion which he had so closely braved, to the sanatory [*sic*] precautions which M. de Lesseps employed, and the application of which he himself directed, but more particularly to the frequent use of chlorures by M. de Lesseps." "Obituary," *Gentleman's Magazine* 97, no. 1 (1827): 648.

[94] "Memorial," TNA FO 352/17A, folder 2 (ff. 129–30).   [95] "Obituary," 648.

[96] Damer, *Diary of a Tour*, 212. Dr. McGuffog was certainly well known by diplomats for the useful connections his practice allowed him to form with Turkish elites. See Jones, *British Diplomatic Service*, 87.

Dr. McGuffog, the chief physician at the British Embassy in the 1830s and 1840s. That such a practitioner would have had patients among the Ottoman elite points to the fact that in major cities in the Middle East, a diverse medical clientele patronized doctors of all stripes. R. R. Madden's *Travels* clearly demonstrate that his patients (and those of other European doctors) were by no means restricted to "Franks."[97] Pouqueville insisted that "the principal physicians of the Turkish empire are a number of crafty Italians," though he also encountered Greek, Jewish, Armenian, and Turkish doctors.[98] Medical professionals and clienteles, as far as we can tell, were surprisingly heterogeneous.[99] In some ways, plague kept communities apart. But in other ways, it brought them together as Britons, French, Austrians, Greeks, Jews, Circassians, Armenians, Turks, and Arabs circulated the same rumors, told the same medical anecdotes, and even relied on the same physicians. Plague and plague prevention cut across social, racial, and confessional boundaries.

If national distinctions did not, despite the opinions of travelers, dictate responses to the plague, the conception among Western Europeans that they constituted a "Frankish" community with unusually strict plague-fighting tendencies was noted and subtly mocked by local Ottoman subjects. Alexander Kinglake appears to be writing a paean to Turkish beauty when he reveals that the object of his affection is deriving amusement by mocking his fear of the plague:

You smile at pretty women – you turn pale before the beauty that is great enough to have dominion over you. She sees, and exults in your giddiness ... presently, with a sudden movement, she lays her blushing fingers upon your arm, and cries out "Yumourdjak!" (Plague! meaning "there is a present of the Plague for you!") This is her notion of a witticism: it is a very old piece of fun no doubt.[100]

It does not require one to read too strongly against the grain to understand that the woman's joke was not simply motivated by a desire to derive amusement from frightening Kinglake, but also carried the intention of implicitly criticizing the self-conscious isolation imposed by the Europeans on themselves. This "joke," perhaps, reveals a real resentment that European travelers so strenuously emphasized the need to purge themselves after physical contact with locals. Seen here, in miniature, the condescending cultural logic behind the quarantine system becomes readily apparent.

---

[97] See Madden, *Travels*, 260–62.   [98] Pouqueville, *Travels in the Morea*, 194.

[99] For more on the cosmopolitan nature of Ottoman medical practice, see Miri Shefer-Mossensohn, *Ottoman Medicine, 1500–1700* (Albany: SUNY Press, 2009), 193–96. Shefer-Mossensohn suggests that even in the Early Modern period it seems likely that non-Muslims outnumbered Muslims in the medical profession, indicating that when this phenomenon appears in nineteenth-century travel accounts, it is not necessarily related to any increasing Western influence on Ottoman politics.

[100] Kinglake, *Eothen*, 33.

7   A Prescription for England's Condition

At the height of the Reform crisis, during the "Days of May" in 1832, mobs in London threatened a run on the Bank of England in response to the king and Lords' continued blocking of a bill to expand voting rights. Britain's constitution was passing through its most traumatic upheaval in the modern period, and revolution seemed closer than ever. The "Iron" Duke of Wellington threatened what many saw as an antidemocratic coup; the Whig government, meanwhile, whose status was in question, appeared to be in an intractable power struggle with the House of Lords. It was a crisis that had been building for months, as the Reform Bill had ricocheted around the Palace of Westminster (shortly itself to go up in flames).

According to many doctors, it was not only Britain's political constitution that held the nation in thrall in the spring of 1832 but also an "epidemic constitution," poisoning the very air that Britons breathed. In a coincidence acknowledged by medical historians, yet often overlooked in political histories, the reform crisis and the first British cholera epidemic overlapped almost completely. And that epidemic saw the resurfacing of one of the strangest legacies from the work of the seventeenth-century doctor Thomas Sydenham – the idea that in the midst of an epidemic, an invisible poison in the air could transform the ordinary British atmosphere into a malignant, foreign cloud.[1]

In Sydenham's work, plague, rather than cholera, was the origin of what he called an "epidemic constitution." And yet throughout the nineteenth century, this seemingly bizarre idea applied to a whole range of maladies. "The prevailing disease swallows up all other disorders," explained a writer in New York's *Medical Repository* in 1821. "During the prevalence of an epidemic plague, typhus, dysentery, and other diseases of this class, every indisposition of a febrile sort readily assumes the character of the prevailing disorder." In such a time, "a specific virus" in the atmosphere "assimilates

---

[1] On the importance and longevity of perceptions of cholera as a "cloud," see Projit Bihari Mukharji, "The 'Cholera Cloud' in the Nineteenth-Century 'British World': History of an Object-without-an-Essence," *Bulletin of the History of Medicine* 86, no. 3 (2012): 303–32.

the impurities of the air into a poison like itself."[2] Even healthy individuals could not escape this influence. During a plague epidemic, suggested an article in the *Edinburgh Medical and Surgical Journal*, individuals "who escape a positive and marked attack of the epidemic" nevertheless felt phantom "pains in the groins and arm-pits, as if they were to be attacked by buboes."[3]

Epidemic disease touched everyone; it took precedence over the customary epidemiological state of a nation. In applying this idea to cholera, the doctor G. W. Lefevre (describing the course of the disease in St. Petersburg, Russia) showed just how thoroughly cholera could transform the customary medical landscape. "It was observed of this malady," he wrote in 1831, "as Sydenham observed of the plague, that there was during its prevalence what he styled a *Constitutio Epidemica*; or that all kinds, or the greater part at least, of the reigning distempers were converted into this prevailing epidemic." Should the cholera hit Britain, he warned, "imprudence and excesses of the table" which might, in the normal course of things, lead to "an ordinary bowel affection, would in the present case generate a Cholera Morbus."[4]

The bubonic plague exerted its own, more amorphous, epidemic atmosphere over the medical imaginary of early nineteenth-century Britain. Though historians often associate the plague with early modernity, in the nineteenth century, it became a vehicle through which concerns about national health were refracted and amplified. As a memory, as a metaphor, and as a piece of news, plague haunted the dreams of nineteenth-century medical administrators, just as it preoccupied the travelers to the Middle East whose works were discussed in the last chapter. That chapter discussed the many ways in which the barrier of quarantine generated a means of "reading" Ottoman progress, stasis, and exoticism through the lens of the plague. Here, I demonstrate that plague

[2] This appears to be taken from a "Dr. Hosack" and is expanded by the *Medical Repository* author in a footnote, where he notes that the influence of the "epidemic constitution" was so great in the time of plague that the exhalations from dead bodies and the breath of the infected were, alone, enough to infect the whole country. Anon., "Review of Gilbert Blane's *Elements of Logic*," *Medical Repository* 6 (1821): 335–36. The medical writer Joseph Adam invoked the same idea, calling the principle "a well-known law." He further argues that epidemic diseases assimilate other diseases "in proportion to the force of their invasion." See Joseph Adam, *An Inquiry into the Laws of Different Epidemic Diseases* (London: W. Thorne, 1809), 15. For other discussions of this "law," see Robert Venables, "On the Diarrhoeas of the Present Period," *Lancet* 2 (1836–37): 896 (about cholera) and Robert Gooch, "Plague: A Contagious Disease" *Quarterly Review* 33 (1825): 236 (about the plague). It was also applied to yellow fever. See, for example, David Luke Finlay, *Observations on the Remittent (So-Called) and Yellow Fevers of the West Indies* (Dublin: Fannin and Co., 1853), 11.
[3] Anon., "Mediterranean Quarantine Regulations – Plague, Its Origin and Propagation," *Edinburgh Medical and Social Journal* 68 (1847): 206.
[4] George William Lefevre, *Observations on the Nature and Treatment of the Cholera Morbus, Now Prevailing Epidemically in St. Petersburg* (London: Longman, Rees, Orme, Browne, and Green, 1831), 25–26.

formed an equally potent lens for reading the (sanitary) state of the British nation itself.

It is not a coincidence that a major history of the cholera epidemic of 1831 is entitled *The Return of the Plague.*[5] For a government not inclined to act (until the 1840s) against scourges like typhus, typhoid, and influenza, the quarantine laws unequivocally showed that state action against plague was essential. As a referent, plague gave meaning to other major epidemic invader diseases (cholera and yellow fever). As the axiomatic procedure necessitated by a threat of plague, quarantine became the implicit response for epidemic disease more generally. Here, I argue that the fears and precedents set by Mediterranean plagues and the debates surrounding quarantine drove the genesis of public health reform in Britain in a manner that has heretofore been neglected.

Two different conceptions of epidemic disease undergirded the history of public health in nineteenth-century Britain. In the first, epidemics were the exception. In this way of thinking, the plague was utterly distinct – its presence justified extraordinary actions and exotic imaginative associations beyond what was common for other forms of sickness. This line of thinking allowed industrializing Britain to appear, in some ways, as a healthy nation, even as its citizens suffered from typhus, typhoid fever, scarlet fever, smallpox, influenza, poor diets, inadequate sewers, and bad air. From the perspective of nineteenth-century Britons comparing their country with the world outside, these challenges did not detract from the fact that its sanitary state was comparatively good (by European standards), and far superior to the ostensibly plague-riddled world of the Middle East, the supposedly fever-stricken jungles of South America and the "impenetrable" African interior, or the (often sweltering and cholera-stricken) imperial world of South Asia.

But epidemic disease was not *only* a separate category. A second register of thinking cast it merely as the extreme edge of a broad spectrum of ill health. Many public health campaigners felt an obligation to harness the associations and obligations of the plague and apply them to many other ailments afflicting industrializing Britain. Hence Thomas Southwood Smith's insistence that "the plague exists constantly in London," a statement that was only true if one accepted Smith's consistent (if idiosyncratic) assertion that typhus fever was simply an English version of bubonic plague.[6] By affiliating the fight against dirty water, bad air, and common diseases with a much more dramatic sounding fight against the plague, campaigners sought to add urgency to a task that was

---

[5] Michael Durey, *The Return of the Plague: British Society and the Cholera: 1831–2* (Dublin: Gill and Macmillan, 1979).

[6] Thomas Southwood Smith, "Plague – Typhus Fever – Quarantine," *Westminster Review* 3 (1825): 514.

portrayed all too often (according to no less an authority than Benjamin Disraeli) as "a policy of sewage."[7]

Campaigners mobilized these two distinct understandings of epidemic disease to strengthen their arguments and often mingled them together. On the one hand, it was essential to retain the urgency and "otherness" associated with epidemic diseases if one sought to use their reputation to change the level of tolerance toward of "normal" pathologies. On the other hand, the optimistic, progressive aspects of anticontagionism encouraged doctors to try to puncture the sense of mystery and distinctiveness surrounding epidemics. Charles Maclean, we have already seen, claimed to have vanquished the plague as well as contagionism, and that formulation was not uncommon among his medical fellow travelers.

Both visions of epidemic disease filtered into public consciousness. Both shaped approaches to ill health at the level of the individual as well as the state. This chapter investigates the broad intersection of epidemic medicine and public health reform. It suggests a narrative through which plague and Mediterranean quarantine lie at the center of new understandings of the state's responsibility for public health. The threatening world outside the *cordon sanitaire* was not the only zone to be given shape and meaning by the quarantine system. Indeed, the boundaries between health and disease *inside* nineteenth-century Britain must be understood with reference to sanitary boundaries operating far beyond British shores. Cholera and the reform crisis of 1832 together initiated almost two decades of epidemics, famines, and industrial strife that provoked significant inquiries by writers and politicians about the structure of the early Victorian state: a phenomenon generally characterized as the "Condition of England Question." As policy makers, doctors, reformers, and radicals sought prescriptions for England's condition, they conceived Britain as a social body in which the health of individual bodies shaped the health of the nation. The intervention here is to observe how thoroughly quarantine set the precedents for such a conception; the route to British public health reform ran through the Mediterranean.

In this chapter, then, I first consider the complex lineage of medical thought about the plague and explore how that disease's simultaneously horrifying and indistinct boundaries allowed it to represent a whole range of other diseases and social problems. Second, I investigate the debate concerning the transmission of epidemic diseases that roiled the medical establishment in nineteenth-century Europe. Both contagionists and anticontagionists, I argue, were predominantly inspired by Mediterranean quarantine. Their arguments implicitly

---

[7] Benjamin Disraeli, "Crystal Palace Speech," June 24, 1872. Quoted in Alexander Charles Ewald, *The Right Hon. Benjamin Disraeli, Earl of Beaconsfield, K.G., and His Times* (London: William Mackenzie, 1897), 2:239.

pushed the government to accept a greater responsibility for public health regulation. In this way, both of the first two sections show how imagining the plague and debating the theory behind quarantine laid the groundwork for sanitary reform. The final two sections apply this argument to the events of the 1830s and 1840s, first by delineating the ways in which cholera was consumed as plague and, in the final section, by analyzing how successful agitation for the Public Health Act of 1848 depended on an understanding of domestic health and foreign contamination suggested by the history of quarantine. In adopting a more global framework for understanding the vicissitudes of sanitary reform within early Victorian politics, it is not necessary to abandon London's mud – one must simply acknowledge how inquiries into the smoke, smells, and sewers of Edwin Chadwick's Britain were informed by eruptions of plague in the Middle East just as surely as they were by the stink of the Thames.

Imagining the Plague

Charles Knight's 1854 *English Cyclopaedia* defined *pestilence* as a "general term applied to those diseases of an epidemic character, which affect large masses of the population, and are remarkable for their destruction of human life." The word, the *Cyclopaedia* notes, was "most frequently associated" with "plague and Asiatic cholera."[8] Already in this framing, we come to understand the ambiguities inherent in nineteenth-century medical terminology. Influenza, typhus, and typhoid could frequently become epidemic, affect "large masses of the population," and kill many thousands. Yet were they pestilence? Yes, according to Chadwick, Britain's most famous sanitarian revolutionary, who sought to render all forms of ill health pestilential. But Charles Knight's definition was published the year of Chadwick's fall from his perch atop the General Board of Health, and it shows us a definition still rooted in "exotic" epidemic diseases like cholera and plague. Before the 1831–32 cholera epidemic, that understanding left plague as the preeminent referent to pestilence. But if pestilence was plague, what did the plague mean in a society that had not experienced the disease for more than a century?

That is a difficult question to answer. To nineteenth-century Britons, plague was at once exotic and familiar, a foreign threat and a domestic memory. We have already explored the way in which its presence or absence in the Ottoman Empire seemed to many to be a tangible marker of civilizational progress there. For those who never ventured abroad, its foreign home combined with its fabled history gave it a terrifying reputation. Furthermore, the vagueness of plague as a disease, the variety of symptoms it supposedly produced, the fierce

---

[8] Charles Knight, ed., *The English Cyclopaedia* (London: Charles Knight, 1854), 4:433.

debate about how it spread, and the knowledge of its high mortality rates all granted it metaphorical power.

To be sure, the metaphor of plague is an old one. In the early modern period, plague was also seen as the archetypical "dread disease" and was associated with disorder, societal breakdown, and problematic people.[9] Over the second half of the seventeenth century, most Western European nations experienced their final plague epidemics. By the early eighteenth century, it would have appeared that rigorous quarantine could achieve success but that accidents were still possible. There was no sense that plague was an inherently foreign or exotic disease, as would exist in nineteenth-century medical writing.[10] Moral and civilizational explanations, which would become common a century later, were not yet stressed in an age long before "Ottoman decline" existed as an idea in the British consciousness. To the contrary, Lady Mary Wortley Montague's *Turkish Embassy Letters* (written 1716–18, but published in 1763) depict an Ottoman state that seemed particularly advanced in matters of health – the home of the new technique of inoculation and a group of apparently progressive medical practitioners.[11]

The 1744 plague epidemic in Sicily was the last major outbreak of the disease in Western Europe, and the ensuing sense that the disease happened "somewhere else" altered popular terminology. As Daniel Panzac puts it, after 1750, "the universal plague became the plague of the Levant." From this time on, "Oriental Plague," "Asiatic plague," or in French, "*la peste d'Orient*" were increasingly used instead of simply "plague" or "*peste*" in medical treatises.[12] In fact, the geographic fixity of the disease became one of the few facts about it that seemed certain. Numerous authors attempted to divine the central source of the plague, with Central Anatolia and Upper Egypt considered the most likely candidates. In turn, this increasing tendency to identify the East with the plague

---

[9] See Colin Jones, "Plague and Its Metaphors in Early Modern France," *Representations* 53 (1996): 97–127. Also see Foucault, *Discipline and Punish*, 198–99, and Takeda, *Between Crown and Commerce*, 106–9.

[10] Indeed, as Kevin Siena shows, a long-standing idea that the poor and other social outcasts retained pestilential matter within them persisted into the late eighteenth century. See Siena, *Rotten Bodies: Class and Contagion in 18th-Century Britain* (New Haven, CT: Yale University Press, 2019).

[11] See Lady Mary Wortley Montague, *The Turkish Embassy Letters*, ed. Malcolm Jack (London: Virago, 1994).

[12] Panzac, *Quarantaines et Lazarets*, 93. Junko Takeda suggests this change dates to the early eighteenth century (*Between Crown and Commerce*, 106), though it is unusual to find references to "Oriental Plague" or "Plague of the Levant" before at least the 1770s. Nükhet Varlık gives a valuable reminder to medical historians that the term has shaped the history of medicine as well as the consciousness of historical actors. Given the historical contingency of plague transmission patterns (which changed, as we see in Chapter 9, even in the short period of time covered by this book), we must avoid accepting at face value the idea that the Ottoman Empire was the primary reservoir of plague. See Varlık, "Epidemiological Orientalism," 57–91.

affected notions of the disease itself, heightening its fearsome reputation with the exoticism we explored in the previous chapter.

John Antes, who spent time in Egypt in the late eighteenth century and witnessed serious epidemics of plague in Cairo, found that the easiest way to define the plague was simply to stress its peerless capacity for destruction. "The plague is without contradiction," he wrote, "the most terrible of all disorders the human species is subject to."[13] Alexander Russell, an influential Levant Company doctor who served for many years in the mid-eighteenth century as physician at the Levant Company "factory"[14] of Aleppo, devoted substantial space in his *Natural History of Aleppo* (1756) to describing the horrors of various plagues he witnessed. Russell's work remained a standard and influential piece of plague scholarship well into the nineteenth century. In his use of superlatives to describe plague's awesome power, Russell concurred with Antes: "It is no wonder that the very name of plague among us should strike terror whenever it is mentioned ... the distemper itself is the most lamentable to which mankind are liable."[15]

Russell suggests that, on a collective level, plague's potential to provoke demographic catastrophe rendered it a dread disease, and writers with many different backgrounds concurred that it represented the ultimate form of ill health. The French medical traveler F. C. Pouqueville noted that "the very name alone of the plague presents immediately to the mind the most dreadful of all afflictions with which a country can be visited."[16] Parisian ministers frequently referred to plague by the ominous, generic term "*Fléau-Déstructeur.*"[17] Thomas Hancock calls it "the destroyer."[18] Andrew White, Superintendent of Quarantine of Corfu, terms plague "the snake" and "the dreadful enemy."[19] Plague's etiology may have been a subject of medical contention; about plague's devastating nature and implacably destructive potential, there was no argument.

Gavin Milroy deemed plague, of all epidemic diseases, "the most dreaded because the least known."[20] Yet, in part because of new French and British imperial commitments after 1815 (in the Mediterranean, North Africa, and India) an increasingly wide range of Western Europeans encountered the

---

[13] Antes, *Observations*, 33.

[14] Because Levant Company traders were referred to as "factors," the large building that housed their commercial offices was typically called a "factory."

[15] Russell, *Natural History of Aleppo*, 228–29.   [16] Pouqueville, *Travels in the Morea*, 188.

[17] The term is used throughout ministerial correspondence on quarantine matters in AN (Paris) AE/B/III/210.

[18] Thomas Hancock, *Researches into the Laws and Phenomena of Pestilence* (London: William Phillips, 1821), 11.

[19] White, *Treatise on the Plague*, 16.

[20] Gavin Milroy, *The International Quarantine Conference of Paris in 1851–2: with Remarks* (London: Savile and Edwards, 1859), 4.

disease: soldiers, colonial bureaucrats, East India Company officials, Levant Company doctors, and individual travelers. Additionally, the British consular apparatus in the Ottoman Empire expanded significantly over the course of the nineteenth century, increasing the extent to which discussions of its plague epidemics were directed back to interlocutors in London.[21] Thus encountered and discussed, plague nevertheless remained difficult to define and describe. There was widespread agreement that in most (though not all) cases of bubonic plague, buboes – large, inflamed lymph nodes – would appear, particularly around the groin. Extreme tiredness and fever were also commonly cited, and death often occurred within a matter of hours. But though it is clear that partisans on all sides of medical argument conceived of a distinct disease called plague, all details appeared to have exceptions. Alexander Russell lamented that:

[Just] as there is no disease incident to mankind that is in its nature more terrible and destructive, so there is none more difficult to describe. Its symptoms are scarcely in all respects alike in any two persons; nay, they even vary extremely in an hour in the same subject. The disease begins often with the most flattering [i.e., misleadingly positive] appearances, and ends fatally in a few hours.[22]

In a similar vein, the traveler William Eton, who became the first British Superintendent of Quarantine at Malta (in 1801), lamented that "the physicians at Constantinople say, the more they study the plague the less they know of it."[23] Pouqueville, the French doctor, called the disease "proteus-like" and noted the difficulty in obtaining an initial diagnosis.[24] This, he suggested, enabled epidemics to spread more quickly. Everyone agreed on plague's suddenness as a universal characteristic, and though they highlighted different symptoms, they concurred that, once infected, an individual might exhibit all manner of signs. This changeability exacerbated the dread of the disease for Russell; in the midst of the transformations he describes, a plague sufferer's face moves quickly from "florid" to a "livid colour, resembling that of a person almost strangled." This was replaced by a "cadaverous paleness" and a "ghastly countenance."[25] The chameleon-like quality of plague endowed it with a lingering sense that there was something unknowable at its heart (Figure 7.1).

[21] On the expansion of Britain's consular system in the Levant, see D. C. M. Platt, *The Cinderella Service: British Consuls since 1825* (New York: Longman, 1971), chapter 4. See also Raymond Jones, *The British Diplomatic Service: 1815–1914* (Gerrards Cross, UK: Colin Smythe, 1983), 87, and Allan Cunningham, "The Dragomans of the British Embassy at Constantinople," in *Eastern Questions in the Nineteenth Century*, ed. Edward Ingram (London: Frank Cass, 1993), 2:1–22.

[22] Alexander Russell, *Natural History of Aleppo*, 229.

[23] Eton, *Survey of the Turkish Empire*, 258.   [24] Pouqueville, *Travels in the Morea*, 193.

[25] Russell, *Natural History of Aleppo*, 230.

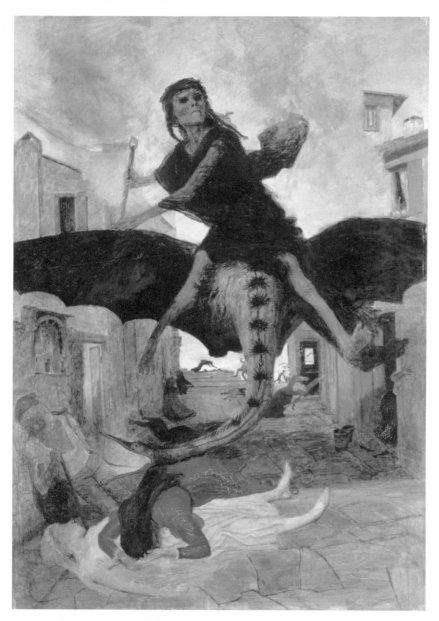

Figure 7.1 Arnold Böcklin, *Plague*, 1898. © Kunstmuseum Basel.
Photograph by Martin P. Bühler.

This combination of fearsome reputation and symptomatic uncertainty gave plague a generic quality that allowed it to stand in for a broad range of other contagions. In all major European languages, noted Patrick Russell, the word "contagion" could refer to "plague itself," while at other times it meant a whole class of diseases, or a substance that transmitted diseases.[26] Under the terms of the 1753 Quarantine Act in Britain, in addition to quarantines in normal operation in the Mediterranean, the king and the PC could declare quarantines against ships from any region of the world if they received intelligence of an epidemic "of the nature of the plague" (a formula repeated by subsequent legislation).[27] As vaguely as it was understood, then, plague set the pattern for epidemic response. More than a century and a half later, an American medical textbook suggested that "the plague is the very type of the infective diseases."[28]

In this way, just as Sydenham's *Costitutio Epidemica* endowed the plague with the capacity to assimilate other pathologies during the time of an epidemic, so the plague subsumed the conceptual understanding of other epidemic diseases. As yellow fever and cholera (the two major "new" epidemic diseases of nineteenth-century Europe) threatened European governments after 1800, they were often addressed with explicit reference to the plague. In Chapter 1, for example, we saw this when Britain's 1805 Board of Health suggested regulations against "the plague of the Levant" could stand in for any other distemper, and again with the Genoese bureaucrat who suggested in 1804 that there was "little difference" between yellow fever and the "true plague." Despite the different symptoms and geographies of these two major epidemic diseases, doctors invested in proving the contagiousness of one often felt it necessary to make claims about the other, so persuasive was the idea that there was one epidemic type defined by the plague.[29]

Nineteenth-century medical conceptions of the plague divested it of specific meaning, yet rendered it full of implication; it was malleable but definitive, archetypical but vague. "There is no disease that has been considered in such different, opposite, and contradictory ways as the plague has been," wrote the

---

[26] Patrick Russell, *A Treatise of the Plague* (London: G. G. J. and J. Robinson, 1791), 201. Patrick Russell was Alexander's brother and another respected medical authority on the plague. On the Middle Eastern careers of both Russells, see J. C. M. Starkey, "No Myopic Mirage: Alexander and Patrick Russell in Aleppo," *History and Anthropology* 13, no. 4 (2002): 257–73.

[27] For examples of such declarations (regarding, in this case, yellow fever epidemics on the East coast of the United States in the 1790s), see Wellcome Ms. 8396.

[28] Wilson, "Plague," 776.

[29] The French contagionist Dr. Bulard briefly disparaged the anticontagionist Nicolas Chervin's research on yellow fever, prompting Chervin to write a blistering treatise slamming Bulard's conclusions regarding the plague (this despite Chervin not having devoted significant research to plague outbreaks at all). See Nicolas Chervin, *Observations critiques sur les expériences proposées par M. Le Docteur Bulard, dans le but de connaître le mode de propagation de la Peste* (Paris: J. B. Baillière, 1838).

French anticontagionist Clot Bey in 1840.[30] "There is no term that has been applied to so many different conditions, that has been used as extensively by historians, *savants*, and poets in a figurative sense."[31] If metaphors of plague and contagion have struck scholars as a fertile field for cultural history,[32] the plague writers who witnessed epidemics were equally aware of their metaphorical potential. In the service of his long-held belief that vanquishing contagionism was part of a project of civilizational advancement, Clot Bey cast the plague itself as an avatar the past.

Despite the symbolic weight placed upon the question of epidemic contagion by Clot Bey and others, participants on both sides of the medical argument tended to cohere around similar suggestions for avoiding plague. Contagionists and anticontagionists alike (as well as those who held a middle position of "contingent contagionism") might emphasize living moderately, avoiding the close air of a sick room, and attempting to mitigate one's fear of disease.[33] Alexander Russell suggested that anyone in close contact with plague patients could maintain good health if they followed his advice "to avoid, as much as possible, all excesses, violent passions, or large evacuations, but not to live more abstemiously, either with regard to eating or drinking, than usual."[34] This idea was clearly based on a Hippocratic tradition, which stressed that moderation, calmness, and cheerfulness could be preventatives against the plague.[35] In this way, the intense divide over questions of etiology (which we will explore in detail in the next section) tends to dissolve when medical writers lay out techniques of prophylaxis. Contagionists would have stressed above all isolating oneself from those who were sick. Anticontagionists, meanwhile, typically emphasized purging corrupt air, warding off strong emotions, and refusing heavy food. For ordinary consumers, these ideas could easily be synthesized.

---

[30] Born Antoine Clot, the French doctor "Clot Bey" became a chief medical adviser to Mohammed Ali, founded a progressive Egyptian medical school, sought to reform medical practice in the Egyptian Army, and was a lifelong opponent of quarantine.

[31] Clot Bey, *De la Peste*, 1.

[32] See, among others, Jones, "Plague and Its Metaphors"; Laura Otis, *Membranes: Metaphors of Invasion in Nineteenth-Century Literature, Science, and Politics* (Baltimore, MD: Johns Hopkins University Press, 1999); Peta Mitchell, *Contagious Metaphor* (London: Bloomsbury, 2012).

[33] Pelling, *Cholera, Fever*, 22. Pelling suggests this "contingent contagionism" was a majority view throughout the 1820s, 1830s, and 1840s. The phrase was used at the time. In fact, the *Medico-Chirurgical Review* explicitly endorsed the idea, referring to "the question of *contingent contagion*, on which so much has been written, pro and con, proving, we think, in a satisfactory manner, that fevers, even within the tropics, are capable of taking on, under particular circumstances, a character of contagion which had nothing to do with their original production." With regard to the plague in particular, however, the *MCR* evinced a much stricter belief in contagionism. See "Fever-Contagion-Quarantine," *Medico-Chirurgical Review* 2, no. 3, New Series (1825): 3.

[34] Russell, *Natural History of Aleppo*, 260.

[35] On the lingering influence of Hippocratic explanations for the spread of plague in the eighteenth century, see Takeda, *Between Crown and Commerce*, 109–16.

To many, it appeared that the extremity of plague could be confronted with the comforting balm of moderation.

In this way, if excess was a concept many used to explain the presence of the plague in the Middle East, British emphasis on moderation seemed to be a reason for immunity at home. Especially if one relied on the second understanding of epidemic disease laid out above, in which it was simply one extreme of a continuum of diseases, the fight against the plague in Britain itself was ongoing, and references to it abounded across popular culture. In William Moncrieff's popular play, *The Pestilence of Marseilles*, a character warns an assembled crowd that "if you value your lives, and don't want to have your town another Marseilles, you'll all of you mount guard like lynxes."[36] Many members of the audience at the Theatre Royale, Surrey (where the play was first performed) might have responded that they had heard that advice before. Anyone, for example, who was interested in home construction might pick up a copy of Richard Rowed's *Comprehensive Plans* to stop "cholera, plague pestilence, and fevers." These ponderous and terrifying diseases, Rowed posited, could be thwarted by following supremely mundane advice such as his precept that "every dwelling-house ought to run a two-inch pipe into the house drains to the kitchen-chimney, to carry off the effluvia."[37] That the fight against contagion was something Britons were responsible for at home should help us understand that the apparently abstract medical debate surrounding the cause of disease had stakes that were familiar to ordinary consumers. It should not surprise us that Charles Maclean was able to rustle up an audience for popular lectures he gave on epidemic contagion in the 1810s.

Bubonic plague remained close to the surface of popular consciousness for other reasons too. British newspapers provided breathless updates of the spread of plague around the Mediterranean during the 1810s – readers of the London *Times*, for example, encountered no fewer than eighteen stories about the plague of Malta during the summer and autumn of 1813. An article in the *Morning Post* reported on a plague at Smyrna that had left so many dead they were lying "in heaps in the streets unburied." The source was "a gentleman who arrived in town yesterday, after performing a quarantine of 40 days."[38] The arrival of plague ships, the responses of southern European countries to plague epidemics in North Africa, and intelligence about epidemics inside the Ottoman Empire derived from British consular reports were all frequent topics in newspapers across the country. In the early nineteenth century, it would have

---

[36] W. T. Moncrieff, *The Pestilence of Marseilles, or, the Four Thieves: A Melo-Drama, in Three Acts* (London: Thomas Richardson, [1829]), 36.

[37] Richard Rowed, *Cholera, Plague, Pestilence, and Fevers Mitigated by Adopting Rowed's Comprehensive Plans for the Improvement of the Health of the Metropolis and Large Towns* (London: James Watson, [1849]), 10.

[38] "Plague at Smyrna," *Morning Post*, August 19, 1813.

taken a very uninformed individual to believe that *Britons* (if not *Britain*) no longer experienced the disease.

Even as a historical fact, the plague was more visible in this period than it had been for generations. The centenary of the 1720 plague of Marseille witnessed a resurgence of interest in the disease in France, some of which spilled across the Channel. Moncreiff's play about this event, for example, was based on a French original written in the wake of the 1820 commemorations. In his preface, Moncrieff helpfully recommends six recently published histories of the Marseille epidemic that were available to British readers.[39] Possibly in reaction to a profusion of texts memorializing the heroic Archbishop Belsunce and the Marseille plague, interest in Britain's own plague-sites grew during the 1820s. The village of Eyam, where, under the leadership of their local reverend, residents had sealed themselves off after the plague arrived in 1665 to save the neighboring towns, was constructed as a kind of British answer to the French story.[40] Morality tales, poems, and histories about Eyam were all written during the early nineteenth century.[41]

Finally, there is every reason to think that the populace was far from convinced that Britain enjoyed any kind of permanent immunity from the plague. In 1836, Thomas Wakley, one-time editor of *The Lancet* and Radical MP, introduced an urgent question in the House of Commons regarding rumors that the plague had broken out near Tottenham Court Road in central London. Charles Poulett Thompson, President of the Board of Trade, was well aware of this rumor and glad of the chance to publicly deny it. Apparently, a well-known doctor who had observed plague in Constantinople had publicized a story that a draper had opened a box of cloth and instantly died from imported contagion, along with seven assistants. No less an authority than Quarantine Superintendent William Pym was brought in to make inquiries, wherefrom it transpired that the draper had died of brain fever and all of his assistants enjoyed good health. The disgruntled Poulett Thomson noted that a deputation of people from the area had visited him at the Council office that morning "in considerable alarm" and that the rumor "could not too soon be contradicted."[42] His frustration with the popular willingness to believe the plague might invade London in the year 1836 is palpable. Though the plague might appear to have resided firmly in the distant past, ordinary people were

---

[39] See Moncreiff, *Pestilence of Marseilles*, v.
[40] See Patrick Wallis, "A Dreadful Heritage: Interpreting Epidemic Disease at Eyam, 1666–2000," *History Workshop Journal* 61, no. 1 (2006): 40–41.
[41] See, for example, Mary and William Howitt, "The Desolation of Eyam," published in the collection *The Desolation of Eyam: The Emigrant: A Tale of the American Woods, and Other Poems*, 2nd ed. (London: Wightman and Cramp, 1828), 10–40.
[42] Hansard, House of Commons Debate, June 7, 1836, vol. 34, cc. 165–67.

clearly willing to believe it remained a potent threat at the brink of the Victorian age.

Debating Contagion

If most doctors in the 1820s, 1830s, and 1840s were contingent-contagionists, willing to admit the operation of some sort of human-to-human transmission in certain cases, does it even make sense to speak of a contagion debate?[43] True enough, many of the positions taken by medical authors in the nineteenth century had been echoed in earlier years. Yet, the debate still has meaning as a phenomenon of the 1810s–1840s. Interest in the question of contagion soared in the course of the nineteenth century (a fact which we might attribute to the expansion of the quarantine system, an increase in Mediterranean trade volume, and the series of epidemics outlined in Chapter 1). This is visible through the bibliography of the 1835 *Cyclopaedia of Practical Medicine*. The editors of this bibliography counted only fifty-four works on the question of epidemic contagion in the 250 years between Fracastorius's *De contagione* and the turn of the nineteenth century (1546–1799) but at least sixty-two works between 1800 and 1833.[44] Furthermore, while earlier authors cited ancient medical authorities but rarely each other, nineteenth-century authors of contagion pamphlets were more often in dialogue. They produced a decades-long conversation that was cantankerous, defensive, and vitriolic.

Even if one focuses only on those medical authorities who self-consciously felt themselves to be debating contagion, it is clear that writers were often talking past each other. They relied on contradictory definitions of basic medical concepts and proposed idiosyncratic schemes of classification for different diseases. Thomas Southwood Smith, for example, defined "the presence of an epidemic atmosphere" as the "generally admitted" criterion that allowed epidemics to be transmitted, a vision that would render the quarantine of foreign localities

---

[43] To divide the medical community even into "contagionists," "contingent contagionists," and "anticontagionists" is to ignore the vast diversity of explanations for epidemic disease mooted by medical writers in the nineteenth century. This includes advocates of "animalcular" transmission, proponents of "zygmotic" origins of illness, and those who dabbled in "cognate fungus theory." On these and other systems of classifying disease transmission, see Crook, *Governing Systems*, 202.

[44] "Select Medical Bibliography," in *Cyclopaedia of Practical Medicine*, ed. John Conolly, John Forbes, and Alexander Tweedie (London: Sherwood, Gilbert, and Piper, 1835), 4:37–39. Indeed, as Margaret Delacy has recently shown, the doctrine of contagion itself was slow to gain acceptance in Britain. Notwithstanding an awareness of Fracastorio's work, it took significant effort in the course of the eighteenth century by a particular group of medical advocates to make contagion a commonly accepted explanation for the origin of disease. See Margaret DeLacy, *The Germ of an Idea: Contagionism, Religion, and Society in Britain, 1660–1730* (New York: Palgrave, 2016), and DeLacy, *Contagionism Catches On: Medical Ideology in Britain, 1730–1800* (New York: Palgrave, 2017).

completely superfluous.[45] Charles Maclean went so far as to flatly define an epidemic disease as one that is never contagious.[46] Plague, cholera, and yellow fever were indisputably epidemic, therefore Maclean's framing would seem to end the debate simply by manipulating definitions. Conversely, as we will see in the next chapter, though some British officials tasked with fighting plague (*mahamari*) in India in the 1850s adopted a sanitarian and antiquarantinist approach, they always did so by arguing that the disease they saw could not be plague. Meanwhile, they accepted as axiomatic that plague *was* contagious and that quarantine was required to halt its spread.

Not only did medical writers embrace contradictory definitions of basic concepts but they also relied on sets of "alternative facts." This points us to another revealing characteristic of this debate: medical evidence mobilized during it was almost exclusively in the form of historical case studies. David Barnes, appropriately, calls arguments about the contagion question "rigorously anecdotal."[47] In this way, contagion debaters were essentially writing some of the most detailed and argumentative early histories of medicine long before the history of medicine was an academic discipline. The contagionist historian J. P. Papon provided an illustration of this point in 1800, when he wrote that to come to accept contagion theory "it is sufficient to gather together [the histories] of what doctors employed by boards of health have done when numerous trials have shown the wisdom of their defensive system. The subject is thus purely historic: it suffices, in treating it, to read much and to read well."[48] And yet, partisans on both sides could easily read within their respective echo chambers. Contagionists and anticontagionists wrote their own (contrasting) histories of yellow fever outbreaks, of the plagues of Malta, Corfu, and the Ottoman Empire, and of epidemics in the ancient and medieval worlds.

Within such histories, different anecdotes and facts were given prominence to undergird the position of the author. But even the same anecdotes could generate divergent positions. As the totally disinterested surgeon Thomas Hodgkin mused, the tale of the members of one family all dying of an epidemic disease could be read differently, depending on one's position in the contagion debate. Presented with such a tale, Hodgkin noted, "the simple statement of the fact looks so much like the execution of a confessedly contagious malady, that the contagionist regards it as almost conclusive and notes it in triumph." But to an

[45] T. Southwood Smith, *The Common Nature of Epidemics, and Their Relation to Climate and Civilization* (Philadelphia: Lippincott, 1866), 72.

[46] This definition actually derived from the eighteenth century, when the doctor William Grant had posited "an absolute distinction between 'contagious' and 'epidemic'." Pelling, *Cholera, Fever*, 19.

[47] The idea is explored in David S. Barnes, "Quarantine and the Role of Surveillance in Nineteenth-Century Public Health," in Nkuchia M'ikanatha and John Iskander, eds., *Concepts and Methods in Infectious Disease Surveillance* (Oxford: Wiley-Blackwell, 2014), 26–30.

[48] Papon, *De la Peste*, 1:41–42.

194   Imagining the Plague

anticontagionist, a pattern of transmission among closely linked people would suggest something different. Such an individual, Hodgkin noted, would assume "that the different members of the family may have been similarly exposed either from residing in a suspected district or by similarity in their avocations leading them to similar exposure."[49] Defenders of contagion, for example, considered it absolutely conclusive that the plague of Malta ended after Sir Thomas Maitland ordered the inhabitants of Valletta to withdraw to a less crowded encampment in the countryside where the healthy and the sick could be totally separated: "such then is the portrait of CONTAGION; and the disease which follows such a course is CONTAGIOUS," insisted Augustus Bozzi Granville.[50] Yet to anticontagionists, the change of atmosphere and the improved living conditions outside of Valletta appeared to be the conclusive factors.

For the most part, despite what partisans on each side might have thought, the evidence for both the contagiousness and the noncontagiousness of epidemic diseases was evenly balanced in the early nineteenth century. Current understandings of these diseases help explain how there could have been so much ambiguity. Of the three epidemic diseases most debated, bubonic plague and yellow fever are today considered to spread by primarily by animal rather than human vectors. And, while cholera is considered to be contagious, its bacteria spread through the water and through contamination from excrement, not from touch or from breath. With this in mind, it should be easy to see how the contagion debate seemed so impossible to resolve.

The impossibility of determining "facts" in this context became especially frustrating to politicians when it came to details that had bearing on actionable quarantine policy. The arguments of Britain's most voluble nonmedical opponent of quarantine – the Radical MP John Bowring – often returned to the supposed fact that no lazaretto employees at Malta had caught the plague.[51] Yet, according to the records of another anticontagionist, at least three expurgators had been struck in Malta during the expurgation of plague ships there in 1821 and 1841.[52] A series of letters from 1840 between Alexandre Gouin, then French Minister of Commerce, and the Marseille *Intendance* shows that the *Intendance*'s archive contained details of several expurgators catching the plague but, due to their comparative antiquity (episodes in 1720 and 1726) or unique circumstances (a Marseille expurgator sent to Alexandria to fumigate a ship there in the midst of a plague epidemic), Gouin refused to accept them as valid.[53] This was the kind of question for which voluminous records existed. Yet, here, as so often in the

---

[49] Undated lecture notes of Thomas Hodgkin, MD (probably from the early 1830s). Wellcome PP. HO.D.D56, Box 21.
[50] Granville, *Letter to Robinson*, 21. Emphasis original.
[51] Bowring, *Observations on the Oriental Plague*, 23–24.
[52] Milroy, *Quarantine and the Plague*, 64–67.
[53] See, in particular, Alexandre Gouin to the Intendants, March 18, 1840, ADBR 200 E 208.

contagion debate, the harder one pushed on facts, the more inconclusive they seemed. In 1838 Giorgio Cattaneo of Genoa's *Sanità* quoted a recent example of two previously healthy individuals developing the plague eighteen days after the arrival of their ship, which had suffered one death from the plague *en route* to Genoa.[54] However, after canvassing numerous doctors, the French anticontagionist Louis Aubert-Roche (who had treated the plague himself while in Egypt) published a treatise in 1843 that insisted no evidence showed plague had an incubation period longer than eight days.[55]

While the differences in case histories and contradictory assertions must have been maddening to nonmedical observers, they alone do not explain the passions generated by the contagion debate. Nor does an actual divergence in theoretical principles. If it is a misleading characterization to say that contagionists believed touch alone was the cause of disease transmission,[56] and if even the most ardent anticontagionists conceded that contagion functioned for some diseases, how was the level of disagreement sufficient to warrant the vitriol the debate produced? The answer is quarantine itself. If quarantine edicts generated intermittent protest in the course of the eighteenth century, the regular operation of the system from the late eighteenth century onward generated an unprecedented level of protest. With no analysis of actual expenses, John Bowring assessed that quarantine cost British commerce millions of pounds. As a utilitarian rationalist, Bowring found this particularly offensive because he viewed faith in the system to be irrational: equivalent to "the belief in ghosts, witches, and other marvels."[57] In casting the quarantine system as a conspiracy concocted by superstitious Continental Catholics and bureaucrats, some British critics of the practice come across as nineteenth-century equivalents of today's Brexiteers. And just like today, some anticontagionists believed they could have their cake and eat it too. Charles Maclean, for example, estimated that quarantine's annual cost to the government ran to about £27,000 a year in the early 1800s (exclusive of the costs of the abandoned Chetney Hill Lazaretto) and that a further annual sum of £144,800 constituted the cost to commerce.[58] Conspicuously missing from

---

[54] See G. Cattaneo to the Sardinian Secretary of the War and Marine Department, August 1838 (day missing), in *Correspondence Relative to the Contagion of the Plague*, 168–69.

[55] Louis Aubert-Roche, "Enquête sur les quarantaines de la Peste," *Annales d'Hygeine Publique* 33 (1845): 242. A survey of opinion undertaken by Aubert-Roche revealed some specialists put the outer limit at three days and others "several months." See Aubert-Roche, *Réforme des Quarantaines*, 65–66.

[56] The contagionist J. P. Papon, for example, suggested the plague could spread by touch, by way of contaminated merchandise, or by way of "pestilential emanations" emitted by infected persons and things. See Papon, *De la Peste*, 2:1–2.

[57] John Bowring, *Autobiographical Reflections of Sir John Bowring* (London: H. S. King, 1877), 203.

[58] See Maclean, *Evils of Quarantine Laws*, 30 and 33. Maclean abandoned precision and advanced arguments that prefigured Bowring's, however, when he wrote that the ostensibly broader cost of quarantine in "preventing agriculture, commerce, navigation, and manufactures" was "above

such estimates, however, as Bowring (at least) was willing to concede, was an estimate of the losses to British commerce if all ships originating in British ports suffered from retaliatory quarantines on the Continent.

To reiterate, I am suggesting that a person's attitude to quarantine served as the primary marker of difference between anticontagionist and contagionist doctors. Erwin Ackerknecht seems to gesture to this point when he notes that the contagion debate was "never a discussion on contagion alone, but *always on contagion and quarantines.*"[59] To Ackerknecht, quarantine simply grounded the contagion debate in practical terms. But the system did not just endow the contagion debate with practical relevance – it brought it into existence. Indeed, it was the one topic about which it was clear that contagionists and antic-ontagionists could have a debate without talking past each other. In this way, neither Ackerknecht nor the subsequent historians of medicine who have challenged the strictness of his dichotomies have properly accounted for the role of quarantine in provoking, animating, and grounding the debate about epidemic etiology. Nor have they recognized the role of the Mediterranean. Historians who have written about the contagion question have pushed it ever later into the nineteenth century, the better to coincide with the cholera epidemics. Yet, even the authors who debated contagion in the 1840s, 1850s, and 1860s did so with reference to an understanding of epidemic disease derived from earlier debates about plague and Mediterranean quarantine. In this way, then, to study doctors' participation in debates about contagion, we need to do more than investigate whether they supported classically "quarantinist" (con-tagionist) or "sanitationist" (anticontagionist) policies in their own countries. We must also take into account their attitude toward the quarantine laws and disinfection policies in effect at Europe's frontiers. Finally, we should expand our understanding of who constituted a participant in this debate. In the 1840s, for example, several Mediterranean quarantine officials themselves began to weigh in, suggesting modest reforms while humbly defending the practice they had long governed.[60]

---

all calculation." Maclean argued that Britain would gain so much by abolishing the quarantine laws that the Continental powers would be forced to repeal their own rules simply to keep up. Maclean, *Evils of Quarantine Laws*, 34.

[59] Ackerknecht, "Anticontagionism between 1821 and 1867," 567. Emphasis original.

[60] See, for example, Luigi Gravagna, *Rapporto officiale fatto al Sopra-intendente alla quarantena di alcuni casi di Peste* (Valletta: G. B. Mompalao, 1841); G. B. Schembri, *Ragionamento pratico-sanitario sopra varie osservazioni riguardanti la Peste-Bubonica, e metodo con cui s'arresta, s'attacca, e si estingue in questo Lazzaretto di Malta* (Malta, 1842); and Amédée Moulon, *De la peste orientale et de la nécessité d'une réforme dans les quarantaines* (Trieste: Jean Maldini, 1845). Gravagna was a doctor employed by Malta's Board of Health, Schembri had served as Captain of Malta's Lazaretto, and Moulon was a member of the Board of Health of Trieste. Even earlier, Jacinto Roger, the physician at Spain's Port Mahon lazaretto, had written a treatise which had strongly defended quarantine in the cases of cholera and yellow

The apparent intractability of this debate created a frustration evinced by both contagionists and anticontagionists. As much as many anticontagionists sought to portray themselves as avatars of new, empirical medical theories in contrast to the blind adherence to a contagionist tradition, many took pains to suggest that logic (and not medical experience) could resolve the debate in their favor. Charles Maclean told Parliament in 1819 that the contagiousness of plague was a question "entirely ... of fact, not of physic."[61] Here, he was drawing on eighteenth-century *contagionist* plague writers who had adopted the same wording.[62] The conception is not so different from J. P. Papon's idea (quoted above) that history, rather than medical knowledge, could prove plague's contagiousness.

The implicit concession of expertise created an opening for governmental involvement in the contagion question. Medical science had proven itself inadequate. As an author in the *British and Foreign Medical Review* opined, "such a contrariety of opinion upon one of the few questions in which our profession is consulted by the legislative power is peculiarly unsatisfactory."[63] Satisfactory or not, the transfer of the contagion question to the political realm entailed a difference not only in who the arbiters were but in what methods were used. All told, argued the French anticontagionist Louis Aubert-Roche, by the 1840s, the philosophy underlying sanitary administration had ceased to be "an administrative and scientific" issue and had been "transformed into a political and national question."[64] In both Britain and France, bureaucrats in the 1830s and 1840s began to attempt to create clarity through inquiries that would examine the circumstances surrounding the arrival of every plague ship that had arrived in a European port and use that to arrive at a reasonable estimate of an incubation period.

Such efforts represent an increasing usurpation by the state (in the late 1830s and 1840s) of questions that had previously been left to doctors, medical colleges, and boards of health. But if some doctors resented this, it was a situation they had, in many ways, brought on themselves.

While the strict division of anticontagionists and contagionists into political categories of "liberal" and "conservative," respectively (a central pillar of

fever. On Roger, see Arrizabalaga and García-Reyes, "Case of Nicasio Landa," 180. Gravagna's work was reviewed in the *British and Foreign Medical Review* alongside much more famous participants in the contagion debate, such as Arthur Holroyd, Clot Bey, and Arsène Bulard. See Anon., "Bulard, Clot-Bey, Davy, Ségur-Dupeyron, Williams &c. on Contagion and Quarantine," *British and Foreign Medical Review* 16 (1843): 289–308.
[61] 1819 Select Committee Report, 97.
[62] See Patrick Russell, *Treatise of the Plague*, 203. Russell is, himself, quoting an article in the *Explainer* from 1722, which also uses the phrase "rather a question of fact, then of physic" to characterize the dilemma of epidemic contagion.
[63] "Bulard, Clot-Bey, &c.," *British and Foreign Medical Review*, 290.
[64] Aubert-Roche, *De la Réforme des Quarantaines*, 3.

Ackerknecht's pioneering study of the contagion debate), stumbles over numerous counterexamples, it is clear that authors across the spectrum of etiological opinion inclined toward political solutions. Calls for more standardization of quarantine or, alternatively, new sanitation schemes that could render quarantine unnecessary, both attempted to elicit greater government interest and greater funding for medical security.

This inclination toward questions of state policy encouraged some medical writers to conflate matters medical and political in their work. Charles Maclean, for example, was so frustrated that the Select Committee appointed to study the doctrine of contagion in 1819 was not persuaded by his arguments that he channeled his rage into a searing indictment of the British polity as a whole. The resulting *Specimens of Systematic Misrule* (1820) opens with the unsubtle Shakespearean epigraph ("something is rotten in the state of Denmark"). Maclean proceeds to identify the root cause of Britain's "destitution, sickness, mortality, and crime" as the 488 seats in Parliament controlled by the "oligarchic ascendancy," which, in his view, determined Parliament's rejection of his medical arguments.[65] In this way, Maclean blends the strength of his feeling about plague's etiology into a typical pre-1832 attack on the unreformed Parliament.[66]

Boyd Hilton has perceptively noted that metaphors about fever permeated political discourse in the first half of the nineteenth century.[67] The reverse is also true; ideas about the nature of the state permeated medical writing about contagion and quarantine. Among British and French liberal anticontagionists, this attitude often centered upon the idea that the lazaretto institutionalized arbitrary government.[68] The power of life and death that boards of health could wield over those detained in quarantine seemed to encapsulate despotism itself. John Bowring wrote that:

If there be a spot in the world placed beyond the control of public opinion, it is a Lazzaret. Believed, as it is, to be an invention for public security, the tyranny, the

---

[65] Maclean, *Specimens of Systematic Misrule*, vii and xii.

[66] Michael Brown argues that Maclean's motivation in writing the book was the Peterloo Massacre, which had occurred one year earlier. See Brown, "From Foetid Air to Filth: The Cultural Transformation of British Epidemiological Thought, ca. 1780–1848," *Bulletin of the History of Medicine* 82 (2008): 520. In my opinion, Maclean's anger about his treatment by the Home Office, Board of Trade, and Select Committee on Contagion were more than enough to explain the political nature of *Specimens*.

[67] Boyd Hilton, *A Mad, Bad, and Dangerous People? England 1783–1846* (Oxford: Oxford University Press, 2006), 338.

[68] By way of comparison, for a recent work emphasizing the relationship among Enlightenment ideas about science, ideas about the nature of the state, and the debate over epidemic transmission (in the American context), see Thomas Apel, *Feverish Bodies, Enlightened Minds: Science and the Yellow Fever Controversy in the Early American Republic* (Stanford, CA: Stanford University Press, 2016).

extortions, the injuries which are inflicted within it, escape all animadversion. Discussion as to its organization, its laws, its judicature, seems wholly excluded.[69]

Bowring, whose anticontagionism was closely linked to free trade activism, was content to rail against the quarantine laws and leave the finer points of alternative public health regimes to others. Yet, to break down the walls of the lazaretto and to accept broader public health regulation as the responsibility of the state required enormous expense. As we will see below, it was essential to the task of the sanitarians to incorporate the outward logic of quarantine – its division of the world into competing landscapes of health and disease – and turn it inward to the pathologies they diagnosed in the nation itself.

Again, the contagion debate was vituperative, yet it also produced a subterranean consensus in favor of greater state action against disease, with doctors on both sides of the debate endorsing similar interventionist principles. For example, many contagionists argued for the reform of lazarettos (rather than their abolition) on lines that were coincident with sanitarian ambitions. As early as the eighteenth century, the reformer John Howard's plan for a healthier lazaretto emphasized open spaces, running water, and better air circulation. Like many who rejected his belief in contagion, Howard expressed a desire to learn about plague anew by observing plague patients in the Mediterranean, and "not from the Theories of Persons who have never visited Patients in that distemper."[70] Outside of occasional contagionist defenses of institutions like the Royal College, there is absolutely no reason to associate contagionism and a resistance to empirical medicine, as anticontagionist advocates tended to imply.

Furthermore, many contagionist doctors were no less energetic supporters of public health reform in the 1830s and 1840s than their opponents. Augustus Bozzi Granville, for example, was an early advocate for sewer reform. R. R. Madden emphasized that bad ventilation and poor sewer construction could make the plague "highly contagious," when, in ordinary circumstances, he believed, it was difficult to transmit.[71] The same explosion of statistics that inspired Edwin Chadwick's major 1842 *Report into the Sanitary Conditions of the Labouring Population of Great Britain* were widely acknowledged by contagionists as well as anticontagionists to show an association between poverty and disease. Compressed populations and the lack of adequate sewers for carrying off effluvia could foster the spread of contagion just as they could foster the presence of an infectious atmosphere. As G. B. Schembri, of Malta's quarantine administration, wrote, poverty was the underlying cause of most plague deaths. This was not for the sanitarian reason that poor homes suffered from more environmental defects and an excess of pestilential atmosphere, but

[69] Bowring, *Observations on the Oriental Plague*, 12.
[70] John Howard to an unknown correspondent, May 20, 1789, Wellcome Ms. 7948/5.
[71] Madden, *Travels*, 270.

because the poor tended to disobey isolation orders "preferring to run the uncertain risk of dying from the plague to the certainty of dying from hunger."[72]

Poverty, bad sanitation, and overcrowded cities, then, were acknowledged to augment epidemic threats on all sides of medical argument. The intractability of the contagion debate, the medical literature it generated, and the consistent inquiries it provoked in national legislatures and commissions of medicine all served to legitimize the growing consensus that the state was obligated (thanks to the precedent set by quarantine) to intervene to a greater extent in matters of public health. The fusion of approaches from both the contagionists and the anticontagionists in the course of the first cholera epidemic aided this process to an even greater extent.

The 1832 Cholera Epidemic and the Legacy of the Plague

As an item of foreign news alone, the plague could not have shaped metropolitan health policy nearly so significantly as it did. And yet, cholera provided the plague with a potent entry point into the British body politic. On its own, cholera has been accorded a crucial role in initiating British public health reform, including by Victorians themselves.[73] This conception was challenged by Margaret Pelling, who influentially has argued that cholera was "a distraction, rather than an impetus, to reform." Instead, she argues, we should eschew the "shock value" of cholera in seeking to explain the genesis of public health reform and focus on more quotidian "fevers" that killed hundreds of thousands of nineteenth-century Britons.[74] Pelling's work is an important reminder that the stuff of ordinary Victorian days should matter as much as the substance of unusual Victorian nightmares. But here, I argue that if cholera is a distraction, it is so because to complete our understanding of the origin of Victorian public health, we need to look outward at the Mediterranean context and backward to Britain's epidemic history. Plague was the precedent that shaped the reaction against cholera, the association that lent it its "shock value," and the guiding inspiration for its general consumption.

For a start, we know this because plague explicitly provided the rationale for declaring cholera a national emergency. Under the 1825 Quarantine Act, cholera was not specifically named as a disease that could justify quarantine –

---

[72] Schembri, *Ragionamento Pratico-Sanitario*, 6–7.

[73] See Briggs, "Cholera and Society," 86. Briggs notes a current of opinion that cast cholera as the "ally" of the sanitarians in inspiring further reforms. To that point, the Peelite MP Sir James Graham disdained the prospects of a bill regulating burials in London advocated by Chadwick by saying "in the midst of cholera, it might have been carried." Quoted in Peter Mandler, *Aristocratic Government in the Age of Reform* (Oxford: Oxford University Press, 1990), 264. The proposed Metropolitan Internments Bill ended up passing by a wide margin.

[74] Pelling, *Cholera, Fever*, 4–6.

the act was written with plague as the primary focus, with a specific section that mentioned yellow fever. So, under the long-standing practice of the British state, cholera could only be met with quarantines after the king and Privy Councilors indicated they considered the danger from the disease to be similar to the threat of the plague (which they did in June 1831). In this way, from the pinnacle of the British state, the symmetry between cholera and plague was considered official policy. Noting that government officials, pamphleteers, and diarists frequently resorted to plague metaphors and analogies when describing the cholera epidemics, Michael Durey finds the comparison "startling, if, on reflection, quite understandable."[75] Is it so startling? As we have seen, the plague had a capacity to represent *all* epidemic diseases and was a growing topic of interest in the news and in popular culture. Given the recent plague epidemics in the Mediterranean detailed in Chapter 2 (the plagues of Malta, Corfu, Noja, and Mallorca all occurred less than twenty years before cholera arrived in Britain), and given the extent to which the distinct nature of cholera was poorly understood, it would have been far more startling had Britons *not* made the comparison in 1831. Cholera's potential arrival provoked existential fears about an epidemic on the scale of the 1665 plague or larger.[76]

The quarantines instituted in 1831 as British administrators prepared to meet this first cholera epidemic further indicate the extent to which it was treated as an invasion of the plague. After draconian quarantine rules expanded the detention of ships at British ports to include ships from the Baltic in the summer of 1831, Britain's already crowded "floating lazarettos" experienced an enormous influx of traffic. Across the nation, in that summer alone, a total of 2,556 ships performed quarantine. This can be compared to a seasonal average, in the years leading up to 1831, of 839.[77] Quarantine lengths, fumigation procedures, and categorizations of which trade items were "enumerated goods," were all lifted directly from the plague-centric quarantine practice long followed in British ports and based on Mediterranean precedent. The diarist Charles Greville complained that the massive augmentation of quarantine that summer "requires more ships and lazarets than we have, and the result is a perpetual squabbling, disputing, and complaining between the Privy Council, the Admiralty, the Board of Health, and the merchants."[78] To cope with the increase of traffic, Stangate Creek, the largest quarantine site in Britain, tripled

---

[75] Durey, *Return of the Plague*, 2.
[76] See Morris, *Cholera 1832*, esp. chapter 2, on what he calls the "crisis atmosphere" (14) as cholera approached.
[77] See *Quarantine: Return to an Order of the Honourable House of Commons* (London: House of Commons, 1831), 1–5.
[78] Charles Greville, *The Greville Memoirs*, ed. Henry Reeve (London: Longmans, Green, and Co., 1874), 2:157.

its staff from 66 to 199.[79] The infrastructure of British quarantine was central to the nation's response to cholera in more ways than one; in the second epidemic (1848–49), for example, Liverpool's small quarantine site of Bromborough Pool was transformed into an isolation hospital for cholera patients.[80] All told, in Britain as well as on the Continent, the defense against cholera simply refocused the plague-based quarantine system in new directions. In November 1830, for example, Austria extended its antiplague military frontier along its border with Russia in response to the new threat.[81] Prussia, in turn, hastily mobilized a military force to guard its own military frontier, comprising some 60,000 troops. Anyone passing through one of the twelve "temporary stations" was fumigated with nitric acid and bathed in fortified water.[82] In this way, cholera did not provoke completely new infrastructure, so much as it accomplished the expansion of long-standing antiplague sanitary cordons across new terrain.[83] In many European states, the quarantines planned in response to the 1831 epidemic were the most ambitious in the course of the nineteenth century. And though they failed, they showed the lingering and singular power of antiplague defenses in setting the generic pattern of responding to an invader disease.

The precedent of plague and the practice of quarantine were mobilized not only because they were the clearest referents available but also because, for a long time, the exact identity of cholera as a distinct disease remained in doubt. Although British doctors in Bengal had treated cholera patients when the disease first became epidemic in the 1810s, it was unclear that the disease moving through central Asia and into Russia at the end of the 1820s was the same ailment. Some believed the malady was not a new one at all but an already-known disease that had been given a new name.[84] In the spring of 1831, as the rapid advance of the epidemic through central Asia to the fringes of Europe convinced many that Britain itself would be struck, the PC (in consultation with the Royal College of Physicians) dispatched two doctors to Moscow to study the disease and produce a rubric of recommendations from which the government could formulate a response. Drs. David Barry and William Russell both had experience dealing with epidemic disease (Indian

---

[79] "A Return of the Number of Officers and Mariners at the Different Quarantine Stations on the 5th January of 1831 and 5th January of 1832 with the Rates of Pay and the Rates of the appointment of the Officers," TNA PC 1/2659.
[80] See the table on mortality at Bromborough Pool in 1849, TNA PC 1/2659.
[81] See Richard Ross, *Contagion in Prussia, 1831: The Cholera Epidemic and the Threat of the Polish Uprising* (Jefferson, NC: McFarland, 2015), 15.
[82] Baldwin, *Contagion and the State*, 43–44.
[83] On this point, and regarding northern Germany, see Richard Evans, *Death in Hamburg: Society and Politics in the Cholera Years, 1830–1910* (London: Penguin, 2005), 257.
[84] See James Kendrick, *Cursory Remarks upon the Present Epidemic* (London: C. J. G. and F. Rivington, 1832), 6–8.

cholera as well as Spanish yellow fever), and the first questions to which they turned were questions of identity.

Russell had already seen cholera patients during his time in India. It did not take him long to come to the "unqualified conviction" of the Russian disorder's "perfect identity with the Indian spasmodic cholera."[85] Despite this diagnosis, as Russell and Barry examined patients, they continued to check for the symptoms of plague. In their second report back to the PC, they began by taking pains to emphasize that the disease they saw was not the plague, having observed no "glandular swellings, nor carbuncles, nor petecchiae."[86] Barry and Russell were clearly aware that any invader epidemic disease would be interrogated for its relationship to the plague and were anxious to establish that cholera was a distinct disease. That said, the long tradition of using quarantine to prevent the plague guided the questions they asked Russian doctors. What kinds of goods were considered capable of harboring the contagion that caused the disease? How effective was isolation? What were typical incubation periods and how did the state of the atmosphere in St. Petersburg seem?[87]

In ports hit by cholera elsewhere in the world, British consuls drew analogies between the new disease and the plague. John Barker, the consul in Alexandria, noted that European and Muslim elites had adopted the same "shutting up" policies common during plague epidemics, and that, all told, he himself was highly confident in "the usual precautions adopted in the time of the plague."[88] Treating the cholera as the plague immediately imposed a specific interpretation of cholera as a disease charged with moral significance and weighty associations. Like plague, for example, cholera became firmly linked to the "East"; the term *Asiatic cholera* was often used to refer to the new disease. Also like plague, the disease became known for its uniquely horrifying symptoms; another name for it was "blue cholera" (in reference to the bluish state of the desiccated skin of cholera victims).

The facts of this first cholera epidemic have been extensively described in the historiography – accounts from medical history, social history, literary studies, and popular history have presented the terror and drama of this arrival of a new disease and used it to cast light on broader fissures

---

[85] Dr. Russell to the Clerk of the PC, July 1, 1831. Published in *Official Reports Made to Government by Drs. Russell and Barry on the Disease Called Cholera Spasmodica* (London: Privy Council, 1832), 20.

[86] Second Report by Drs. Russell and Barry to Charles Greville, July 16, 1831. Printed in *Papers Relative to the Disease Called Cholera Spasmodica in India, Now Prevailing in the North of Europe* (London: Winchester and Varnham, 1831), 27–28.

[87] All of these questions were posed by Drs. Russell and Barry in a questionnaire they sent to a Dr. Rehman, July 14, 1831. Printed in *Papers Relative to the Disease Called Cholera*, 71–72.

[88] Extracts of letters from August and September 1831 (presumably by John Barker, consul at Alexandria). Quoted in *Papers Relative to the Disease Called Cholera*, 68.

and dilemmas in British society on the eve of the Victorian period.[89] Yet, the full implications of cholera's interpretation as a variant of the plague have yet to be understood. Let us return, then, to a fevered Britain in 1830 and 1831. It was a country whose citizens both dreaded "the return of the plague" and resented efforts at control. Privy Councilors, invested with the solemn responsibility of protecting the kingdom solely by virtue of the Quarantine Act, worried, dithered, and delayed. In addition to dispatching Drs. Barry and Russell in the summer of 1831, they consulted a range of British doctors and diplomats who had observed the disease first-hand. The questions they asked understandably focused on developing a strategy of response, yet there was no medical consensus on basic issues like cholera's incubation period, the types of goods it could infect, and the nature of its transmission. Even its symptoms were presented with a vagueness and drama derived from the tradition of the plague. According to a Dr. Keir, who observed the disease in Moscow, "it most commonly began by a feeling of general uneasiness," shortly to be followed by "giddiness" and "a sense of oppression in the stomach."[90] Doctor after doctor stressed that within an hour patients might go from hale, healthy, and hardy to blue, desiccated, and dead (Figure 7.2).

By the early summer of 1831, the mixed response from the medical community on crucial questions of cholera's etiology left the PC unsure of how to act.[91] The fact that it was assumed that the PC would be the focus of deliberations itself shows a clear sense that this disease was certainly "of the nature of the plague" and liable to the Quarantine Act. And, as a nationwide threat, it was instantly politicized. Charles Greville noted in his diary that "the Tories would even make [the disease] a matter of party accusation against the government, only they don't know exactly how. It is always safe to deal in generalities, so they say that 'Government ought to be impeached if the disease comes here.'"[92] Members of the PC sweated under the political pressure. As guardians of the nation's health, yet perplexed by a novel illness, they turned repeatedly to the Royal College of Physicians (RCP), which responded with further ambiguity. Despite the willingness of its aristocratic president, Sir Henry Halford, to accommodate the PC, the full college refused to endorse a firm position on the question of the contagiousness of goods and merchandise. As a result, the PC enforced a strong quarantine on Baltic shipping, hoped for the best, and

---

[89] See Norman Longmate, *King Cholera: The Biography of a Disease* (London: Hamish Hamilton, 1966); Asa Briggs, "Cholera and Society"; Morris, *Cholera 1832*; Durey, *Return of the Plague*; Mary Poovey, *Making a Social Body: British Cultural Formation, 1830–1864* (Chicago: University of Chicago Press, 1995), chapter 3; Pamela Gilbert, *Cholera and Nation: Doctoring the Social Body in Victorian England* (Albany: SUNY Press, 2008).

[90] Extract from Dr. Keir's "Report." Printed in *Papers Relative to the Disease Called Cholera*, 10.

[91] See Durey, *Return of the Plague*, chapter 1, "Preparations," esp. 10–14.

[92] Greville, *Greville Memoirs*, 2:152.

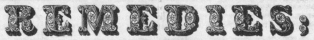

TO THE INHABITANTS OF THE PARISH OF
CLERKENWELL.

His Majesty's Privy Council having approved of precautions proposed by the Board of Health in London, on the alarming approach

OF THE

INDIAN CHOLERA

It is deemed proper to call the attention of the Inhabitants to some of the Symptoms and Remedies mentioned by them as printed, and now in circulation.

Symptoms of the Disorder;

Giddiness, sickness, nervous agitation, slow pulse, cramp beginning at the fingers and toes and rapidly approaching the trunk, change of colour to a leaden blue, purple, black or brown; the skin dreadfully cold, and often damp, the tongue moist and loaded but flabby and chilly, the voice much affected, and respiration quick and irregular.

REMEDIES;

All means tending to restore circulation and to maintain the warmth of the body should be had recourse to without the least delay.

The patient should be immediately put to bed, wrapped up in hot blankets, and warmth should be sustained by other external applications, such as repeated frictions with flannels and camphorated spirits, poultices of mustard and linseed (equal parts) to the stomach, particularly where pain and vomiting exist, and similar poultices to the feet and legs to restore their warmth. The returning heat of the body may be promoted by bags containing hot salt or bran applied to different parts, and for the same purpose of restoring and sustaining the circulation white wine wey with spice, hot brandy and water, or salvolatile in a dose of a tea spoon full in hot water, frequently repeated; or from 5 to 20 drops of some of the essential oils, as peppermint, cloves or cajeput, in a wine glass of water may be administered with the same view. Where the stomach will bear it, warm broth with spice may be employed. In every severe case or where medical aid is difficult to be obtained, from 20 to 40 drops of laudanum may be given in any of the warm drinks previously recommended.

These simple means are proposed as resources in the incipient stages of the Disease, until Medical aid can be had.

THOS. KEY,
GEO. TINDALL,} *Churchwardens.*

Sir GILBERT BLANE, Bart. in a pamphlet written by him on the subject of this Disease, recommends persons to guard against its approach by moderate and temperate living, and to have in readiness the prescribed remedies; and in case of attack to resort thereto *immediately* but the great preventative he states, is found to consist in a *due regard to Cleanliness and Ventilation.*

N.B. It is particularly requested that this Paper may be preserved, and that the Inmates generally, in the House where it is left may be made acquainted with its contents.

NOV. 1st, 1831.

T. GOODE, PRINTER, CROSS STREET, WILDERNESS ROW.

Figure 7.2 Cholera notice from Clerkenwell, in London, 1831. Courtesy of the Wellcome Library. (CC BY license)

punted the most important medical dilemmas to a series of commissions. The first of these can be considered the Russian expedition of Drs. Russell and Barry. The second was a canvas (conducted by members of the RCP) of the opinions of East India Company doctors who had treated cholera victims in

Bengal. The third commission to be tasked with coming up with a response to the disease was a new board of health, formed in late June 1831. This was composed of five government bureaucrats and administrators (including Sir William Pym, previously mentioned as the Superintendent of British quarantine) and six medical members (largely chosen from the upper echelons of the RCP). This was eventually superseded in the autumn of 1831 by another new group (the Central Board of Health), with more representation from doctors who had actually observed cholera victims (including Russell and Barry, now returned from Russia).

Despite early hopes, none of the medical commissions were able to agree on a specific treatment regimen. Describing the testimony of the Indian doctors, the RCP noted that because of "the small success of any treatment in the earlier appearance of it, a feeling of disappointment, and almost despair, seems at times to have dispirited the medical officers, and they are described (from the hopeless state in which they found their patients) as changing from one extreme of practice to another." In the end, the RCP felt unable to recommend to provincial physicians one method of treatment.[93] Epidemic pessimism, sudden attacks, and extreme symptoms all worked to solidify the association between cholera and the plague. Seeing their aim as more to stir up (appropriate) panic than to calm nerves, the elite doctors formulating cholera policy emphasized the utter difference between cholera and any disease a Briton might have encountered before. "After striking a person apparently in good health like lightning," wrote Sir Gilbert Blane, "it never quits him till throwing his whole frame, vitals, body, and limbs, into a state of suffering more violent than the English malady, it destroys life in a few hours, frequently in a single hour or less."[94]

Although the epidemic resulted in an increase of state power, the state itself entered the critical period with a very muddled health administration (with authority divided between the new health board, the PC, and the Customs Service, which administered quarantine). In the height of the summer of 1831, Privy Councilors faced two dilemmas. First, a huge fleet of British ships (700–800 strong) was being kept from departing the Baltic coast with a cargo of flax and hemp, two items that had long appeared on lists of "enumerated goods" capable of carrying contagion. Given the RCP's failure to agree that merchandise could not transmit cholera, this was an administrative nightmare, especially on top of the extra quarantine given to the ships that *were* allowed to proceed to the British coast. Second, as the new board of health

---

[93] Dr. Keir's "Report" and statement by Henry Halford, President of the Board of Health, in *Papers Relative to the Disease Called Cholera*, 6 and 19.

[94] Gilbert Blane, Henry Halford ct. al., *Cholera Morbus: Its Causes, Prevention, and Cure; with Disquisitions on the Contagious or Non-Contagious Nature of This Dreadful Malady*, 3rd ed. (Glasgow: W. R. M'Phun, 1831), 15.

planned a slew of stringent sanitary rules should the epidemic arrive (in particular, mandatory isolation and purification procedures for infected houses), disturbing news filtered in of cholera riots in Prussia, Russia, and Hungary in response to draconian rules imposed there.

Having observed the violent reactions that these restrictions on movement had elicited in Eastern and Central Europe, the members of Britain's Central Board of Health drafted final recommendations (issued by the PC as an Order in Council for October 20) that stepped back from the more stringent regulations proposed in the summer. Given that the disease was then on the north German coast, Central Board members wearily sensed that its arrival was inevitable, thanks to smugglers operating between Germany and Britain. To minimize the risk, the Board adopted regulations it hoped would be perceived as directed toward the general good. No forced removals, it was decided, were worth the unrest they would provoke. Still, if family members refused to let a sick relative be transported to a cholera hospital, they were to be quarantined together, the house denoted with a painted mark reading "SICK." Even after all inside had recovered, "CAUTION" was to be painted on the door until a local board agreed the danger had passed (usually twenty days). Such local boards would be appointed "in every town and village" and include local magistrates, clergymen, "principal inhabitants," and two medical practitioners (one of whom "should be appointed to correspond with the Board of Health in London"). Large towns would be divided into districts, each superintended by a district committee.[95] Between infected towns and districts and healthy ones "all intercourse . . . must be prevented by the best means within the power of the magistrates, who will have to make regulations for the supply of provisions." Inside the districts, there was to be a drive for "extreme cleanliness" and enforced fumigation of infected residences. Each district was encouraged to "appropriate a public hospital" to receive cholera patients, with the Board of Health recommending military barracks as particularly good candidates for such a site.[96] Districts, magistrate committees, and patrols – again, the formula for governing during cholera was more or less directly lifted from the report of the 1805 Board of Health and its plague-centric vision of responding to a disease imported from the Mediterranean (discussed in Chapter 1). Indeed, a current description from the UK Parliament's website regarding British administrative bodies tasked with

---

[95] Order in Council, October 20, 1831. Printed in *Official Reports*, 15–17.

[96] Ibid., 16–17. This last suggestion might appear unremarkable – a local barracks was a large building and the nation was not at war. Yet, the decision it is indicative of the extent to which cholera challenged the nation in an existential manner. A converted barracks appealed not simply because it was convenient, but because an epidemic seemed to require a *national* response and military barracks were one of the few types of buildings associated with the nation that was in a number of towns.

public health terms the 1831–32 Central Board of Health a "reconstituted" body, which had initially met in 1805.[97]

The historian Charles Rosenberg suggests that an epidemic has a "dramaturgic form" which involves "a plot line of increasing and revelatory tension." The plot follows a common "move to a crisis of individual and collective character" and "the quality of pageant" that mobilizes communities "to act out propitiatory rituals." All epidemics, then, feature a response defined by its "public character and dramatic intensity."[98] This model certainly fits the first cholera epidemic in Britain. It crossed the North Sea in October, and by the end of the month, it struck down a sufferer in Sunderland. Despite efforts by Sunderland authorities to conceal the presence of the disease (out of the legitimate fear of internal quarantines), the central government announced the arrival of cholera in Britain in November 1831, and little by little, the epidemic atmosphere engulfed the nation.

This first cholera epidemic killed approximately 32,000 people in the UK (a comparatively small number at a time when the UK population was around 25 million). For our purposes here, the detailed course of this first cholera epidemic matters less than the sense that it constituted an unambiguously *national* challenge, derived from its connection with plague. The experience of managing the epidemic helped solidify the understanding that public health was a subject that (at least when the chips were down) demanded state intervention. It also fostered novel forms of taxation (a further precedent for the Public Health Act of 1848); under the terms of the Cholera Prevention Act of 1832, if the Privy Council deemed certain sanitary improvements to be desirable for preventing cholera, local justices of the peace could draw on parish poor rates to fund sanitary improvements. Though this Act's provisions were limited to times when cholera was epidemic, it helped make such forms of taxation acceptable (prefiguring provisions of the 1848 Public Health Act). While the Cholera Prevention Act mattered little for the 1831–32 epidemic (which was already starting to wane), it was recognized at the time that a new precedent was being set. For example, in the parliamentary debate over the Scottish version of the bill, in February 1832, the moderate Whig, John Campbell, lamented that "the general adoption of the compulsory system of relief, would work much more evil toward Scotland, than the operation of the disease itself. If once this system was introduced, it would never be got rid of."[99] Meanwhile, other MPs doubted the bill's principles for different reasons. Robert Peel was similarly skeptical about instituting a permanent system of

---

[97] www.parliament.uk/about/living-heritage/transformingsociety/towncountry/towns/tyne-and-wear-case-study/introduction/cholera-in-sunderland, accessed February 2, 2019.

[98] Charles Rosenberg, *Explaining Epidemics and Other Studies in the History of Medicine* (Cambridge: Cambridge University Press, 1992), 279.

[99] Hansard, House of Commons Debate, February 15, 1832, c. 404.

levying taxes to fund sanitary improvements, but in times of cholera, supported an even more far-reaching scheme of direct funding from the public purse in London rather than a parish-based plan; "The whole country had the deepest interest in the subject ... We were all as much interested in preventing the spread of contagion in Bethnal Green as in Cumberland and Westmoreland."[100]

The sense that each Briton (at least potentially) owed something to the state in the service of warding off cholera can be seen in Parliament's order for a general fast day in March 1832. Perhaps God would be more inclined to alleviate a national affliction if presented with nationwide sacrifice and prayer. In the end, the comparatively small death toll from this epidemic obscures the hundreds of thousands of Britons who were touched by the disease through their prayers, the sermons they heard, the gossip they exchanged, the taxes they paid, and the news they read. As Mary Poovey and (more recently) Pamela Gilbert have suggested, however, a complementary line of inquiry acknowledges the extent to which cholera fostered a growing sense of the British population as a coherent "social body."[101] The epidemic connected the health of festering slums to the health of the grandest houses. But as we acknowledge this point, we should recognize the extent to which cholera completed a logic already suggested by quarantine – the sense that the nation was a single sanitary unit, and an epidemic threat to some within it was a threat to the whole. Indeed, this was the very premise of the long-standing British tradition that quarantine was only called for against a disease that was "of the nature of the plague." The response to cholera was shaped by a century and a half of quarantine practice, through epidemics hypothetical as well as real, through a long-remembered and constantly reinforced sense of a nation that was vulnerable, not to cholera, but to the plague. *Vibrio cholerae* found its fateful point of entry to the British "social body" well demarcated by *Yersinia pestis*.

Quarantine failed to stop cholera (though it may have delayed its arrival in 1831), and separation, isolation, and domestic quarantines did not appear to have impeded the epidemic's progress inside the UK. This perceived failure (in Continental Europe as in Britain) ensured that defenders of quarantine practice came under increasing pressure from the 1830s onward.[102] In the 1820s, mainstream British political opinion was unwilling to consider a complete end to the quarantine laws. In the wake of cholera, however, a parliamentary consensus began to develop in which quarantine was increasingly seen to be an ineffective practice, one with which Britain engaged only to oblige Continental

---

[100]   Hansard, House of Commons Debate, February 14, 1832, Vol. 10, cc. 339–40.
[101]   Poovey, *Making a Social Body*, chapter 3; Gilbert, *Cholera and Nation*.
[102]   Hardy, "Cholera, Quarantine," 251.

allies. Cholera marks such a strong inflection point in the history of quarantine because the disease itself was contextualized as the successor of plague. And yet, while cholera may have hastened the demise of the quarantine system, the 1831–32 epidemic became a conduit through which the logic, precedents, and procedures of quarantine shaped domestic sanitary politics over the 1830s and 1840s.

Turning Dirt into Plague

The "Condition of England" question formed an especially suggestive back-drop for an increasing focus on epidemic disease and a treatment of ill health as a crisis that bound the nation together. In the same chapter of *Chartism*, in which Thomas Carlyle coined the phrase "Condition of England," his diagnosis of the British state is explicitly written in terms of a national disease:

Glasgow Thuggery, Chartist torch-meetings, Birmingham riots, Swing conflagrations, are so many symptoms on the surface; you abolish the symptom to no purpose, if the disease is left untouched ... The virulent humour festers deep within; poisoning the sources of life; and certain enough to find for itself ever new boils.[103]

With this framing, "Condition of England" thinking lent itself to a medically inflected search for root causes. In the course of the 1830s and 1840s, advocates of public health reform were conducting a similar analysis of the root causes of poverty and disease in Britain. Increasingly, a new generation of anticontagionist miasmatists they began to consider their preeminent enemy to be "filth," broadly conceived.

In the wake of the first cholera epidemic, then, the second-generation applied anticontagionism of the sanitarians diverged from the earlier theorizing of anticontagionists like Maclean. First-generation anticontagionists stressed climate as the cause for pestilential diseases – diseases that, from a French and British perspective, were limited to warmer climes and to imperial spaces. They considered factors like air temperature, wind, and humidity to be far more important than muck, overcrowding, and lack of infrastructure. Yet cholera helped change the balance. If a plague could arrive in Western Europe, then parts of the West itself must (it seemed) be pestilential. In this way, Michael Brown's framing of an anticontagionist movement that moved "from foetid air to filth" is particularly helpful.[104]

Sanitarians contrasted their ambitious mission with quarantine's exclusive emphasis on external threats. Yet, they retained from the precedent of quarantine an understanding that any consideration of health in Britain must be

---

[103] Chapter 1 of Carlyle's *Chartism* is titled "Condition-of-England Question." See Thomas Carlyle, *Chartism*, 2nd ed. (London: James Fraser, 1840), 1.

[104] Brown, "From Foetid Air to Filth."

national in focus. One fever-nest could corrupt the sanitary balance of the whole, just as, according to the logic of quarantine, a single bale of cotton or unfumigated letter could compromise the health of a continent. Though quarantine was lambasted for its limited reach, its conceptual basis implied a relationship (based on contagion) among all sanitary units. It was such a useful foil for public health reformers like Southwood Smith because its totalizing ambition (a kingdom free of epidemic contagion) was similar to the sanitarians'. But, it was also a useful precedent, which impelled discussions about "public health" toward larger frameworks that encompassed the whole nation. Southwood Smith's focus, argues Michael Brown, whether his topic concerned sanitary reform or intervention on an individual body, was "systemic malfunction."[105] Chadwick, too, was no mud-grubbing investigator who recommended piecemeal improvements wherever he encountered dirt – he clearly took pride in his famous 1842 *Report*'s comprehensiveness. Christopher Hamlin calls him a "hydraulic thinker," who thought only in terms of vast systems.[106]

To understand the ambition behind this strand of medical thought, it is important to situate oneself within the mindset of early industrial Britain. The underlying message of exposés of ill health, such as Chadwick's *Report*, William Farr's statistical analyses from the Registrar General's Office, or Henry Mayhew's sensationalist reports in the *Morning Chronicle*, was not simply that Britain's poor were living in filth, but that filthy living conditions were a recent result of rapid changes that characterized the early nineteenth century – urbanization, crowded tenement life, and factory labor. Importantly, sanitarians construed these symptoms not as pathologies of modernity so much as *foreign* impositions on the British body politic. In this way, despite their hatred of quarantine, they took from that system its emphasis on different epidemiological states for different countries. In both contagionist and anticontagionist thinking, Britain existed as a nation whose natural state was good health. For advocates of quarantine, that meant firming up the border and quickly isolating any outbreaks of ill health within. For anticontagionists, conversely, it meant a stress on domestic ill health as positively un-British. "How many acres of Sierra Leone," demanded a reviewer of Chadwick's work, "are, to our shame, existing at this moment in our metropolis in the shape of churchyards?"[107] This rhetoric, in which something as unremarkable and ubiquitous as church graveyards was imbued with the pestilential reputation of Britain's West African colony, shows how firmly the strict sanitarian dichotomy of health and ill health could be conflated with

---

[105] Brown, "Foetid Air to Filth," 538.   [106] Hamlin, *Public Health and Social Justice*, 4.
[107] Review of Chadwick's *Report, Quarterly Review* 71, no. 142 (1843): 422.

a dichotomy of national versus foreign.[108] Thomas Beggs, for example, wrote a representative description of cholera during the second epidemic, which emphasized that its birthplace "was among the swamps and jungles of India. True to its origin, it principally reveled in the crowded and neglected districts of our large towns."[109] Anticontagionists, in particular, saw zones of pestilence as foreign appendages to be operated on and transformed by the knife of the surgical bureaucrat.

And yet, many of these same reformers were simultaneously arguing for the demolition of quarantine barriers against the outside world and attempting (when discussing foreign epidemics) to demystify rather than dramatize epidemic disease. This curious kind of "double-think" is apparent from a typical anticontagionist interpretation of nosology, which held that many diseases classified as distinct were only considered to be so because of climatological variations. The theory is encapsulated in Southwood Smith's assertion that "plague is typhus fever modified by the climate of the Levant. Typhus Fever is plague modified by the climate of England."[110] Smith's intention was to raise the sense of threat from typhus rather than to diminish the threat of the plague. His neat formulation had the dual advantage of making communication with the non-European world less threatening *and* making the sanitary deficiencies of Britain itself seem worse. It also established a firm way of linking the long-standing practice of guarding against imported epidemics through quarantine at the frontier to the new fight against "fever nests" inside Britain's borders. While major sanitary reformers sought the repeal of the quarantine laws, then, they wholeheartedly took up quarantine's impulse toward comprehensive protection against epidemic disease, its demarcation of zones of purity and pollution, and its implication that a central goal of state policy should be insuring that Britain reconfirmed its status as a healthy nation.

Most proximately in the 1830s and 1840s, the aim of the sanitary reformers in the new Health of Towns Associations was to make the familiar strange and to borrow from the exoticism of epidemic disease to accomplish that goal.[111] That Britain could be struck with cholera rendered this type of argument even easier. Plagues could and did arrive in Britain itself, and the urgency and fear they inspired, reformers argued, should be channeled to salutary ends. In the

---

[108] Erin O'Connor makes a similar point in *Raw Material*, suggesting that this quotation shows a fear that England was being transformed into Africa. I am indebted to this observation, but contextualize that strain of thought as part of a broader emphasis in the rhetoric of public health reformers that sanitary problems were foreign impositions. See O'Connor, *Raw Material: Producing Pathology in Victorian Culture* (Durham, NC: Duke University Press, 2000), 30.

[109] Thomas Beggs, *The Cholera: The Claims of the Poor upon the Rich* (London: Charles Gilpin, [1849]), 1.

[110] Smith, "Plague – Typhus Fever – Quarantine," 514.

[111] Erin O'Connor persuasively calls this process "making plague." See O'Connor, *Raw Material*, 29.

midst of the second cholera epidemic, for example, Thomas Beggs demanded:

How is it that we are stirred into activity by an invasion of cholera? That we feel so much alarm? It is proved that the mortality from attacks of cholera, during its visitation in 1831–2, was not greater altogether than the average annual mortality occasioned by typhus ... And yet we sit down with the latter, and become reconciled to its existence, *because it is common and always with us.*[112]

It was morally indefensible, insisted Beggs, for public officials to tolerate local diseases while they professed an obligation to fight imported epidemics like cholera. In fact, the central charge of Beggs's pamphlet is that when cholera slackened and epidemics ended, the urgency behind sanitary reform was forgotten. This seemed particularly unjustifiable given the confidence sanitarians had that environmental improvements could ward off disease. In 1832, the anonymous author of "A Letter on Spasmodic Cholera" urged broad and permanent sanitary reforms to stave off the epidemic. "While pestilence is on foot," the author demanded rhetorically, "are we justified in passively succumbing to its influence, and, with a paralysing fatalism, make [*sic*] no decided effort for the public preservation, when human means *have been, and are, available?*"[113] The challenge for the Chadwickians was maintaining urgency in the intervening years; the dichotomy between "foreign" epidemics and a presupposition that health was the just and natural condition of the metropole was essential to this task.

Armed with new statistics (largely thanks to Farr's work at the Registrar General's Office), such anticontagionist crusaders could point to identifiable problems and begin to link them with potential environmental solutions. Chadwick's *Report*, for example, and its appendix on metropolitan interments depended on a detailed statistical epidemiology that reinforced a localist position about the connection among fever mortality, bad drainage, and metropolitan graveyards. Such connections were optimistic, at the most basic level, because they allowed for the possibility of intervention where before there was none. "It is not in human power to take from any disease the property of contagion, if this property really belongs to it," noted Southwood Smith, "but it is in our power to guard against and prevent the effects of any contagion, however intense."[114] Thus, it was not necessary to disprove contagion theory to recognize the clear correlations evident in recent statistical work and to begin to take action. To be clear, Southwood Smith was completely convinced that contagion did not spread epidemic disease. But he pitched the sanitarian case above the level of typical medical disagreements in a broad call for legislation

---

[112] Beggs, *The Cholera*, 4. Emphasis original.
[113] Anon., *A Letter on Spasmodic Cholera* (London: Highley, 1832), 51. Emphasis original.
[114] Smith, *Common Nature*, 69.

to address the "universal effects of overcrowding, filth, and atmospheric impurity."[115]

The first articles in Britain to enunciate the "sanitary idea" as a policy were written by Southwood Smith in the *Westminster Review* in 1825. That fact has been noted by various historians of public health. What has not been emphasized, however, is that Southwood Smith wrote them to intervene in the debate over the 1825 Quarantine Act; they are almost entirely concerned with the question of the contagiousness of the plague.[116] In their wake, Smith was singled out in Parliament by a defender of Britain's quarantine laws as an unhinged acolyte of Charles Maclean.[117] The connection between quarantine and public health reform fundamentally shaped the nature of that reform as the century progressed. As Matthew Newsom Kerr shows, a bias against the construction of fever hospitals among sanitarian reformers sprung from such hospitals' supposed connection to the pest houses and lazarettos they so often campaigned against.[118] However, in their language and in the intellectual tradition they followed, the sanitarians relied on precedents suggested by a quarantine system they abhorred. In 1800, for example, when the French defender of quarantine J. P. Papon suggested a new and stronger health board to serve as an impediment to plague epidemics in an era of war, he advocated "a bureau which will levy taxes on all inhabitants for the sanitary needs of the city," a bureau "which will have an absolute authority in everything which relates to health."[119] It is not a coincidence that the new agency empowered by the 1848 Public Health Act to superintend and investigate the sanitary state of Britain was dubbed the "General Board of Health."

In other ways, as sanitarians and Health of Towns Association members sought to gin up momentum for public health reform in the 1830s and early 1840s, they implicitly used the precedents of quarantine to justify a set of expensive reforms. After all, Huskisson's summary of the 1825 Quarantine Act was that a decision had been made "that the expense of quarantine should be borne by the country at large, and not by any particular class in it."[120] Though

---

[115] Ibid., 76.
[116] See Ruth Hodgkinson, *The Origins of the National Health Service: The Medical Services of the New Poor Law, 1834–1871* (London: Wellcome, 1967), 621. Also Margaret Pelling, *Cholera, Fever*, 6–7. Michael Brown, however, does indeed note that Southwood Smith's articles were written largely in support of the anticontagionist Charles Maclean. See Brown, "From Foetid Air to Filth," 525.
[117] Hudson Gurney lampooned Smith as a "the most zealous" of Maclean's "co-adjutors." Quoted in McDonald, "History of Quarantine," 27.
[118] See Kerr, *Contagion, Isolation, and Biopolitics*, chapter 2.
[119] Papon, *De la Peste*, 2:19–20.
[120] Hansard, House of Commons Debate, March 25, 1825, c. 1216.

some quarantine fees remained, this represents the first time that the central government adopted the principle that, on a continuing basis (rather than for a particular epidemic), the community at large bore responsibility for the maintenance of good health. On top of this, Parliament had earmarked (between 1800 and 1810) around £150,000 for the building of the ill-fated Chetney Hill Lazaretto in Kent and authorized diverting money from the poor rate to sanitary reform in the 1832 Cholera Prevention Act. Granted, these were not the first public expenditures that went toward sanitation or health. It is certainly true that money from the poor rate had been devoted to communal health before – about half of all parishes had appointed a medical officer before 1834.[121] But the enduring principle that epidemic disease prevention necessitated an ongoing and permanent investment by the general community was a product of the early nineteenth century. The new expenditures were for a novel genre of health intervention: *national* health care rather than irregular care provided at the parish level.[122]

The post-1848 Public Health Act General Board of Health (GBH) itself employed the ambiguity of disease transmission to rely on the contagionist principle that the health of one impinges on the health of all even as its members considered environmental improvements to be the crucial determinants of health and the path to broader social good. As James Hanley has demonstrated, understandings of public benefit as a concept changed in the face of sanitarian agitation. In the mid-1850s, a legal precedent was set that local boards of health could rate households in the rough vicinity of proposed sewer lines (even if they were not to be connected to the new line), on the grounds that an "indirect benefit" would accrue to everyone in a district where the health was improving.[123] The ill health of one was a danger to all; epidemic disease provided a cord that linked the state of the most degraded sewers of the kingdom to the sanitary state of the whole. In their arguments about quarantine, the members of the GBH (particularly Southwood Smith and Gavin Milroy) developed a vision of sanitation explicitly in answer to the quarantine system's impulse toward separation and isolation. Much of the rage anticontagionist sanitary reformers seem to have felt against quarantine was down to its limited nature and ambition; to justify demolishing the lazaretto it was necessary to bring disinfection out into society and to expand its ambitions. The GBH considered an extraordinary range of issues: cholera epidemiology, drains,

---

[121] Hodgkinson, *Origins of the National Health Service*, 680.

[122] Ruth Hodgkinson finds important precedents for the expenditure of public money on healthcare in Jeremy Bentham's advocacy for a Minister of Health and a service of preventative medicine during the 1820s. But singling out these two thought experiments from other precedents obscures the fact that in the 1820s and earlier, the central government was *already* claiming a clear role in the maintenance of public health. See Hodgkinson, *Origins of the National Health Service*, 621.

[123] See Hanley, *Healthy Boundaries*, chapter 3.

cemeteries, cesspools, workhouse nutrition, and the salutary power of light in residences.[124]

At this point, deep into a history of public health reform in the 1840s and beyond, one might wonder how we can have gotten so far from Mediterranean quarantine. Yet, there is a deep affinity between the sanitarian idea that forgotten cemeteries, districts, and individuals could impinge on the health of the nation and the logic of quarantine – the sense that lazarettos could arrest germs in the clothing of obscure travelers who were returning to the body politic and thereby preserve the health of an entire nation (or continent). The British government had already endorsed the national importance of the health of certain individuals at least as early as 1825, when it held that it was the duty of taxpayers to finance (partially) the decontamination of ships at the border in the Quarantine Act. The form of the "board of health" as a function of urban administration derived from centuries of quarantine practice in the Mediterranean. Finally, the powers of action granted to local boards of health were grounded in arguments advanced during the quarantine-centric contagion debate. Bubonic plague as generic "pestilence" loomed over all discussions of the sanitary demerits of early Victorian Britain. If historians of public health have not emphasized the connection to long-standing debates about quarantine, the members of the new, post-1848 General Board of Health certainly did. One of the first major reports they produced (in 1849) was a critique of quarantine practice.[125] Positioning themselves within and against the tradition from which their role had sprung was an essential task of these new agents of sanitary bureaucracy.

The significance of this connection in terms of the history of public health reform is enormous. Public health was not an inevitable part of the "Condition of England" question, but it became so because of the threat of epidemic invasion. Inspired by a legacy of plague fighting, public health reformers attempted to locate the sources of insalubrity within that would allow invader diseases to take hold. As Britain positioned itself at the 1851 International Sanitary Conference as a supporter of looser quarantine requirements, the reformation of public health policies at home was a crucial piece of the puzzle. In this way, the 1848 Public Health Act was an international statement as well as a domestic one; to its authors, it said something about the sort of country Britain aspired to be.

---

[124] See, for example, General Board of Health, *Report of the General Board of Health on the Measures Adopted for the Nuisance Removal and Disease Prevention Act and the Public Health Act* (London: W. Clowes, 1849). Also General Board of Health, *Report of the General Board of Health on the Epidemic Cholera of 1848 and 1849* (London: W. Clowes, 1850).

[125] See General Board of Health, *Report on Quarantine* (London: W. Clowes, 1849). There was a *Second Report on Quarantine* in 1852, primarily devoted to quarantine's (in)utility for yellow fever. According to J. C. McDonald, the GBH also planned a report on the plague, but this never came to fruition. See McDonald, "History of Quarantine," 33.

Part IV

Old Patterns, New Cordons

8 Quarantine and Empire

Andrew White, a veteran of the Egyptian Campaign and Peninsular War, continued to serve the British government in the Mediterranean as the Empire expanded in the region after the Napoleonic conflagration. Having served as a medical inspector for the British military, White later rose through the ranks to become Deputy Inspector-General of Hospitals for the entire British Army. His *Treatise of the Plague* (1846) reflected back on what he viewed as perhaps the most significant event of his career: the plague of 1816 in the Ionian Islands. In the course of that epidemic, as one of the highest ranking doctors in imperial administration, White assumed the novel position of "Superintendent of the Plague," charged with eradicating the disease from the new colony. His treatise of three decades later ponders the singular challenge he faced in those circumstances:

There is this peculiarity in plague in which it differs from all other diseases, and, I had almost said, from everything in common life – that there is scarcely any circumstance connected with it which can be called trifling, or of no consequence. Matters which, to the eye of a common observer, merit little or no attention, are to those versed in the police management of the plague, fraught with the most important consequences.[1]

A proper plague superintendent, wrote White, must possess both indefatigable zeal and a capacity for cutting through the lies and evasions of those in infected districts. The requisite qualities were "patience, constant activity, unwearied perseverance, and a strong mind."[2]

White, in other words, felt himself to be the quintessential British imperial "man on the spot," whose unsentimental attitude to "plague police"[3] (plague policy) succeeded in containing the epidemic of 1816. Given what he saw as the natural duplicity of his colonial charges, White complained that it was "a very difficult matter during an attack of plague to get at the real truth of many circumstances which occur."[4] He found himself very much up to the task, and

---

[1] White, *Treatise on the Plague*, 41.   [2] Ibid., 41.
[3] Although this phrase might sound especially ominous to modern ears, it was relatively widely used in the first half of the nineteenth century to mean any policy of action related to the plague.
[4] White, *Treatise on the Plague*, 15–16.

having performed successfully during his time in Corfu, White conceived his treatise as source-text for those imperial bureaucrats confronting similar circumstances elsewhere in Britain's empire. In short, he appeared to view the problem of plague management as an encapsulation of imperial government itself. Power and knowledge fused in the plague superintendent's arsenal; there was no local detail or piece of gossip in which his office should not be interested. The free rein of sanitary administrators during an epidemic was, White held, essential to the rapid extinction of the plague.

I argued in the last chapter that Britain's own public health system owed much to the experience of (and arguments over) the Mediterranean quarantine system. As a global power, however, Britain's evolving policies on public health and the quarantine system cannot be examined without reference to the broader empire. What consequences did Britain's participation in Mediterranean quarantine have on imperial policies regarding disease control? If the patterns, precedents, and arguments surrounding quarantine helped shape the response to epidemic disease in the metropole, did they do the same in the colonies? To what extent was plague management associated with imperial power, and how does this connection help us understand the ideological implications of contagionism and anticontagionism? These are my questions here.

A first and indispensable recognition is that the sanitary relationship between Britain and its Empire was reciprocal. It was, after all, primarily in imperial spaces that British administrators contended with yellow fever and plague. Cholera, the last of the epidemic triumvirate, first became epidemic in Bengal under the auspices of the British Empire, and Anglo-Indian doctors achieved significant recognition as authorities on that disease as it menaced Western Europe.

It is impossible to conceive of the entire Empire as one sanitary space, but it is certainly possible to chart striking continuities within it. As David Arnold has shown, over the course of the eighteenth century, there arose a growing tendency to see tropical imperial landscapes as "deathscapes."[5] This is the period in which British imperial control expanded inward from coastal enclaves in India and parts of Africa, when political economists and slave traders confronted the extreme mortality experienced on the Gold Coast, and when planters and enslaved people first began to die in large numbers from yellow fever in the Caribbean. The expansion of imperial territory resulted in an impulse to understand, record, and control a colonial environment largely considered to be biologically threatening; Arnold explores the genre of "medical topography," which flourished in the late eighteenth and early nineteenth centuries.[6] Medical topographies were essentially geographical compendia,

---

[5] David Arnold, *Tropics and the Traveling Gaze*, 42.   [6] Arnold, *Colonizing the Body*, 21.

which chronicled types of landscape and weather patterns with reference to their medical ramifications.

Such work sought to make unfamiliar landscapes comprehensible in terms Britons could understand and make use of. And yet, the impulse to tame the landscape and render it familiar coexisted with a new way of conceiving imperial health, in which tropical, colonial spaces became sanitary units in their own right, subject to invasions from the outside world and in need of protection – not simply "a land of encircling death" for white Britons.[7] It is little surprise that after a decade in which "medical topographies" peaked as a genre (particularly topographies of India), we see an expansion of the impulse to impose quarantines.

The dilemmas the British and French faced in considering the issue of colonial quarantine impinged on broader questions within the imperial project. To the extent that Europeans paid more than lip service to the nature of their "civilizing mission," the amelioration of a colony's sanitary state was a potential point of demonstration, at least in principle. Yet, to the extent that colonies were naked expressions of economic acquisitiveness (and quarantine impeded commerce), imperial public health projects consistently ran up against unique limitations of motivation and perceived expense. They could also be a focus of major discontent; the coercive British practices deployed to regulate the plague in colonial Bombay during the third plague pandemic in the 1890s inspired significant anticolonial agitation, such as the assassination of W. C. Rand, Plague Commissioner of Pune, in 1897.[8]

Earlier in the nineteenth century, we see a mixed picture of both coercion and neglect in matters of public health; plague is an imperfect, but consistent dividing line between those two impulses. Furthermore, imperial practice contained symmetries with both contagionist and anticontagionist approaches to disease. When it came to plague, British imperial power served as a vehicle for spreading Mediterranean quarantine practice across the globe, but, particularly with other diseases, imperial officials sometimes hesitated to introduce full-scale quarantine in colonies. Quarantine's tendency to discriminate, divide, and sequester certainly went together with many imperial techniques. It was far easier to order a massive internal cordon around a city or to force the removal of sick people to isolation hospitals in an imperial context than it was in Britain itself. Across the imperial world and throughout the nineteenth century, the

[7] The phrase comes from Arnold, *Tropics and Traveling Gaze*, 42.
[8] On coercive practices and the Indian response during the third plague pandemic, see Rajnarayan Chandavarkar, "Plague Panic and Epidemic Politics in India, 1896–1916," in *Epidemics and Ideas*, ed. Terence Ranger and Paul Slack (Cambridge: Cambridge University Press, 1992); David Arnold, "Touching the Body: Perspectives on the Indian Plague," in *Selected Subaltern Studies*, ed. Ranajit Guha and Gayatri Chakravorty Spivak (Oxford: Oxford University Press, 1988); Arnold, *Colonizing the Body*, chapter 5.

presence of plague triggered an automatic assumption that quarantine was the appropriate response.

Yet, in many ways, the anticontagionism of quarantine's opponents was most closely aligned with imperial ambition. It was far easier and more palatable to blame an epidemic on the "filthy" living conditions of imperial subjects than it was to accept responsibility for spreading (or stopping) contagions that were not the responsibility of indigenous people. If quarantine imposed a geography of health and disease that classified Western European nations as healthy and "Eastern" spaces as diseased, the act of colonial appropriation itself appeared to some Europeans as a hygienic boon (Figure 8.1). The anticontagionist rhetoric of demolishing a fetishistic belief in contagion runs together with an imperial discourse of "enlightening" colonized peoples,[9] a point made palpably by Antoine Gros's famous 1804 depiction of the moment when Bonaparte supposedly touched plague victims during his invasion of Syria. A belief in

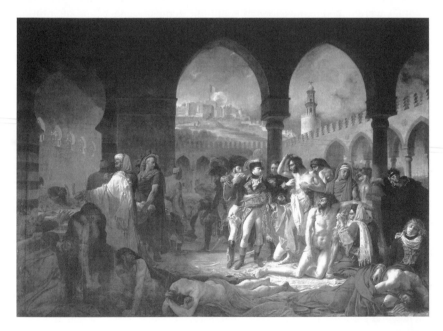

Figure 8.1 Antoine Gros, *Bonaparte Touching the Plague Victims of Jaffa*, 1804. Oil on canvas. Louvre Museum, Paris.

[9] Shula Marks aptly sums up the justification for imperial medical practices by their evangelists as "the triumph of science and sewers over savagery and superstition." See Shula Marks, "What Is Colonial about Colonial Medicine? And What Has Happened to Imperialism and Health?," *Social History of Medicine* 10, no. 2 (1997): 205.

contagion, fear of the plague, and the supposed credulity of colonized peoples are visually united. Here, then, the most famous builder of empires is the most memorable icon of anticontagionism.

European empires in the nineteenth century were epidemiologically complex; it is entirely beyond the scope of a single chapter (or book) to address the manifold efforts to contain epidemic disease within them. Rather than a synoptic analysis of all forms of imperial isolation, here we explore in broad terms the ramifications of the "European sanitary system" on the imperial periphery and simultaneously consider how actual efforts to contain epidemic diseases when they occurred around the Empire shed light on the broader history of quarantine. Overall, I argue that Mediterranean practice and precedent dominated imperial thinking about the plague elsewhere in the British world, and that the competing traditions of anticontagionist and contagionist views of epidemic disease created persistent tensions as imperial officials sought order first and sanitation second.

Epidemic Administrators in Mediterranean Colonies

Officials from France and Britain - Western Europe's two major expanding imperial powers in the first half of the nineteenth century – encountered epidemic disease intimately, even as most individuals in the metropole saw it as a foreign threat. The logic of quarantine suggested that rigorous procedures could guarantee immunity, that countries could secure their interior by policing their border. But growing imperial commitments – often on the "wrong side" of the *cordon sanitaire* – challenged a global dichotomy of "healthy" and "sick" countries. European colonies in the Caribbean suffered some of the highest yellow fever rates in the world. British and French generals in Egypt, between 1798 and 1807, had to contend with plague outbreaks among their troops. British doctors confronted cholera's first transformation into a fast spreading epidemic in Bengal in the 1810s. Finally, Britain's Mediterranean Empire, augmented by the Napoleonic Wars, fell under immediate sanitary stress as the nineteenth century dawned – from Gibraltar's yellow fever epidemic in 1805, to the plagues of Malta (1813–14) and the Ionian Islands (1816). These imperial encounters transformed dread diseases – cholera, yellow fever, and plague – from hypothetical enemies into intimate foes. Administrators were often caught flat-footed, and it is in just such a position that we find the fledgling colonial administration in Malta in the spring of 1813.

As with many epidemics, origins are difficult to ascertain. The most common explanation for the arrival of plague in Malta involves the reception of a Maltese brig (variously called *The San Nicola* or *San Niccolo*), sailing from Alexandria under a British flag. After arrival in Malta's quarantine harbor in early April 1813, it was revealed that two crew members had died *en route*, and numerous others had fallen ill. The ship was ordered to sit dormant in the harbor while the sanitary authorities deliberated, and after some days, it was ordered to depart again. By the end of the month, however, the plague emerged in the house of a shoemaker in Valletta and proceeded to spread rapidly around the island.

Making matters more difficult, this epidemic arrived not only while the Napoleonic Wars were still raging, but at a time of protracted upheaval within Malta's sanitary bureaucracy. The colony's first Superintendent of Quarantine under British rule, William Eton, had been appointed in 1801 after personally writing to Britain's war leaders to tout his experience in observing European lazarettos.[10] Eton attempted to restore order to Malta's sanitary administration,[11] yet quickly became embroiled in political intrigues. Caught scheming with Vincenzo Borg, a Maltese individual who opposed the British administration, Eton retreated to England on indefinite sick leave.[12] During this period, the remnants of the Health Office that had governed the Lazaretto of Malta under the Knights of St. John, occasionally assisted by a temporary board of health composed of British administrators, ensured the quarantine laws never totally lapsed. Yet, even if this arrangement had preserved Malta from epidemics so far, suggested a British administrator in 1810, it was far from perfect.[13] Eventually Sir William Pym was dispatched to succeed Eton. His service in Malta, however, amounted to only a few months before he, too, left the islands.[14] By the time the plague broke out in Valletta, then, Malta had no resident Superintendent of Quarantine, no clear center of authority in sanitary measures, and a murky bureaucratic chain of command.

How was it that the plague had apparently jumped from a brig sitting in the quarantine harbor to the house of a shoemaker in Malta's capital? The clearest answer has been the suggestion that Salvatore Borg was either a smuggler himself or a receiver of goods smuggled off the ship by lazaretto guardians.[15] A popular story contained the ostensibly damning piece of evidence that Borg's last words as he died on May 4 from the plague were "Oh the linen, the linen!"[16] On May 5, confronting rumors that the plague had broken out, the British government published a proclamation declaring that the remaining

---

[10] See Lord Hobart to Charles Cameron, May 14, 1801, NAM 2/1/1.

[11] See, for example, the letters of William Eton to Count Marchesi, July 8, July 10, and July 14, NLM LIBR 845.

[12] Despite his absence, Eton apparently continued to draw his £800 salary until 1810. See Hildebrand Oakes to Lord Liverpool, October 15, 1810, NAM GOV 1/1/7. John Booker notes that some have considered Eton to have been a Russian spy. See Booker, *Maritime Quarantine*, 335.

[13] See Oakes to Liverpool, October 15, 1810, NAM GOV 1/1/7.

[14] See Oakes to Liverpool, May 1, 1812, NAM GOV 1/1/7. Pym went on to become Superintendent of Quarantine for the entire UK, as we have already seen.

[15] See Cassar, *Medical History of Malta*, 175–80.

[16] See "Bulard, Clot-Bey, &c.," *British and Foreign Medical Review*, 292.

members of the Borg family had been removed to the lazaretto and that any possible epidemic had been curtailed.[17] This, it quickly turned out, was false optimism. Only two days later, more deaths had already occurred, and as May wore on, the government began to publish ever longer daily lists of those who had died from the plague.

Officials struggled to impose order. "First: That any person who shall change his place of residence, without special permission from the Council of Health . . . shall be liable to the punishment of Death." So began a proclamation issued by Hildebrand Oakes, the beleaguered Civil Commissioner for Malta, at the height of the epidemic.[18] Eight other (ordinarily reasonable) activities were deemed capital offenses in the same order. Initial measures had been milder, including the closing of shops after the early evening and a general curfew each night. In late May, officials escalated their demands in the face of widespread flouting of the rules and alarmingly high death tallies.[19] Because of the difficulty of finding corpse-carriers after the plague reached epidemic proportions (with hundreds dying each week during June, July, and August), convicts were pressed into this service. Dressed in sheets and hoods in a costume apparently drawn from a popular account of the 1720 Marseille plague, the convicts sowed widespread terror, and many of them were accused of raping and pillaging despite promises of military supervision.[20] In the end, so many of these convicts died from the plague that more were imported from Sicily. By the height of the summer, at least one hundred individuals were dying every day as the disease spread across the island (Figure 8.2).

Serious disagreements between Hildebrand Oakes (the Civil Commissioner) and a temporary board of health arose over the stringency of procedures. This can be seen in a confusing array of proclamations ordering different forms and passes to be carried by the population. Frustrated officials in Valletta responded desperately to the ensuing chaos: "All passes of whatever description," they decreed on July 11, "which have been hitherto issued shall cease to be valid from Wednesday evening next, the 14th instant."[21] Instead, individuals with a license to move would be marked by a red scarf worn on their right arms (mystifyingly, the government considered this device harder to counterfeit than a pass).

By the beginning of August, in another public proclamation, the government admitted that attempts to govern the movement of the Maltese population had failed to address "the fatal progress of the plague." Consequently, they ordered "the general and absolute retirement" of all citizens of Valletta and Floriana.[22] In

[17] See Proclamation by F. Laing, May 5, 1813, NAM GMR 01.
[18] "Notificazione: August 1, 1813," NAM GMR 02.
[19] "Notificazione: May 29, 1813," NAM GMR 01.
[20] See Cassar, *Medical History of Malta*, 183.   [21] Proclamation, July 11, 1813, NAM GMR 01.
[22] Proclamation, August 2, 1813, NAM GMR 02. Valletta is Malta's capital, and Floriana is a dense suburb just outside Valletta's gates.

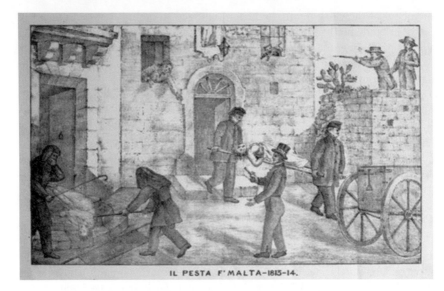

IL PESTA F'MALTA-1813-14.

Figure 8.2 Engraving showing the chaotic impact of the plague in Malta during 1813 and 1814. Courtesy of the *Times of Malta*.

the end, the arrival of Sir Thomas Maitland as the first official Governor of Malta in the fall of 1813 coincided with the beginning of the epidemic's extinction. Maitland ordered the entire population of all suspected districts to withdraw to specially constructed military encampments in the center of the island until the disease ended. Though it now appears the worst was already over, at the time, Maitland's actions were considered to be responsible for the end of the plague.[23]

Over the course of the epidemic, then, there was a clear move toward greater severity. Officials shifted from optimism that the disease could be eradicated with minimal disruption to the grim certainty involved in uprooting individuals from their normal lives. It is clear that during the time of the plague, the logic and vocabulary of quarantine was turned inward to the resident population of Malta. Passes, clothing, and badges signified the right to move; letters, money, and goods were passed through fumigating agents. In essence, the island was converted into a giant lazaretto, not least when most of its citizens were forced to perform lengthy quarantines in tents to achieve the final eradication of the disease.

The response to the Maltese plague was influenced by past British procedure; many of the elements of the 1805 Board of Health's plan for a plague-stricken

---

[23] Maitland's plague procedures also helped to create his reputation for high-handed government that made him into a polarizing figure on Malta and earned him the nickname "King Tom."

Britain were enacted in Malta, including the division of the island into "districts" and the appointment of teams of magistrates and constables to enforce order and obtain information. The devastating legacy of plague in Malta and the perplexing administrative issues it evoked, in turn, rebounded back to the metropole. Again, the plague of Malta became a recurrent point of reference in debates about the quarantine laws of Britain itself.[24] As we will see later in this chapter, it was also a central precedent for colonial officials in India attempting to respond to plague there.

The 1816 plague in Corfu and Cephalonia added a further dimension to the British experience with epidemic disease; it was particularly difficult to control an epidemic during a time of political unrest. Plague arrived in Corfu in the midst of a two-year period of constitution-drafting. In one of the more unusual arrangements imposed by the Congress of Vienna, Britain had been granted the Ionian Islands as a protectorate, though they were simultaneously considered to be an independent state. In 1815, Thomas Maitland, still the Governor of Malta, was given the additional title of "Lord High Commissioner of the United States of the Ionian Islands" and immediately set about drafting a constitution that retained most of the power in the hands of the British administration.[25] This constitution was finalized in 1817, meaning its production coincided with the arrival of the plague.

As we saw at the beginning of this chapter, Andrew White prided himself on his reliance on empiricism and practicality, in keeping with the military-medical tradition from which he emerged.[26] Plague policy, he wrote in his memoirs, needed to be vigorous: "It is an established maxim in the police treatment of plague that half measures will never exterminate this dreadful enemy. The snake may be scotched, but not killed. The road is straight-forward, and we must not deviate from it."[27] Following the example Maitland had set on Malta, White ordered the removal of suspected individuals to remote encampments and the rigid separation of the population into groups of "positively diseased," "highly suspicious," "simply suspected," and "under observation."[28] But at every point, he found his orders confounded by

---

[24] See Granville, *Letter to Robinson*, 19. Also John Hennen, *Sketches of the Medical Topography of the Mediterranean: Comprising an Account of Gibraltar, the Ionian Islands, and Malta* (London: T. and G. Underwood, 1830), 632–37. For both, the plague of Malta is a prime example of the efficacy of quarantine measures and the basic truth of the contagious theory of epidemic disease. For a more skeptical take on the role of isolation in ending the epidemic, see Milroy, *Quarantine and the Plague*, 71. Well into the 1850s, the plague of Malta continued to be a central bone of contention in debates about quarantine. See T. Spencer Wells, "On the Practical Results of Quarantine," *Association Medical Journal* 2, no. 89 (1854): 231.

[25] See Thomas Gallant, *Experiencing Dominion: Culture, Identity, and Power in the British Mediterranean* (Notre Dame, IN: University of Notre Dame Press, 2002), 7–8.

[26] White is a classic example of the "military medical officer" described by Catherine Kelly in *War and the Militarization of British Army Medicine*.

[27] White, *Treatise on the Plague*, 16.   [28] Ibid., 19.

individuals concealing their illness or refusing to give full information to medical inspectors. Unlike at Malta, where the propensity for rule-breaking was ascribed to a Maltese reluctance to take the epidemic seriously, White attributed the failure to follow the protocols to the willful political machinations of "wicked Lechfimists." The residents of the town of Lefkimi, ran the suggestion, were incessantly conspiring, often for reasons of "ill-will" or "party." It thus appears that agitation against encroaching British authority led to a lack of cooperation on the part of the population. The social dissolution inherent in a time of plague allowed, here at least, for an early form of anticolonial agitation to take root. Particularly in this kind of imperial plague management, complained White, "it is a very difficult matter . . . to get at the real truth of many circumstances which occur."[29] His partial (and brutal) solution was to order those who gave incorrect reports of the disease into quarantine with actually diseased individuals.

In Malta and the Ionian Islands, then, a number of British administrators confronted plague epidemics during a formative period of public health policy. When we set them alongside the military officials who had to manage the health of British armies fighting the French in Egypt, when plague was rife, we begin to realize just how frequently a disease that might seem like a premodern fable was a modern and recurrent problem for early nineteenth-century officialdom. As politicians and sanitary campaigners discussed public health policy in the 1830s and 1840s, this history of colonial plague control was of central concern, with the episode of Malta's epidemic often taken as a recent object lesson. As we see in the next section, the attempt to resist disease in the Mediterranean helped to disseminate the logic of quarantine around the British imperial world.

Fighting the Plague in Mid-Nineteenth-Century British India

The management of the plague in Britain's smallest colonies (Malta and Corfu) shaped the response to the disease in India, its largest. This section considers how the control of imperial subjects during Mediterranean epidemics intersects with administrative techniques in vast territories where the spread of disease seemed to be beyond the capacity of British medical care. As in the Mediterranean and in Britain itself, we see a variety of expedients built upon a distinction fashioned (and contested) between epidemic diseases and "normal" ill health, and also upon a history of imperial medicine, which gradually tended to fuse an impulse to quarantine and a campaign to sanitize. We can consider India as a test case of British approaches far beyond the watchful gaze of European diplomats committed to the maintenance of the "European Sanitary System" in the Mediterranean. If the practice in ports like Liverpool

---

[29] Ibid., 15.

was enough to provoke a Continent-wide quarantine on British ships in 1825 (as we saw in Chapter 5), India was not part of the sphere of concern. And yet, even as skepticism about the Mediterranean system mounted in the 1830s and later, British officials were ever ready to use quarantine as a tool to prevent the spread of plague across the Indian subcontinent. Indeed, though he deploys the term in a different context, John Chircop's suggestive idea of the Mediterranean as "Europe's imperial medical archive" is extremely pertinent here;[30] Anglo-Indian officials were eager to learn from Mediterranean experience.

A central issue of concern was whether an outbreak should be considered "a local fever of extreme malignity, or whether it is a *plague*, the spread of which may justly be dreaded."[31] Accordingly, on an occasion when an outbreak's identity was under dispute, an official who resisted the diagnosis of plague concluded that "with such views ... it does not fall to me to propose or recommend any strict quarantine regulations or cordons, which would be indispensable in the case of contagious plague."[32] Thus, while officials occasionally took pains to classify certain outbreaks as extreme forms of typhus rather than the plague, there is evidence of an implicit acceptance of the clear link between the plague and quarantine. The above statement – indicating that quarantine would be required in any plague epidemic – was written in India only a year after the sanitationist luminaries of the metropolitan General Board of Health published their *Report on Quarantine*, denying the utility of the practice *even* in the case of plague.

The intersection between Mediterranean precedents and Indian practice can be seen most clearly when it comes to medicine along the coast. In 1832, a decade after plague outbreaks had apparently ceased to move across the islands of the Mediterranean, a gruesome and devastating epidemic developed in the south of what is now Iran. The British-controlled trading port of Bushire, an *entrepôt* for much of Britain's India trade and the seat of an East India Company office, was particularly hard-hit.[33] On receiving the news from the crew of a recently arrived brig, officials at Bombay Castle resolved that they would establish a lazaretto, make provision for a floating "pest hospital" in the

---

[30] John Chircop, "Quarantine, Sanitization, Colonialism and the Construction of the 'Contagious Arab' in the Mediterranean, 1830s–1900," in Chircop and Martínez, *Mediterranean Quarantines*, 210.

[31] J. H. Batton to J. Thornton, January 1, 1850. Quoted in C. Renny, *Medical Report on the Mahamurree in Gurhwal, in 1849–50* (Agra: Secundra Orphan Press, 1851), 39.

[32] Renny, *Medical Report*, 20.

[33] At least 40,000 people died of plague in this epidemic. In 1877, as plague once again menaced western Iran, the devastating toll of the 1832 Bushire epidemic was discussed as a precedent for the need for a government response. See Firoozeh Kashani-Sabet, "'City of the Dead': The Frontier Polemics of Quarantines in the Ottoman Empire and Iran," *Comparative Studies of South Asia, Africa and the Middle East* 18, no. 2 (1998): 51–58.

case of positive disease, and in all ways apply "the Malta quarantine rules to this Presidency."[34] The government resolved to write to the Maltese government to obtain a formal list of said rules as early as possible (a copy was duly received in the course of the summer).[35] Prior to the arrival of those rules, it was discovered that a Lieutenant Haines, then serving in Bombay with the Indian Navy, would "be able to give much information on the subject, as he passed his Quarantine in the Lazaretto of Malta, and made those observations on the Manner of Conducting the duties which will be found very useful in the arrangement now required."[36] British administrators were so enthusiastic that someone in their midst had first-hand experience of Mediterranean quarantine that it was suggested that Haines should either serve on a new extraordinary Quarantine Committee or superintend the entire response.[37] This episode demonstrates the extent to which Mediterranean procedures were widely acknowledged to be the "gold standard" of epidemic control. Furthermore, the imperial link between Malta and India allowed the rituals of Mediterranean quarantine to spread around the world – not simply by the exchange of paper, but by the fact that the same people often served in different corners of the British Empire.

Throughout the plague of Bushire, East India Company officials at the Navy Board, the Marine Board, and the Governor's office closely coordinated their response. "Any expence [*sic*]" was to be considered acceptable given the extraordinary threat and the need "to protect the millions under our rule from the ravages of this horrible pestilence."[38] Once the disease reached India, administrators feared its progress would become unstoppable. For this reason, Charles Malcolm, the Superintendent of the Navy, recommended a "positive interdiction of all trade with the [Persian] Gulf." Without this, Malcolm wrote, "I see no possibility of keeping the evil off, as hundreds of boats from that quarter annually frequent our habours and posts."[39] As the summer wore on, few ships even made the trip, but at least one brig was burned on the orders of the hastily configured board of health. On this occasion, Lord Clare conceded that the board should have applied for special permission but deemed the action to be justified "even if illegal." This, because "it would be better for Government to be subject to the cost of damages than to run the risk of bringing the Plague into this country."[40] If quarantine administrators in Western Europe

[34] Colin Halket, William Newnham, and James Southerland to the East India Company Court of Directors, June 12, 1832, BL IOR F/4/1350/53605.
[35] Minute by Lord Clare, apparently June 15, 1832, BL IOR F/4/1350/53605.
[36] Charles Malcolm to Lord Clare, June 13, 1832, BL IOR F/4/1350/53605.
[37] See L. R. Reid to the Supt. of the Navy, June 15, 1832, BL IOR F/4/1350/53605.
[38] Halket, Newnham, and Southerland to the East India Company Directors, June 12, 1832, BL IOR F/4/1350/53605.
[39] Charles Malcolm to Lord Clare, June 13, 1832, BL IOR F/4/1350/53605.
[40] Minute by Lord Clare, July 2, 1832, BL IOR F/4/1350/53605.

feared the vocal mercantile lobby and the moderating impulses of central governments, imperial administrators faced fewer obstacles in ordering draconian plague-fighting techniques. If we view plague as a problem of disorder, it is clear why officials like Clare would consider "the cost of damages" so insignificant in comparison with the actual arrival of an epidemic.[41]

Furthermore, British administrators in the Bombay Presidency saw their front-line role as conveying a responsibility to warn different coastal governments throughout the Indian subcontinent. "It is peculiarly incumbent on the Bombay Government," wrote Clare, "to issue strict rules and regulations to guard the country against the invasion of this Terrible Foe as all the other Governments of the Country will naturally look to us from our proximity to the Persian Gulf."[42] He further suggested that all medical reports received from the Persian Gulf should be forwarded to "The Governments of Bengal, Madras, Ceylon, and the Portuguese Government" with the eventual regulations also sent to "the Dutch and all other states" so that an India-wide quarantine might effectively be achieved.[43] Even in the patchwork of states that made up early nineteenth-century India, the threat of epidemic disease pushed officials toward cooperation. The medical logic of quarantine demanded a shared approach, and the umbrella of the British Empire allowed the patterns, rules, and instincts of Mediterranean quarantine to move quickly to India. Either through their efficacy or by sheer luck, the plague of Bushire did not cross the Arabian Sea.

As British officials slowly realized, however, the plague *already existed* as a slow-burning endemic disease deeper in the subcontinent's interior: both in sporadic outbreaks in Rajasthan and in recurrent epidemics in mountain villages in the Himalayas. Unsurprisingly, the uneven approach British administrators took to these small epidemics was entangled within the broader history of imperialism in India; prior to the 1830s, the diseases were largely ignored. Yet once they were "rediscovered" (for a variety of reasons, as we will see below), British officials and Indian doctors again connected the epidemics to plague in the Middle East, and again, they relied on Mediterranean precedent to confront them.

Initial lack of interest played a role in a long-delayed British response to these outbreaks, but so did the fact that the identity of the diseases remained in doubt for a number of years. During a limited series of outbreaks in Kutch and Kathiawar beginning in the 1810s, reports suggested that some of the infected

---

[41] That said, as Aparna Nair has shown, the impulses of British officialdom during the (less pressing) 1802 plague panic surrounding British and Indian troops traveling to India from Egypt were considerably more relaxed, and the very limited quarantines that were introduced then were only partially applied. See Aparna Nair, "An Egyptian Infection: War, Plague, and the Quarantines of the English East India Company at Madras and Bombay, 1802," *Hygiea Internationalis* 8, no. 1 (2009): 7–29.

[42] Minute by Lord Clare, June 12, 1832, BL IOR F/4/1350/53605.   [43] Ibid.

exhibited swollen glands and rashes around the groin. This account left many convinced that the disease was plague.[44] Although the fever had a high mortality and a rapid diffusion (moving as far as Sindh before vanishing), it did not prompt significant action by East India Company officials. Given that it occurred after a three-year famine and in areas relatively far from Company control, it was easy to ignore.[45]

Yet, the apparent unconcern melted away when epidemics occurred closer to the frontiers of the expanding British presence in northwest India. Another contagious fever broke out in 1836, in the Rajasthani city of Pali, which featured high mortality and glandular swelling. From Pali, it quickly spread to the larger city of Jodhpur, from which it spread even further. Given that this disease appeared to be moving far more rapidly than previous epidemics and smoldered only miles from the small East India Company province of Ajmere (Ajmer), British officials were much more alarmed. Although James Ranken, the author of an official report on the Pali epidemic, doubted that the disease was plague, he noted that this was unequivocally the impression of the administrators who responded to it: "Medical Officers ascertained it to be infectious, and considered it to be plague."[46]

British pressure induced local elites to cooperate with the East India Company and to enforce major barriers to trade and travel from areas that might potentially have been infected.[47] Many observers immediately identified the disease with Mediterranean epidemics past and present, calling it "the contagious plague of Egypt"[48] or "the plague of Egypt and Malta."[49] A skeptical James Ranken criticized this widespread assumption but noted that it formed the clear basis for the initial plan at the higher levels of the British administration. Sir Charles Metcalfe, the Lieutenant-Governor of the Northwest Provinces, Ranken suggested, relied fully on Maltese precedents, as he "seems to have taken for his guide Sir Thomas Maitland's regulations, and Mr. Tully's account of their practical efficacy, in excluding or extinguishing Plague in the Mediterranean islands."[50] Ranken criticized Metcalfe's plan as a misguided "modification of arrangements which had proved so

---

[44]   David Arnold suggests this was more likely to have been typhus to plague, in contrast to later epidemics of *mahamari*. Arnold, *Colonizing the Body*, 313.

[45]   See C. R. Francis, "Endemic Plague in India," *Transactions of the Epidemiological Society of London* 4 (1881): 407. Also Frederick Forbes, *Thesis on the Nature and History of the Plague as Observed in the North Western Provinces of India* (Edinburgh: Maclachlan, Stewart, and Co., 1840), 1–2.

[46]   James Ranken, *Report on the Malignant Fever Called the Pali Plague* (Calcutta: Bengal Military Orphan Press, 1838), 1.

[47]   "The Lieutenant Governor of the North Western Provinces of Bengal enjoined the Princes of Joudpore and Oudeypore [*sic*] to prevent the spread of the disease by blockading the places belonging to them in which it prevailed." Ibid., 2.

[48]   Renny, *Medical Report*, 13.   [49]   Ranken, *Report on the Malignant Fever*, 5.   [50]   Ibid., 7.

successful in insular situations ... made applicable to a continental country divided only by arbitrary boundaries."[51] Nevertheless, in the Northwest Provinces and across India, the Maltese precedent continued to appear as the gold standard.

During the Pali epidemic, the connection to the Mediterranean was heightened by the belief that not only was this disease *identical* to the plague of Egypt, but that it literally might be the same epidemic then raging there (Egypt experienced its last major plague epidemic in 1835–36). Because cloth-printers were among the first groups to be struck by the Pali Plague, a theory emerged that bales of cotton imported to India from Egypt had carried the disease with them. One author raised the persuasive objection that it was unlikely for such bales to have passed through the port of Bombay without spreading the plague, only to do so in the far more remote terrain of Pali.[52] That said, the possibility was impossible to discard entirely, and no doubt the sense that the plague could be directly tied to the devastating epidemic then ravaging Egypt added to the urgency of containing it in 1836.

As the map in Figure 8.3 shows, the quarantines set up both by British administrators and Indian Princes were extremely ambitious undertakings involving large numbers of troops. And despite his (minority) belief that the disease was not the plague, James Ranken came to consider the massive, quarantinist response to have been the *responsibility* of a government convinced the disease they were dealing with was the famed plague of the Levant, the "greatest scourge of mankind." "The same principle," Ranken wrote, "which would require [a] functionary to order a man suspected of murder to be apprehended and detained for examination, must have actuated him in treating the epidemic as Levantine Plague, until it proved of a different character."[53] A suspicious disease, this logic ran, should be treated guilty until proven innocent. Even for Ranken, quarantine appeared to be the natural approach to "Levantine Plague."

That said, the practical responses undertaken by British authorities very much depended on the scale of the perceived threat and the ambitions of the local administrators in the zone of disease. The extreme mobilization of military cordons, disinfection stations, and goods inspectors during the 1836 Pali Plague stands in contrast not only to the potential plague outbreaks in Kutch and Kathiawar between 1815 and 1821 but also to the cholera epidemics of the 1810s, which British imperialism clearly had a role in spreading, but which provoked no large-scale quarantines in India. Such selective attention continued as the years

[51] Ibid., 7.   [52] Francis, "Endemic Plague in India," 408–9.
[53] Ranken, *Report on the Malignant Fever*, 21.

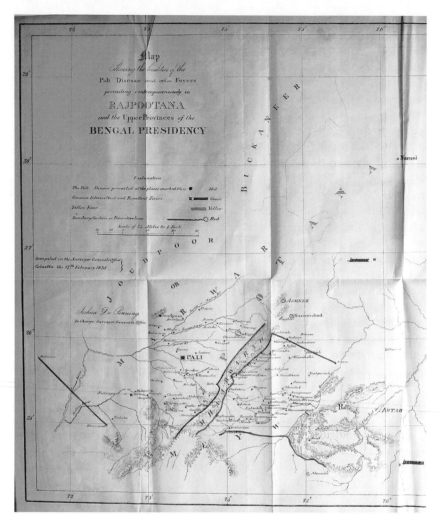

Figure 8.3 James Ranken's map of military quarantines imposed during the 1836 plague epidemic in Pali. Courtesy of the Wellcome Library. (CC BY License).

went on. It is worth noting that just as the presence of bubonic plague appeared to justify unprecedented scale and organization of temporary public health infrastructure, the presence of plague in sites along the frontiers of British control may also explain administrators' willingness to endorse massive quarantines. As Alan Lester has argued, especially within imperial frontier regions, panic could often serve a strategic purpose to "render uncertain zones of sovereignty on colonial frontiers more solid."[54] These plague panics were probably not strategically planned, but perhaps they felt particularly easy to succumb to, as the combination of plague and imperial borderlands formed a potent intersection between two varieties of anxiety.

Apparently, it was in the same year as the Pali Plague (1836) that British officials first became aware of epidemic outbreaks in an entirely different region of Northern India: Himalayan villages in the area of Garhwal. This disease, known locally as *mahamari* ("great death"), was reputed to be highly fatal, and a connection with the plague was suspected. British observers appear to have been just interested enough in 1836 to file an official report, but no other action was taken. As the medical officer C. R. Francis reported later in the century, it was only in 1849 that the government was provoked to investigate further: "so severe had [the disease] now become, that the inhabitants were fleeing from their homes in terror, and the annual revenue was not forthcoming."[55] Interest in the disease was thus based at least in part on a sense that plague was only a problem when isolated deaths turned into financial loss for the East India Company. At the same time, there was a fear that this plague might descend from the heights of the Himalayas and spread desolation throughout British India. As the commissioner of Kumaon ominously warned the Secretary to the Government of the North West Provinces in January 1850, "the plague is undoubtedly coming lower and lower every year."[56]

The twin fears of lost revenue and lost lives were enough to provoke action, and the medical officer Charles Renny was sent to the mountain villages where *mahamari* had struck hardest to examine its nature and make a full report. Like Ranken's interpretation of the disease that hit Pali, Renny took pains to emphasize his opinion that *mahamurree* (as he called it) was not the plague. Interestingly, he justified this through strict contagionism; having treated patients with the disease and emerged unscathed, he concluded it could not be the plague. In addition, he wrote, the temperature in the mountain villages was colder than those at "which it is known that the plague is destroyed or suspended in Europe and Africa."[57] Renny adopted a miasmatist explanation for the disease, blaming the filth, poverty, and poor diets of the Garhwali villagers for their susceptibility to the "infectious" (though not contagious) distemper. Renny's opinion that *mahamari* was not the plague was shared by almost no one else at the time and was dismissed by later writers in favor of an

---

[54] See Alan Lester, "Empire and the Place of Panic," in *Empires of Panic: Epidemics and Colonial Anxieties*, ed. Robert Peckham (Hong Kong: Hong Kong University Press, 2015), 25.

[55] Francis, "Endemic Plague in India," 396.

[56] J. H. Batton to J. Thornton, January 1, 1850. Quoted in Renny, *Medical Report*, 37.

[57] Renny, *Medical Report*, 12 and 14–15.

official line that the disease was identical with the plague of the Middle East and Mediterranean. To Renny, despite its high fever and the buboes on its sufferers, the disease more closely resembled British typhus than Egyptian plague (two diseases, we should recall, that Thomas Southwood Smith had suggested were essentially identical). During an 1847 British typhus epidemic, Renny noted, "glandular enlargements and chronic abscesses" were widespread, and there was no reason, necessarily, to view them as proof of plague.[58]

Nevertheless, the official recommendations he wrote reflected both contagionist and anticontagionist influences. "The first obvious means of counteracting the spread of sickness," he declared, "would be the removal of the sick instantly from the healthy."[59] Renny went on to recommend the disinfection of homes (in many cases, by burning them and offering compensation), a more extreme version of actions contemplated by the General Board of Health in a metropolitan British context around the same time. Indeed, the language adopted by imperial officials evokes a sense of the same possibilities and limits assumed by advocates of sanitary reform in Britain. In comments on Renny's report, several eminent Anglo-Indian medical figures expressed a skepticism that the "inveterately filthy" habits of the Garhwalis could change in short order, but that "it appears to us that much may be done at once by a judicious exercise of authority to improve the construction of their houses, and to require the removal to a distance of the heaps of rotting filth that are allowed to accumulate at every door."[60] In this way, absent the strict partisanship of the contagion debate in Britain, Renny's blend of approaches is a good demonstration that the legacy of that debate was often a fusion of techniques advocated by contagionists and anticontagionists.

By the mid-nineteenth century, imperial policy in the face of epidemics came to constitute a clear medical tradition. Especially by the 1840s and 1850s, references to plagues managed by the British over the last fifty years (in particular, the plagues of Malta and Corfu) came to exceed references to ancient, historic, or foreign epidemics, a trend that enhanced the prestige of quarantine. Relying on this tradition provided clarity in response to the ambiguities posed by plague. As W. S. Stiven, a civil surgeon in the Moradabad district, complained, "all authors who have written on this topic, and their name is 'Legion,' agree in the opinion that the origin of plague is involved in obscurity, and the circumstances on which its propagation depends are obscure."[61] Faced with this lack of clarity, Stiven systematically turned his attention to the best known plague epidemic in the recent British past: the plague of Malta. He succinctly argues that the transmission of plague during

[58] Ibid., 13.   [59] Ibid., 16–17.
[60] Letter from G. Lamb, W. Steven, and J. Thomson to J. Thomason, September 5, 1850. Quoted in Renny, *Medical Report*, 4–5.
[61] Renny, *Medical Report*, 6.

that epidemic appeared contagious to him, and that settled the matter as far as the *mahamari* was concerned. After all, as Stiven saw it, plague was endemic to the Mediterranean region, and the precedents observed in that region should be imported forthwith.[62] Taking his cue from Thomas Maitland, Stiven emphasized "that a 'cordon sanitaire' should be established along all the outlets from the hills of Gurhwal and Kumaon."[63]

The identification between *mahamari* and plague and the consequent necessity of quarantine were fast becoming conventional wisdom. C. R. Francis, retired from service fighting *mahamari* in the 1850s, published a retrospective analysis of the epidemic in 1881, which forcefully argued that the overwhelming weight of medical opinion considered *mahamari* and the plague to be identical. Treating it now as a settled matter that the plague was contagious, Francis observed that in his own experience, contagious transmission had been "distinctly traceable" in several villages under his administration.[64] The plague, so hard to pin down earlier in the century, could be understood by several concrete criteria: a "rapid course," "glandular swellings," and "excessive mortality."[65] Francis also remarked that the disease was notable for its "caprice," a characteristic it shared with cholera. Nosological confidence, it seemed, Francis had in spades, yet he retained a sense of an apparent link among epidemic diseases that marked them out as mysterious and distinct. This makes sense particularly for a doctor writing retrospectively after germ theory had already begun to take hold, but who had completed most of his active career before this point.

Francis's assessment of *mahamari* is most remarkable because, with the hindsight granted to him by retirement, he was able to survey sixty years of plague fighting in India. At least in his narrative, sanitary cordons appear to have been the most effective agents against the disease. Francis suggests that a successful period of interventionist British public health efforts petered to a halt after the mid-1850s, when the disease grew in size and scope. In 1859 and 1860, a resurgent epidemic of *mahamari*/plague killed some 1,000 people, and in 1876–77, a smaller epidemic killed 277 (the death rate for those infected was 95 percent). Francis did not hesitate to equate the disease he had fought in the mountains of Garhwal with the Pali Plague and with earlier epidemics. Furthermore, and with ominous clairvoyance, he noted that the reports of rat deaths prior to *mahamari* outbreaks sounded eerily similar to descriptions in medical reports from Yunnan in China (a local focus of plague that was evolving into the third pandemic just as Francis's article was written).[66]

---

[62] Ibid., 6–7.   [63] Ibid., 27.   [64] Francis, "Endemic Plague in India," 396–97.   [65] Ibid., 399.
[66] Ibid., 401. While Francis's treatise came during a four-year lull in these Garhwali epidemics, outbreaks there would actually continue to the period of the third pandemic itself. See W. J. Simpson, *A Treatise on the Plague* (Cambridge: Cambridge University Press, 1905), 178.

Painted thus, plague appeared to be a global phenomenon, a disease whose wide reach was made more visible through imperial penetration and communication. Yet, despite his endorsement of contagionist theory, Francis assigned blame just where one might expect for an imperial official: on political unrest among colonial subjects. According to this analyst, the plague of Yunnan emerged as a result of a rebellion by local Muslims.[67] The first recorded outbreak of Indian *mahamari*, Francis argued, became epidemic as a result of overcrowding during a religious festival. Even for this committed contagionist, non-Christian religious ceremonies, political agitation, and "dirty" conditions seemed to cause epidemics to emerge out of thin air.[68]

Again, despite the seemingly conclusive victory of contagious interpretations of plague's transmission from the 1850s on, environmental, cultural, and climatological explanations continued to proliferate. In part, this is because anticontagionist critiques of living conditions, individual habits, and even religious beliefs as etiologically significant mapped so easily onto broader assumptions by imperial administrators. Matrices of condescension, coercion, and neglect undergirded so much British policy in India that it is unsurprising that medical administrators should have drawn on socio-cultural explanations even if they were simultaneously committed contagionists. The plague of Malta remained the historical touchstone for British medical administrators. Yet, while the survey above shows that most perused J. D. Tully's narrative of that plague in detail, and were more or less convinced by its author's contagionist interpretation of the plague, the most important lesson they appear to have drawn from it was a norm of decisiveness and practicality. Thomas Maitland's dramatic orders and large-scale encampments of medical isolation served as a model for plague-fighters well into the late nineteenth century and across the world.

Even at the end of the century, when thousands of British and Indian officials contended with the devastating effects of the third pandemic, plague fighting in the Mediterranean served as a more influential "medical archive" than the long history of combating *mahamari* in India. In the autumn of 1896, soon after plague first arrived in India (probably from Hong Kong), the port of Bombay was placed under a general quarantine elsewhere in India and, eventually, Aden. The explicit bureaucratic model the government claimed as a basis was an 1882 episode, in which, for more than six months, the Egyptian Board of Health (along with Malta and the Ottoman Empire) placed a

---

[67] Francis, "Epidemic Plague," 401.

[68] Religious festivals and the associated movements of people remained a central focus of British officials tasked with fighting the plague. See Manjiri N. Kamat, "'The Palkhi as Plague Carrier': The Pandharpur Fair and the Sanitary Fixation of the Colonial State; British India, 1908–1916," in *Health, Medicine, and Empire*, ed. Biswamoy Pati and Mark Harrison (London: Sangam, 2001).

quarantine on all ships from India based on the fear of cholera.[69] In the face of a much wider catastrophe than any Mediterranean plague in the modern era (the third pandemic killed more than 10 million people in India), the Middle Sea nevertheless seemed to be the font of precedents that could serve Anglo-Indian plague administrators.

Is There an Imperial Pattern?

Prior to the third pandemic, the response of British administrators to Indian plague exposes a curious dualism. Even as they sought to prevent the plague from spreading beyond the mountains and hills in which it recurred, they continued to view the entire Indian medical landscape as one of extreme peril and high mortality. As we have seen, the very idea of quarantine carries an assumption that a healthy existence can be secured within a protected border. In a land of epidemic chaos where imperial officials half expected to be struck down at any turn, one would think quarantine would appear as a self-defeating absurdity. By the time of the Bushire epidemic and the Pali Plague in the mid-1830s, the flourishing genre of "medical topography" and the discourses of imminent death that David Arnold draws out in *Colonizing the Body* were in the (recent) past. The largely successful attempts to stop plague from crossing the Indian Ocean coincided with new views of a kind of "normal" balance within an insalubrious India that the British were prepared to accept.

In this way, the narrative followed above of officials anxious to eliminate epidemic disease coexisted with toleration and neglect of severe threats to Indian livelihoods. During the 1860s and 1870s, as British administrators sought to prevent the spread of *mahamari* from the Himalayas into the rest of the country, they also (infamously) presided over woefully inadequate responses to famines that killed millions. Indeed, C. R. Francis began his article on *mahamari* with a lurid invocation of the "colossal scale" on which India exhibited the "phenomena of nature." He enumerated the "severest scourges known to man" that the subcontinent exhibited, such as "cyclones," "storm-waves," and "hailstones of more than regulation cricket-ball size."[70] Plague and cholera form part of this list, but Francis's view is clear. The latter two epidemic diseases demanded intervention when they threatened to spread

---

[69] On the Egyptian basis of this order, see Mark Harrison, *Public Health in British India: Anglo-Indian Preventive Medicine, 1859–1914* (Cambridge: Cambridge University Press, 1994), 140. On the 1882 episode itself, see *Report on the Administration of the Bombay Presidency for the Year 1881–82* (Bombay: Government Central Press, 1882), 69.

[70] Francis, "Epidemic Plague in India," 391.

uncontrollably, but otherwise, imperial administrators could do no more than throw up their hands at the chaos.

How to resolve this apparent contradiction between imperial severity and imperial indifference? One way is to see that in an era when environmental medicine was attractive to policy makers, a country's state of health was often considered in terms of a national equilibrium. Quarantine carried the aspiration of stability, and the risk was that a new onset of disease would disrupt the precarious balance – something that could come to pass by granting free pratique to ships from more unhealthy regions of the world. India may have been beset by the world's "severest scourges," but at least during the Bushire epidemic, in the midst of the Pali Plague, and against *mahamari*, British administrators believed that the risk of "atypical" threats was strong enough to devote resources to combat it.

Across the imperial world, even where quarantines were not actually applied, numerous colonial officials saw past British quarantine practice as an important precedent. In 1839, for example, a judge in Mauritius wrote to the Colonial Office to seek more information on Britain's quarantine laws, for the purposes of improving the island's sanitary defenses. This request eventually reached Quarantine Superintendent William Pym, whose opinion was transmitted by Lord Greville. Britain's quarantine laws, wrote Greville, "have been established chiefly against the Plague, a disease not to be dreaded excepting by the Mediterranean Colonies."[71] As such, outside of the Mediterranean, the colonial world had no need for quarantine in Greville's mind. Yet, the stream of colonial requests to incorporate Mediterranean practice into local legislation *did* create momentum for spreading quarantine around the Empire. A year later, Lord Bathurst of the Colonial Office attempted to discourage Van Dieman's Land (Tasmania) from instituting expanded quarantine laws, distinguishing between a regularized system (which he viewed as inappropriate) and a reactive use in the case of specific epidemic threats, which, he conceded, was essential.[72]

Quarantines that were temporarily imposed in the midst of epidemics could be quite severe. In 1820, when an epidemic disease struck Mauritius (correctly assumed at the time to be cholera exported from India during the epidemic of the 1810s), the government of the Cape Colony enacted a quarantine not simply on ships from Mauritius (which were relatively rare), but on "all vessels coming from the Eastward."[73] According to the Acting Governor's instructions, the directive included all ships from India, and even China. Such ships would be released if they had (verifiably) not called at Mauritius, but only after

---

[71] Lord Greville to the Colonial Office, November 7, 1839, TNA PC 7/5, ff. 310–12.

[72] Lord Bathurst to J. Stephen, February 12, 1840, TNA PC 7/5, ff. 323–24.

[73] Sir Rufane S. Donkin to Lord Bathurst, January 31, 1820. Published in *Records of the Cape Colony*, ed. George Theal (Cape Town: Government of the Cape Colony, 1902), 13:13.

examination of the health of the crew. Meanwhile, the zone of sea open to fishing was contracted in anticipation of a large new quarantine harbor. In announcing these rules, the Acting Governor drew closely on Mediterranean language and normative ideas of quarantine justice: "And it is hereby made known, that, according to the general Law of All Civilized Nations, any infringement of the necessary Quarantine Regulations, renders the Offender liable to the punishment of Death, without any form of Trial."[74] Evidently, a stringent quarantine not only contributed to the preservation of health, but also to the colony's conformity to the standards of "civilized nations." The language evokes the terminology used only five years later by Continental boards of health to criticize the British for ostensibly abolishing quarantine in the fracas surrounding the 1825 Act.

In the Caribbean, for example, medical officers in each port had discretion to order the removal of individual ships deemed excessively pestiferous, though given the ubiquity of yellow fever in the region, quarantines against it were unusual. Here as elsewhere, much about imperial quarantine depended on the disposition of the individuals in positions of command. Were they Maitlands or Macleans? Certainly, the reputation of the former was most readily acceptable to imperial bureaucrats as a point of reference. Yet, given the death rates that regularly saw extreme mortality from fever (primarily malaria) among white troops in Caribbean garrisons,[75] the incentive to quarantine even a ship with seriously ill crew members was significantly smaller than in other parts of the imperial world. By the 1850s, for example, a "Central Board of Health" was meeting at Kingston, Jamaica. At the same time, as a report from one of its members and another Jamaican doctor shows, medical opinion among British officials in Jamaica militated against the regular imposition of quarantine. Noting the arrival of the *William Jardine*, a ship arrived from Trinidad with yellow fever on board, the two doctors noted that while opinion on yellow fever varied, it was united as to the principle of "its not being contagious or infectious in the ordinary acceptation of these terms." Quarantine, as a result, was considered to be "both unnecessary and cruel."[76]

Thus far, Kingston's Central Board of Health appeared to be governed by conventional anticontagionism. Yet, the same doctors recommended that, going forward, should a ship in the port of Kingston be infected with disease,

---

[74] Proclamation of Acting Governor Rufane Shawe Donkin, February 1, 1820. Published in Theal, *Records of the Cape Colony*, 13:15.

[75] Fevers were far and away the major killer among British troops. Among those who died from fever-based diseases, 90 percent were killed by malaria and the remainder from yellow fever and typhus. See Richard Sheridan, *Doctors and Slaves: A Medical and Demographic History of Slavery in the British West Indies, 1680–1834* (Cambridge: Cambridge University Press, 1985), 13.

[76] Report by Dr. Dempster and Dr. Bowerbank. Quoted in Gavin Milroy, "Yellow Fever in Jamaica – Quarantine," *The Lancet* 62, no. 1570 (1853): 325.

the healthy members of the crew should be "landed and kept on shore" while the sick would be forcibly removed to a hospital. During periods of pestilence, the board recommended that ships should moor off the coast at some distance from each other, that unnecessary communication with the shore should be limited, and that crew members should sleep in the open air of the deck to prevent contamination from the close air below.[77] Here was a kind of "quasi-quarantine," with communication discouraged rather than forbidden. The guiding rationale was the miasmatic idea of avoiding contaminated atmosphere, though a contingent contagionism is also present. Beyond such efforts, however, British officials never seriously considered building a lazaretto or instituting regular quarantines in the colonies of the Caribbean.[78]

This was not the case in Britain's pre-1776 American colonies. Though most extant quarantine structures in major Atlantic ports like Baltimore, Philadelphia, and New York postdate independence, the first quarantine regulations in the US seem to have been the Massachusetts Bay Colony's prescriptions against ships arriving from yellow fever–stricken Barbados in 1647.[79] Although the precise linkage between tropical mosquitoes and yellow fever was not confirmed until the twentieth century, the fact that the disease that killed so many in the summer was quiescent in colder months led to seasonally applied quarantines that merchants trading along America's Atlantic seaboard were able to accommodate.

These examples, drawn from around the British Empire and across a wide swath of time, indicate the reach and consequence of Mediterranean quarantine. As a practice, not an institution, it remained open to revision and reinterpretation, and its prominence in fomenting imperial responses to impending medical catastrophe further cemented its status as a norm-encouraging precedent. As both geopolitics and medical science evolved over the mid-century decades, the Mediterranean paradigm survived as a body of official record and a collection of bureaucratic instruments. I conclude the section by noting a notable variation.

Cholera, rather than yellow fever or plague, became the impetus for some of the later quarantine establishments constructed in the British Empire. In 1832, during the first wave of cholera in Britain and Ireland, the government of Lower Canada created a new quarantine station on Grosse Île, outside Quebec City. In the same year and in the face of the same threat, Sydney's North Head Quarantine station opened. Most of the ships detained at Sydney (at least initially) actually had an outbreak of contagious disease onboard, but although

---

[77] Ibid., 325.

[78] Mark Harrison perceptively notes the contrast between the British lack of a defensive response to yellow fever in the Caribbean and some Britons' criticisms of the Ottoman Empire for not responding more proactively to the plague. See Harrison, *Contagion*, 22–23.

[79] See Harrison, *Contagion*, 22.

the station had been opened during a panic over cholera, there was no tradition here of restricting quarantine to cases of the "big three" epidemic diseases (plague, cholera, and yellow fever); between 1837 and 1840, for example, some fifteen ships from Britain and Ireland were quarantined because of the presence of typhus, with journalistic hand-wringing about "fever ships" adding to the pressure to act harshly.[80] Typhus was not uncommon on ships in the nineteenth century, so though quarantine stations such as Grosse Île and North Head were not mobilized against *all* arrivals from one particular area, they did detain thousands of immigrants. Suggestively, both quarantine stations shared a similar (grim) afterlife. The Grosse Île Quarantine Station in Quebec achieved notoriety just over a decade after its opening as a detention point for Irish immigrants fleeing the potato famine and was the site of almost 5,000 deaths. Similarly, the North Head Quarantine station found a rationale as a detention point for all immigrants to Australia. Both stations lasted into the late twentieth century.

It is through the long lives of such later institutions of quarantine around the British world that we can see how dramatically practice and meaning was transfigured outside of the Mediterranean. Away from a region beset by a seemingly intractable epidemiological divide (the ostensibly plague-ridden Ottoman polity facing plague-free Europe), administrators in imperial spaces like Sydney or Quebec faced a world where the primary threat to domestic sanitary equilibrium was represented by a generic unknown, with potentially unhealthy ships of immigrants the clearest focus of anxiety. From a system focused on regions of the world to an intermittent practice selectively applied to individuals, imperial quarantine began to distinguish among kinds of people rather than points of origin. Outside the Mediterranean, and later in the century, quarantine became a discriminating tool rather than a universal system.

---

[80] Katherine Foxhall, "Fever, Immigration and Quarantine in New South Wales, 1837–1840," *Social History of Medicine* 24, no. 3 (2011): 624–25.

9   Mutually Assured Deconstruction

Over the course of the 1840s, the quarantine system underwent a radical shift. Despite numerous lazarettos posting all-time highs in terms of quarantine traffic, the number of days of mandated detention was on the decline in ports across Europe. By the end of the 1840s, in much of Europe, it was possible for the first time in about a century to travel from most ports in North Africa, Anatolia, and the Middle East to Western Europe without any kind of sanitary detention. The "universality" of the system as it existed since the late eighteenth century had been undone. On the one hand, this change was inspired by a major epidemiological shift, in which the plague itself began to decline in the Ottoman Empire in the late 1830s. The sanitary disequilibrium that had explained quarantine's existence, observers marveled, was apparently vanishing. On the other hand, the transformations of the 1840s witnessed the displacement of quarantine as a feature of European ports and European travel onto the non-European world and onto colonized peoples: in particular, to new quarantine sites in the Red Sea.

In some ways, the changes of this period are hard to spot, which is why it does not stand as a major marker in many histories of specific quarantine sites. Although most Mediterranean lazarettos continued to function, after the early 1850s, they were mobilized into action only in the service of extraordinary events. While boards of health differed on whether to enforce quarantine against ports infected with cholera, across Europe, quarantine still applied in cases of plague or yellow fever in the port of departure. Yet, as these diseases receded, this became ever rarer. The end of quarantine can also be harder to identify when examined from the level of national legislation. After all, in Britain, the Quarantine Act of 1825 technically remained in force, in the cases of plague and yellow fever, until 1896. Despite the great hopes of its organizers, a consensus has emerged among historians of medicine that the International Sanitary Conference of 1851 did little to change quarantine.[1] According to this narrative, quarantine withered away over a half-century. Such a framing, however, ignores the radical changes of

---

[1] For a recent expression of this view, see Crook, *Governing Systems*, 202.

the 1840s and 1850s. The dominoes fell quickly; a system that had, over several centuries, grown into an implacable barrier between East and West, that had fostered collaboration and controversy, that had detained hundreds of thousands, essentially ended in the course of a decade. By 1851, there was a Continent-wide resolve after the first International Sanitary Conference that quarantine for most ships with clean bills of health would be ended. While the agreement of the conference was officially ratified by only two of the twelve nations that had participated,[2] the fact of the agreement's presence bolstered a consensus that it was possible to end universal quarantine without suffering retaliation.

Limiting quarantine to ships with foul bills of health (as most ports did just before or just after the 1851 conference) almost ended quarantine altogether. Charles Maclean's assessment that 90 percent of ships traveled to Europe with clean bills of health was made before the plague began its long retreat from the Middle East. As early as 1824, Maclean made clear that he considered the limitation of quarantine to ships with foul bills to be "a change which amounts nearly to a total abolition of the system."[3] By the late 1840s, the proportion of ships with clean bills must have been close to 100 percent. To change quarantine from a system that ensnared everything that moved across the Mediterranean, East to West, to a system applied only in times of plague and yellow fever was to fundamentally transform it from a universal feature of Mediterranean travel and trade into an occasional anomaly. Here, while I consider the afterlife of the quarantine system in the 1850s and 1860s at some length, I argue that 1851 marks the end of an era. In its wake, we see the transformation of quarantine from a system that figured detention based on point of origin to a tool deployed according to preconceptions and stereotypes about the health status of individuals.

Aside from the influence of anticontagionism, there were two major reasons that Western authorities were comfortable ending quarantine on ships from the Middle East and North Africa. First, again, as the 1840s began, a sense grew among Western diplomats, doctors, and politicians that plague had begun to disappear from areas in which it had seemed entrenched. Second, the Ottomans themselves had instituted quarantine in major coastal cities in 1839 (Egypt had instituted a lazaretto and a board of health even earlier, in 1831). For the last decade of "universal quarantine" in the West, the practice was, in fact, truly a cross-Mediterranean enterprise. Confident it was now safe to shift the burden to Ottoman and North African ports, European politicians who had previously been reluctant to reduce quarantine requirements dropped their previous opposition.

---

[2] Piedmont-Sardinia and France. See Bon, "Cholera Epidemics," 47.

[3] From Maclean's summary of proposed changes to the quarantine laws after the 1824 Select Committee Report. See TNA SP 105/142, f. 377.

Given the extent to which Western political and cultural evaluations of the Ottoman state were linked to the presence of the plague and shaped by the barrier of universal quarantine, one might expect the end of that system to have marked an improvement in Western opinions. Certainly, from the perspective of Ottoman diplomats, the alliance with France and Britain during the Crimean War (1854–56) represented a high point of relations with Western Europe.[4]

Yet, quarantine's geography of suspicion remained in place in other ways. Despite the sudden waning of the plague in most of the Ottoman Empire, and despite the granting of free pratique to ships from the southern and eastern coasts of the Mediterranean, the second half of the nineteenth century witnessed a "hardening of attitudes" toward the Ottoman regime paired with a much more inflexible, pseudo-scientific racism.[5] In the late nineteenth century, Western condemnation of the Empire grew in response to the violence in the Balkans during the era of nationalistic revolts.[6] At the same time, British and French penetration of the Ottoman economy increased, especially after the 1875 debt default and 1881–82 creation of the Public Debt Administration; the decades following the abolition of universal quarantine represent the nadir of Western respect for the Ottoman regime.

The tightening of racial, political, and imperial categories in the late nineteenth century went along with a broad transformation in the global practice of quarantine; before 1851 and the end of quarantine for most ships with clean bills of health, travelers and crew members of European origin formed the majority of those subjected to the practice. In the latter part of the nineteenth century, the balance shifted. Now, with bodies rather than geographies the target of quarantine laws, non-Westerners formed the clear majority of those who experienced medical detention. Later in the nineteenth century, International Sanitary Conferences began to impose quarantines for Indian Muslims *en route* to the *Hajj*. During the third plague pandemic, which (with some major exceptions) largely hit port cities in the Global South, quarantine continued to be a response inflected by racism. Immigrants and refugees around the world were often subjected to quarantines in ports of arrival.

In this chapter then, we move from a consideration of the end of quarantine as a Mediterranean system to a consideration of its global afterlife. With the

---

[4] See R. H. Davison, "Ottoman Public Relations in the Nineteenth Century: How the Sublime Porte Tried to Influence European Public Opinion," in *Histoire économique et sociale de l'Empire ottoman et de la Turquie, 1326–1960*, ed. Daniel Panzac (Leuven: Peeters, 1995), 593–602.

[5] The phrase comes from James Mather, *Pashas: Traders and Travelers in the Islamic World* (New Haven, CT: Yale University Press, 2009), 9.

[6] On this phenomenon, see Davide Rodogno, *Against Massacre: Humanitarian Interventions in the Ottoman Empire, 1815–1914* (Princeton, NJ: Princeton University Press, 2012), and Michelle Tusan, *Smyrna's Ashes: Humanitarianism, Genocide, and the Birth of the Middle East* (Berkeley: University of California Press, 2012).

beginning of the International Sanitary Conferences, we see a shift in power away from boards of health and upward to central governments. The world those boards built, however, set precedents that lingered. The new sanitary regimes that arose in the 1850s and 1860s demonstrate the deep influence of the early nineteenth-century system on the birth of international health.

The Ottoman State in the Face of the Plague

The institution of quarantine in the Ottoman Empire in 1839 was the result of a complicated negotiation in which varying interests were counterposed: a reluctance to adopt a Western framing of epidemic disease, a sense that patterns of disease transmission might make quarantine redundant, a resistance among certain conservative Islamic scholars who opposed pre-emptive attempts to prevent epidemics, and a desire to respond to the one-sidedness of European quarantines by imposing delays on foreign ships. Quarantine offered Ottoman reformers an opportunity to insist on a policy that would make the government appear modern, proactive, and reformist to the outside world. It represented, too, an opportunity to subject Western European ships to the same treatment, when arriving in Ottoman harbors, that ships departing from those harbors had long experienced in the West. After Mohammed Ali's regime in Egypt instituted quarantine in Alexandria in 1831, the ports of the Ottoman heartland were some of the only ones around the Mediterranean to send forth ships subject to quarantine elsewhere but impose none in return, a fact which the Ottoman court had long been aware of. As early as 1806, in fact, Sultan Selim III had made an abortive attempt to institute quarantine in Anatolia.[7]

This context strengthened the hand of Hamdan bin Osman Hoca, an influential advisor of Mahmud II. Exiled from French Algeria for his political writing in 1833, Hamdan had personally witnessed the destructive power European incursions had already exerted on the Mediterranean's southern coast, and quarantine formed part of an administrative arsenal he wanted the Ottoman state to build in response. Although European observers of the 1838–39 reform tended to ascribe it to pressure exerted by European states, Birsen Bulmuş has demonstrated that Hamdan's political acumen and long advocacy for the institution of quarantine were decisive. In the prelude to the Tanzimat reforms, Mahmud II was persuaded by Hamdan's program in the late 1830s, when he concluded that the population of the Empire was being "wasted" by incursions from the plague.[8] Bulmuş rightly emphasizes the irony in Britain's use of quarantine for centuries in its own ports and the sudden criticisms of the proposals introduced in the Ottoman Empire by Britons in the late 1830s.[9]

---

[7] Bulmuş, *Plagues, Quarantines*, 97.   [8] Ibid.,109.   [9] Ibid., 112.

Bulmuş makes a persuasive case that Ottoman rather than European impetus lay behind the eventual institution of quarantine. A survey of quarantine practice in other ports affiliated to the Ottoman state (though outside its direct control) confirms the sense that Mahmud II's regime had a variety of precedents to draw on from across the Muslim world. The Beys of Tunis, for example, had intermittently issued quarantine decrees for incoming ships from at least the late eighteenth century. During the devastating 1818–20 plague, Mahmud (Bey from 1814 to 1824) instituted particularly strenuous quarantine measures under the conviction that the disease had been spread by Algerian traders. This epidemic was to prove the last in Tunisia's history, and throughout the next three decades, the health of that province compared favorably with that of the rest of the Ottoman Empire.[10] As early as 1793, the Moroccan Sultan Moulay Slimane instituted a terrestrial sanitary cordon against Algeria during a plague epidemic there, albeit with the urging of various European consuls.[11]

In Egypt, irregular quarantines imposed toward the beginning of Mohammed Ali's reign were followed with a permanent quarantine at Alexandria instituted at the end of the 1820s. Ali financed the construction of a lazaretto and named the Italian contagionist Dr. Grassi chief of the new service. In the 1830s, this reform provoked howls of discontent from European travelers ensnared by the quarantine. Many cast scorn on the idea that Egypt could benefit from a lazaretto when Upper Egypt was considered to be one of the chief suspects as the "foyer" of contagion from which plague spread outward. But, despite the frustrations of many Western travelers and the catastrophic failure of Ali's quarantine system during the plague of 1835, the system also had Western supporters. The British military traveler C. Rochfort Scott, for example, praised the lazaretto as an example of Ali's ambitious modernization program and claimed that despite its failure to stop the 1835 epidemic, there were at least six occasions when it had prevented plague epidemics from spreading beyond infected parties of travelers.[12] Grassi himself counted ten times that the plague had reached the Lazaretto of Alexandria between 1831 and 1837 alone and noted that eight of those invasions were stopped inside the lazaretto walls. The two that were not, insisted Grassi (including the 1835 epidemic), could be explained by "the non-adoption of similar regulations" elsewhere in Egypt.[13] While British intervention in 1840–41 crushed some of Ali's planned public health infrastructure, the lazaretto continued to operate at full capacity.

---

[10] For more on quarantine and public health in late eighteenth- and nineteenth-century Tunisia, see Nancy Gallagher, *Medicine and Power in Tunisia*.

[11] Malika Ezzahidi, "Quarantine in Ceuta and Malta in the travel writings of the late eighteenth-century Moroccan ambassador Ibn Uthmân Al-Meknassi," in Chircop and Martínez, *Mediterranean Quarantines*, 112.

[12] Scott, *Rambles in Egypt*, 1:44–45.

[13] Quoted in T. S. Wells, "On the Practical Results of Quarantine," *Association Medical Journal* 2, no. 89 (1854): 833.

Between 1840 and 1843, for example, some 5,240 individuals performed quarantine there.[14]

Clot Bey, who was generally close to Mohammed Ali, opposed the institution of quarantine unsuccessfully. This was not for lack of trying; Clot personally injected himself with blood from a plague victim to prove its noncontagiousness during the 1835 epidemic (Figure 9.1). He claimed that the Pasha had been captivated by "quarantine mania" under the influence of contagionist doctors.[15] But as LaVerne Kuhnke persuasively argues, like political leaders in the West, Ali adopted policies from both the anticontagionist and contagionist camps, noting their equal plausibility. Ali recognized that the fusion was most likely to create a favorable impression in Europe and so build support for his bid for autonomy.[16] Indeed, a generation earlier, in the 1820s and 1830s, Ali had actively cultivated French and Italian physicians who were

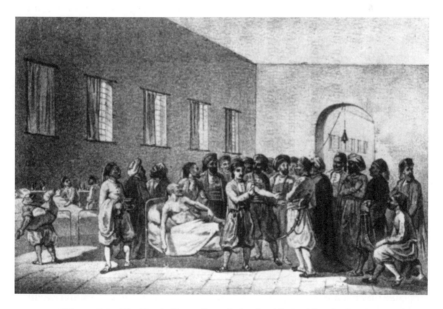

Figure 9.1 Clot Bey's "auto-inoculation" with the blood of a plague victim. Courtesy of the National Library of Medicine.

---

[14] These numbers are based on Clot Bey's summary of statistics presented to him by Dr. Grassi. See Anon., "Mémoire sur la réforme des quarantaines," in *Derniers mots sur la non-contagion de la peste*, ed. Clot Bey (Paris: Victor Masson & Fils, 1866), 17.

[15] Clot Bey, "Résumé sur la contagion de la peste," in *Derniers Mots*, 16.

[16] See LaVerne Kuhnke, *Lives at Risk: Public Health in Nineteenth-Century Egypt* (Berkeley: University of California Press, 1990), 5.

interested in establishing careers in Egypt. Many of these doctors, like Grassi and Clot Bey, were diametrically split on the issue of the contagiousness of the plague, but their ubiquity throughout the Middle East by the 1840s provided a large body of "expert" opinion that European governments consulted again and again during the period of quarantine reform.[17] Such doctors were professional associates, and many began to see themselves as part of one cohesive group of expertise with shared interests, however divided, on the question of plague's contagiousness. This is visible in works by the bitter enemies Clot Bey and the contagionist doctor Arsène Bulard, which both feature literal "casts of characters" – lists of doctors with short summaries of their opinions on the question of contagion.[18]

The conflicting precedents offered by the Western European tradition point to the ambivalent role Western diplomats played during the institution of Ottoman quarantine. Though Bulmuş emphasizes that by 1838, most Europeans tended to oppose Hamdan's quarantine proposal, a longer history would show frequent pressure exerted in the opposite direction. When, in 1831, the Sultan expressed interest in setting up a formal quarantine system, Stratford Canning (the British ambassador) urged the Maltese government to send a rubric of quarantine practice as an example of British sanitary protocol.[19] The Austrians exerted consistent pressure on the Ottomans to introduce quarantine procedures throughout the 1830s, just as Britain and France began their attempts to persuade Austria to join an international conference that would scale back quarantine across Europe. Indeed, as discussed in Chapter 5, in tandem with the Ottoman quarantine proposal of 1838, an Austrian diplomat (Baron d'Ottenfels) signed a treaty with the Ottoman ambassador in Vienna providing for Austrian assistance in setting up the new lazaretto, including the temporary provision of experienced personnel from the Lazaretto of Semlin.[20]

Prefiguring later nineteenth-century developments, in which Europeans would displace Ottoman officials in numerous administrative capacities within the Empire, the central bone of contention in the 1838 proposal was the principle that the new boards of health in Ottoman ports would be entirely composed of Ottoman subjects. In the quarantine eventually promulgated, this proposal had been modified to include mixed boards of Ottomans and Western Europeans. Some, like Lord Palmerston, continued to oppose the reform on the (convenient) grounds that public health in the Ottoman interior ought to

---

[17] See Sylvia Chiffoleau, *Genèse de la santé publique internationale. De la peste d'Orient à l'OMS* (Beirut: Institut Français du Proche-Orient, 2013), 56–65.

[18] See Arsène Bulard, *De la peste orientale* (Paris: Béchet Jeune et Labé, 1839), 306–38, and A. B. Clot, *De la Peste*, xiii–xxiv.

[19] See Greig to CSG, March 31, 1831, NAM CUST 04/1. John Booker demonstrates how this proposal spurred British interest in an international conference to end quarantine from the mid-1830s on. See Booker, *Maritime Quarantine*, chapter 15.

[20] Treaty between Baron d'Ottenfels and Rifaat Bey, October, 1838, HHStA MdÄ AR F50-2.

precede quarantine rules in Ottoman ports. Still a decade away from a public health law in Britain, and given quarantine's venerable age compared to "the sanitary idea" in British legislation, this argument was more than a little hypocritical. Furthermore, British and French representatives on Ottoman boards of health began to use their position as a vantage point for use in overseeing new quarantines on imperial subjects moving around the Red Sea.

John Bowring greeted the news of the Ottoman reforms by opining "Lazzarets in Turkey forsooth!"[21] As an anticontagionist convinced that the geographic range of plague was delimited by the atmosphere, Bowring viewed a quarantine against ships arriving in Turkey as the height of absurdity. Such attitudes were not uncommon; the official policy of the British government was to oppose new extensions of quarantine. But a cannier view of the Ottoman initiative might have recognized it as an opportunity for European powers to scale down their own quarantine system.

As early as 1838, Metternich signaled to the British and French that he was open to an international conference on the matter. This concession, which Metternich noted came well after the first French and British overtures, was explicitly tied to the creation of Ottoman quarantines rather than the needs of commerce. In a letter sent to Baron Langsdorff, the French *chargé d'affaires* at Vienna, Metternich suggested that he had resisted reform because, prior to the 1830s, the Ottomans appeared to remain in the grip of "religious fanaticism," subject to "inveterate prejudices, and a lack of regard that Oriental Governments heretofore held toward the introduction of sanitary precautions." Long an adherent (like most Western Europeans) of the centuries-old canard that all Muslims evinced "fatalism" in front of the plague, Metternich was apparently willing to change his thinking (influenced, no doubt, by commercial ambitions and an eagerness to shift the burden of quarantine). Egypt's relatively new quarantine apparatus, new quarantine administrations in independent Greece, and a decline in epidemic disease throughout the Balkans provided a convenient rationale. Metternich's self-congratulatory conclusion was that Mahmud II had decided "to bestow on his subjects the benefits of European civilization" in the form of quarantine, and he professed himself satisfied that what he had considered an Ottoman predisposition to shun public health "no longer existed."[22] Such a change, as Metternich saw it, was accomplished through the heavy intervention of Austria, with a new Ottoman health administration to be partially staffed by employees seconded from the Lazaretto of Semlin.[23]

---

[21] Hansard, House of Commons Debate, July 23, 1844, c. 1295.

[22] Klemens von Metternich to Baron Langsdorff, July 13, 1838, HHStA MdÄ AR F50-2.

[23] On the importance of Austrian influence on Ottoman medical structures in encouraging Metternich to accept quarantine reform, see Chahrour, "A Civilizing Mission," 702.

Thus, whereas British and French politicians and authors tended to disdain the Ottoman efforts, those policies were crucial in persuading Metternich to join the cause of reform. The Europe-wide Congress, which reformers saw as the key to breaking impasse, was now endorsed by the three strongest Mediterranean powers. Amid upheaval in the Middle East and a dispute between Austria and France over which power would play host, the proposal foundered as the 1840s began. Nevertheless, as we will see below, Austrian participation in this abortive effort gave confidence to both the British and French governments that the rigidity of the system might be mitigated. This conviction only increased as the decade wore on and Western Europeans became aware of another variable that confounded the root assumptions of quarantine: the steady retreat of plague from the Middle East.

Ottoman sources and some Western records constitute reasons for skepticism about the certainty expressed by historians such as Daniel Panzac that the 1840s mark a conclusive disappearance of the plague in the Middle East.[24] Nevertheless, the perception of a major epidemiological shift was ubiquitous among European observers at the time, and it is impossible to overstate the significance of this perception for the development of quarantine reform. Given the extent to which the Middle East had seemed, for so long, to be the heartland of plague, any perception that its sanitary state had changed called for a major revision of the quarantine laws. And in the Middle East itself, the amelioration of plague over the course of the early and mid-nineteenth century upended long-term cycles that had, decades earlier, seemed deeply intractable. In Egypt, Syria/Palestine, and coastal Anatolia, despite its renewed presence during the third pandemic, the 1840s marked a major transformation. While, in a very *longue durée* view, overall mortality declined between early modern epidemics and the plague outbreaks of the 1820s and 1830s, Egypt's 1835 plague was one of the most destructive in its history and also the last epidemic with major demographic effects. A limited outbreak in 1844 was the final plague epidemic large enough to attract international notice, and probably the last epidemic of plague before the third pandemic. Similarly, a large epidemic in 1838 and a series of cases in 1841 constituted the final times European consuls felt called upon to issue foul bills of health from the port of Constantinople. According to Panzac's statistics, this followed some ninety-four years in the period between 1700 and 1841 in which the presence of plague was ubiquitous enough for it to surface in European consular and health board records.[25]

Both the long-term definitiveness of the apparent retreat of plague in this period and the reasons for it are obscure. One possibility is ecological change.[26]

---

[24] See Panzac, *Peste*, esp. 506–7. For a more skeptical note, see Nükhet Varlık's forthcoming monograph on the long-term trajectory of plague in the Ottoman Empire.

[25] Panzac, *Peste*, 198–99.

[26] Panzac tends to favor the decisive role of quarantine but does suggest that longer-term environmental factors must have contributed to the diminishment of the plague. See Panzac, *Peste*, 509–10.

Indeed, as Alan Mikhail has demonstrated, one of the reasons plague seemed so intractable in late eighteenth-century Egypt, at least, was the way in which plague's epizootic origin and large-scale demographic effects meant it was a part of broad environmental cycles alongside other ecosocial events – famines, droughts, and economic fluctuations.[27] Yet, while long-developing changes in these cycles and new trends in the distribution of rat-flea populations probably made a difference, the fact that, at least according to observers at the time, plague appeared to disappear so suddenly means short-term considerations are also important. In the case of Egypt, LaVerne Kuhnke notes the implausibility of attributing the transformation to sudden changes in diet, ecology or bodily immunity after 1844. Other than incredible luck, the only possible cause, as she sees it, is the increasingly regular institution of quarantine, both in Egypt's ports and also during epidemics.[28] The close chronological coincidence between the expansion of Egyptian quarantine practice during the 1835 epidemic and the institution of quarantine in other Ottoman ports in 1839 increases the likelihood that it contributed to the epidemiological changes in this era.

While we should be skeptical of accepting wholeheartedly the narratives both of quarantine officials anxious to show success and Western figures eager to dismantle the quarantine laws, on the level of anecdote, it is very difficult to doubt that the new quarantines prevented several epidemics that would otherwise have killed thousands. The commercial writer John Davy, for example, recounts a case of an Egyptian merchant vessel landing at a new lazaretto in Constantinople with plague on board. This, he notes, was after at least three years, during which the Ottoman capital had been completely free of plague. After its arrival on June 8, 1841, Abdullah, a healthy guardian, and Mehmet Hussein, a healthy porter, were sent onboard to disembark passengers and their goods to the lazaretto. By June 22, both had died, and on being examined by Dr. Davout Oglou (the lazaretto health officer), buboes were revealed on the groins of both men. "May it not be concluded as a thing certain" asked Davy, that "if these two men had not communicated with the persons and effects brought in the infected vessel, they, in common with the whole population of the city and its suburbs, amounting, it is estimated, to about 800,000 souls, would have remained free from the disease?"[29] Left hanging, of course, is the question of what might have happened to many of those 800,000 souls if the quarantine facilities had not recently been established.

The retreat of the plague occurred during the end of the Mohammed Ali crisis – during the unruly dénouement of the Egyptian invasion of Syria,

---

[27] Alan Mikhail, "The Nature of Plague in Late Eighteenth-Century Egypt," *Bulletin of the History of Medicine* 82, no. 2 (2008): 249–75.
[28] Kuhnke, *Lives at Risk*, 154–56.   [29] John Davy, *Notes and Observations*, 2:334.

Lebanon, and Cyprus. Again, this crisis ended decisively in favor of the Sultan thanks in part to British support in the wake of the Anglo-Ottoman trade agreement of 1838. The retreat of the Egyptian armies left an unsettled set of local grandees, mayors, and warlords to restore calm; a chaotic ambience that one might imagine was fertile terrain for the *expansion* rather than the retreat of the plague. And yet, the devolution of power among numerous conflicting local authorities in an era when a growing local acceptance of the logic of quarantine seems to have resulted in the proliferation of sanitary authorities (some of these a result of the Ottoman quarantine program instituted in 1839 and staffed both by Ottoman and European doctors). Equally important and unrelated to sanitary control in particular: the political chaos undoubtedly posed restraints on movement throughout much of the Middle East as the rules surrounding what letters, passports, and papers one needed to travel from one city to another continually changed.

The diaries of the Jewish philanthropist and traveler, Sir Moses Montefiore, give a helpful window into this complex milieu. Montefiore, traveling through the Holy Land in summer 1839, had to negotiate several quarantines alongside other impediments to travel. His journey was interrupted by reports of brigandage, a plague epidemic, and an evolving military situation. Detained and examined by a sanitary officer at Jaffa, Montefiore's party was *again* placed under quarantine (this time for a period of seven days and a threat of a forty-day detention on the appearance of any disease) after completing the short journey to Mt. Carmel.[30] The testimony of this one traveler should point us to hundreds of similar impediments to movement that were not preserved in written records. All told, the Middle Eastern milieu between 1838 and 1842 seems to have been one in which there were significant checks on movement. Perhaps, then, this period saw longer term ecological shifts coinciding with a momentary arrest of the normal mobility within the region, a dynamic that could well have hastened the retreat of the plague.

Universal Quarantine Comes Apart

Historians of the plague have generally not seen the 1840s as a major marker in periodizations of the disease. In part, this is because the disease continued to make sporadic appearances in outlying regions of the Ottoman Empire – epidemics into the 1870s in Mesopotamia, Yemen, and the Libyan port of Benghazi received considerable attention among Western diplomats, doctors, and politicians.[31] Furthermore, the final episodes of Ottoman plagues occurred

---

[30] See Sir Moses and Lady Montefiore, *Diaries of Sir Moses and Lady Montefiore*, ed. Louis Loewe (London: Jewish Historical Society of England, 1983), 1:186–92.
[31] See John Simon, "Annual Report of the Medical Officer to the Pricy Council and Local Government Board for the year 1874," quoted in *Papers Relating to the Modern History and*

concurrently with the first stirrings of plague in Yunnan Province in China, epidemics that would explode by the final decade of the century into the destructive third plague pandemic.[32] Finally, while large-scale plague epidemics mostly disappeared, cholera, typhus, and influenza epidemics continued to occur. All of those caveats, however, do not detract from the fact that perceptions of a cessation of plague outbreaks in the major Ottoman and Egyptian cities lining the Mediterranean coast mattered decisively in creating the momentum to end mandatory quarantine over the course of the 1840s.

The relative speed with which Western diplomats and bureaucrats began to perceive epidemiological change can be explained by the efficiency with which boards of health exchanged medical information. The regular reports received by the *Intendants* at Marseille regarding the state of health throughout the Ottoman Empire enabled them to reduce quarantine lengths substantially in 1842, owing to "the satisfactory state of the public health in the various countries of the East for several years past."[33] Several years later, Gavin Milroy reported that "since the year 1839, it appears that there has been no case of plague observed at Constantinople. The board of health of that city attributes this exemption altogether to the quarantine measures, that have been adopted of late years."[34] Milroy himself was skeptical. Yet, it was clear that while the cause and extent of the retreat of the plague (then as now) remained mysterious, it was an essential part of the background against which European boards of health began to reduce their required detentions. So, too, from a British perspective, was an increasing sense, even among contagionist doctors, that the plague's incubation period was shorter than most voyages to Northern Europe. Dr. Grassi, a staunch defender of contagion theory and the utility of the quarantine he ran at Alexandria, put an upper limit of ten days before plague would reveal itself. Dr. Madden could both agree forcefully with Dr. Grassi's perspective and argue that (as a British reviewer put it) "on this side of Gibraltar, no quarantine at all is necessary."[35]

In 1847, in the wake of a French Academy of Medicine report into the contagion of the plague, France reduced quarantine even further, with British observers noting they did so almost entirely on the grounds of Egypt's

Recent Progress of Levantine Plague (London: George Eyre and William Spotiswoode, 1879), 3.

[32] On these nineteenth-century plague epidemics in Southwestern China that eventually led to the third pandemic, see Carol Benedict, *Bubonic Plague in Nineteenth-Century China* (Stanford, CA: Stanford University Press, 1996).

[33] Intendants to Alexander Turnbull, December 9, 1842. *Correspondence Relative to the Contagion of Plague*, 111. For an example of a travel narrative from this pivotal period, which reveals how fast European observers noted that plague was beginning to retreat from Egypt, see W. H. Yates, *The Modern History and Condition of Egypt, Its Climate, Diseases, and Capabilities* (London: Smith, Elder, and Co., 1843), 136.

[34] Milroy, *Quarantine and the Plague*, 21.

[35] *Medico-Chirurgical Review* 34, no. 68 (1841): 594.

newfound salubrity. A customs official, summarizing the French reforms for the benefit of the Privy Council, began by noting (somewhat mystifyingly) that "the Plague has ceased to manifest itself at Alexandria for upward of 27 years and for upward of five years in the rest of Egypt."[36] Once the general cessation of plague in the Middle East became clear, the apparent longer term immunity of particular centers seemed all the more probative (though this report of Alexandria's immunity conspicuously ignored the major plague outbreak of 1835).

The reform of quarantine was sanctioned even by powers that had not signed on to the proposed international convention in 1838. The British consul in Rome informed the Foreign Secretary in 1843 that the quarantine imposed in the Papal States' ports of Ancona and Civitavecchia was subject to an imminent reduction and that "reductions are continually made by a courteous application from the consulate."[37] This was a far cry from the situation only a few years earlier, when consular pleas would have been unlikely to accomplish much, and the Italians were seen by the French and British as stubbornly unwilling to reduce the length of detention.

Meanwhile, travelers came to expect a reduction in quarantines as a matter of course. John Gardiner Wilkinson, author of one of the most popular British guidebooks to Egypt, noted that in 1847, the "full quarantine" at Malta for returning passengers from the Middle East was twenty-four days, but that it "will be probably soon be less than at present."[38] Thus, while the mid-1840s represented a high point of traffic in Malta's lazaretto, an expectation grew quickly that the status quo was due for imminent change.

From 1841, the British government shirked its own rules, which still required ships proceeding from the Ottoman Empire with clean bills of health to be quarantined in British ports, when the PC allowed the P&O company the right to land its new steamers at Southampton having counted their quarantine en route (something that had never been allowed before).[39] The P&O advertised a voyage length of fourteen days, which exceeded the twelve-day duration of Britain's *foul bill* quarantine on ships from Egypt (from 1842), while the clean bill quarantine was (at least by 1843) limited to five days (Figure 9.2).[40] In practice, then, no steamers from Egypt would be subject to quarantine at all. Such an expedient offered travelers much less onerous itineraries than those

---

[36] "Quarantine in France," April 24, 1847, TNA PC 1/2659. This was, obviously, a misunderstanding of Alexandria's experience during several Egyptian epidemics in the 1820s and 1830s.

[37] John Freeborn to the Earl of Aberdeen, April 13, 1843, *Correspondence Relative to the Contagion of Plague*, 130.

[38] Wilkinson, *Handbook for Travelers in Egypt*, xix.

[39] *Bombay Almanac, Directory, and Register for the Year 1842* (Bombay: Times Press, 1841), 54.

[40] See William Pym to Charles Greville, December 24, 1842, and Charles Greville to C. Scovell, September 26, 1843, TNA PC 7/5.

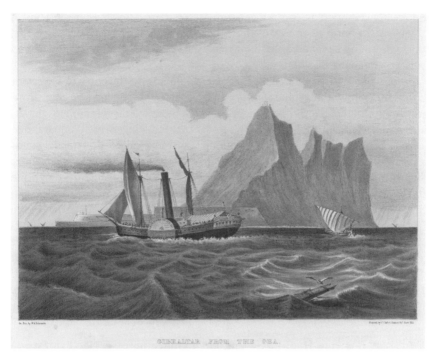

Figure 9.2 The P&O steamship *Lady Mary Wood* at Gibraltar. Engraving by
W. A. Delamotte. The ship was in regular service on the P&O's Mediterranean
routes and carried William Thackeray during part of his 1844 journey to
Gibraltar, Malta, Egypt, and Anatolia. © Royal Museums Greenwich.

with enforced interruption at Malta, Livorno, or Marseille, a fact that inspired
further French agitation for reform. It prompted Dr. Aubert-Roche, for example, to write in the *Revue D'Orient* that Britain had "destroyed" and "abolished" quarantine with its new rule about steamships.[41] This was
a characteristic overstatement, and Aubert-Roche was clearly seeking to
build momentum in France for the repeal of the quarantine laws. It was
a significant change, and it rendered quarantine no longer "universal" in the
way I defined it in this book's introduction. Yet, the P&O had one sailing per
month, its steamships were required to have a medical officer onboard, and this
exception to the rules in no way seemed to the British like the end of quarantine.
Indeed, more than a year later, William Pym suggested to the Privy Council that
it would "be desirable to assimilate as nearly as possible the terms of
Quarantine in this Country to those established in France" (France was

---

[41] Aubert-Roche, "Des Quarantines," 69.

apparently considered to have a generally *lesser* quarantine burden).[42] Thus, it is misleading for historians to suggest that Britain ended quarantine in 1841, when the change applied only to one route. The majority of the system stayed intact until the later 1840s.

Nevertheless, the very idea that any ship could be allowed entry to a Western European port without quarantine indicated that the "tit-for-tat" retaliatory quarantines that had fashioned congruity for so long were beginning to sputter. In the same letter just quoted, Pym argued that reducing Britain's quarantine lengths should now be possible "without any chance of the Italian states retaliating as they did in the year 1825 by placing British vessels under quarantine when arriving in their Ports from the United Kingdom."[43] In the end, the requirements that ships with clean bills of health perform quarantine in Britain were dropped in 1847.[44] Given that the end of the plague in Middle Eastern port cities made foul or suspected bills extremely unlikely, the elimination of clean bill quarantine was essentially the end of the system. The same rule change was accomplished in Malta and many other Mediterranean ports in the years after the first International Sanitary Conference (1851–52). By 1854, a British guidebook could complacently note that thanks to recent changes, "quarantine is practically abolished."[45]

A Board of Health Resigns and a Quarantine Service Protests

The elevated traffic in quarantine stations in the 1840s (even as the length of confinement steadily shortened) meant that the staff associated with lazaretto administrations and boards of health *expanded* just before the end of clean bill quarantine. The result was that a large number of quarantine workers were suddenly threatened with redundancy. During this same moment, the recentering of power from the networks created by boards of health to government ministers in Paris, London, and Vienna (who were intent on ending quarantine) brought significant consternation to many health board members and lazaretto employees. To understand the significance of the end of the quarantine system, we have to consider the change not only from the vantage points of diplomacy and epidemiology but also from the perspective of the workers who had long enabled it to function. In this section, we examine how the powers that health boards had accumulated over the preceding century could dissipate so quickly.

Marseille's *Intendants* were a self-confident bunch, especially in their relations with other Continental boards of health. They developed a proud corporate identity and were fierce defenders of the city of Marseille and its right to

[42] Pym to Greville, December 24, 1842, TNA PC 7/5.   [43] Ibid.
[44] See Booker, *Maritime Quarantine*, 506.
[45] John Murray (firm), *A Handbook for Travellers in Turkey* (London: John Murray, 1854), 12.

remain the sole port of France permitted to undertake commerce with the Levant. France's quarantine laws had last been revised in 1822, and during this process the Marseille *Intendance* sent its own deputation to Paris to help put its stamp on the rules which governed the health of the nation.[46] As we have seen, Marseille's sanitary authorities appear to have seen their city's experience with the plague of the 1720s as having conferred an on them the eternal right (and duty) to protect the rest of France from contagion. Though there is evidence that the Interior Ministers of the Restoration (1815–30) attempted to prod the *Intendants* toward flexibility, they were largely unsuccessful.

The deadlock began to break, however, as France's links to the far side of the *cordon sanitaire* increased after the invasion of Algeria. Furthermore, under the July Monarchy (1830–48), the responsibility for French quarantine shifted from the Interior Ministry to the Ministry of Commerce and Industry. After the early 1830s, the balance of power between Paris and Marseille began to shift. By the middle of that decade, protests against changes to the laws were not enough to stop Parisian ministers from allowing a few select ports to join Marseille in the right to receive ships, cargoes, and passengers from the Levant.

French government ministers, by this time, decided to examine Mediterranean quarantine practice without consulting the *Marseillaise*. Pierre Ségur-Dupeyron, a journalist and bureaucrat we have encountered before, resumed his long-standing interest in quarantine by publishing a major report in 1839 detailing the various procedures in different ports in Europe.[47] Named "Inspector-General of Lazarettos" and "President of the Superior Council of Health," Ségur-Dupeyron constituted an alternative (and reformist) locus of expertise upon which government ministers could rely, and fashioned a new method of calculation. Quarantine policy could be made, he insisted, without relying on divided medical opinion, simply by balancing risk of disease, risk of retaliatory quarantine, and expense. While presumably boards of health considered similar variables, Ségur-Dupeyron's work can be seen as an attempt to make quarantine regulation legible for national ministers, to enable them to take it on themselves. This was in concert with the trend described in Chapter 7, in which governments began to take over for doctors by addressing etiological conundrums through empiricism. By the late 1830s, it was no longer persuasive for the *Intendants* to insist that liberalization would elicit retaliatory quarantines in Italy, Spain, and Austria. In this context, the willingness of the British and

---

[46] Étienne Majastre, the powerful secretary of the *Intendance*, and Alexis-Joseph Rostand, one of its members, appear to have been central to debates over the composition of the 1822 law. For their correspondence with the *Intendance* during the debates on the law in 1821, see ADBR 200 E 343.

[47] P. Ségur-Dupeyron, *Rapport adressé à S. Exc. le Ministère du Commmerce et l'Agriculture sur des modifications à apporter aux règlements sanitaires* (Paris: Imprimerie Nationale, 1839).

Austrians to move toward an international conference convinced successive Ministers of Commerce that they could now push for greater reform in Marseille. In particular, Laurent Cunin-Gridaine, who served as minister from 1839 to 1848 (with one interruption), developed a nakedly antagonistic attitude to the *Intendants* (Figure 9.3).

Immediately after the publication of Ségur-Dupeyron's 1839 report, Cunin-Gridaine instructed the *Intendants* to reduce their required periods of detention and to ease the fumigation rules for Levantine cotton.[48] Less than two weeks later, he wrote again, noting with approval the modest reduction on quarantine for ships coming from Constantinople. This minor victory, however, only whetted his appetite for more liberalization, and he used the precedent of this first concession to press for more fundamental change. In the contentious climate of the 1840s, if the *Intendants* gave an inch, the Minister came back demanding a mile.

Quarantine as practiced at Marseille, Cunin-Gridaine informed the *Intendants*, was out of step with the times. The speed of the new steamboats, he claimed, "has, for some time now, fundamentally changed our relationship with the Levant . . . and the sanitary rules, written in entirely different circumstances, can hardly be

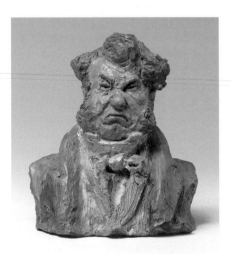

Figure 9.3 The satirical artist Honoré Daumier's 1833 depiction of Laurent Cunin-Gridaine (Minister of Commerce and Industry and chief antagonist of Marseille's Intendance Sanitaire). Painted clay sculpture. Musée d'Orsay, Paris.

[48] See Cunin-Gridaine to Intendants, January 11, 1840, ADBR 200 E 208.

applied today without accepting shockingly unreasonable contradictions."[49] Anticontagionist doctors, such as Louis Aubert-Roche, were ever more eager to trumpet arguments like this, knowing they would be more persuasive to ministers than the details of medical theory. Cunin-Gridaine's apparent certainty that it was safe to dramatically reduce quarantine was influenced by another claim made by Aubert-Roche in 1841: that plague had only ever broken out in the lazaretto after the arrival of a plague ship. In other words, no ship without plague on board had brought plague to Europe.[50] Though this excluded a number of debatable cases (such as Remé Fondant's spontaneous death described in Chapter 4), it implied that more than 99 percent of quarantine could safely be abolished. Empirical statistics like this proved a potent challenge to boards of health in the 1840s in a way they had not before. Cunin-Gridaine proved himself to be adept at spotting any foreign regulations that were more liberal than Marseille's and pressuring the *Intendants* to follow suit. In the same letter quoted above, Cunin-Gridaine noted that he had examined the tables of quarantine lengths from Italian lazarettos and that Livorno required fewer days in quarantine. He ended his letter with the hope that in the future the *Intendants* would "take initiative" themselves in reducing their quarantine requirements.[51]

The next few years would reveal the vanity of this hope. Before Marseille had even agreed (under pressure from Cunin-Gridaine) on the proposal to admit ships from French Algeria in free pratique, the Minister was telling the *Intendants* he saw no reason why Egypt, in years without plague, could not have its ships admitted without quarantine.[52] Ministers were now questioning long-standing practices of the quarantine system, such as the principle of fumigating merchandise. Cunin-Gridaine's temporary successor, Alexandre Gouin, complained that in response to skepticism about the contagious properties of trade goods, the *Intendants* consistently recalled the cases of porters in the 1720s who had died after fumigating merchandise. Such facts, Gouin complained, were marked by "extreme uncertainty." If the *Intendants* wanted to insist on the hazard of imported goods, they had better "consult their archives" and come up with something better.[53]

Returning to the Ministry in January 1841, Cunin-Gridaine demanded once and for all that Marseille end quarantine on ships from Algeria.[54] The *Intendants* responded that this laxity would not only endanger France, but also damage their own reputation. To allow ships to arrive from Africa in free pratique would provoke a reaction from boards of health in Italy and

---

[49] Cunin-Gridaine to Intendants, January 27, 1840, ADBR 200 E 208.
[50] Aubert-Roche's publication to this effect is cited in Wells, "Practical Results," 833.
[51] Cunin-Gridaine to Intendants, January 27, 1840, ADBR 200 E 208.
[52] Cunin-Gridaine to the Intendants, February 15, 1840, ADBR 200 E 208.
[53] Alexandre Gouin to the Intendants, March 18, 1840, ADBR 200 E 208.
[54] Cunin-Gridaine to the Intendants, January 28, 1841, ADBR 200 E 208.

Spain.[55] Though the *Intendance* was forced to back down on this occasion (now having maintained a quarantine on a supposedly integral part of France for more than a decade), its members were right to be concerned about the reaction abroad. When the British consul in Turin invoked French precedents in order to persuade the Sardinian government to loosen rules for ships coming from Gibraltar, he was told "that the Marseilles Board of Health has lost a great deal of its credit of late, owing to the relaxations introduced into its laws, and that this country [i.e., Piedmont-Sardinia] was chiefly influenced in her sanitary system by Naples and Leghorn."[56] This was a far cry from the state of affairs only a few years earlier when Genoa and Marseille were in as harmonious a concord as two boards of health could be, and other Italian boards looked to their example. While Britain and France continued efforts to reduce quarantine, the Italian states appeared to be a redoubt of the old severity. As late as 1850, for example, the Naples Board of Health threatened to place all ships from Malta under quarantine because Malta had allowed the French steamer *Télémaque* into free pratique on its arrival from Southern France, at a time when Naples was trying to pressure the French to quarantine arrivals from North America.[57]

The *Intendants* were not willing to accept this loss of status without a fight. In addition to pleading with ministers about the danger of losing credibility among foreign boards of health (and floating the possibility that French ships might be detained in Italy), they contrived other strategies. One was to simply ignore requests to reconsider their rules,[58] or even to take active measures of retaliation against those calling for further reform. When Mohammed Ali's French medical advisor Clot Bey published a treatise claiming that he had observed abuses occurring in the Lazaretto of Arenc, the *Intendants* sued him for libel.[59]

Throughout this contentious period, the *Intendants* attempted to sustain the normal patterns of communication and the mutual enforcement of common European standards, despite their government's efforts to impose unilateral reform. In the winter of 1841–42, when the Maltese Board of Health announced its plan to reduce quarantine for ships from the Levant, the *Intendants* communicated their severe displeasure, and Malta backed down. This episode however, reached the ears of the Foreign Affairs minister who, in turn,

[55] See Cunin-Gridaine to the Intendants, February 19, 1841, ADBR 200 E 208.

[56] Augustus Foster to Lord Palmerston, May 11, 1840, *Correspondence Relative to the Contagion of the Plague*, 171.

[57] William Temple to Gov. O'Farrall, June 23, 1850, NAM CSG/03/707.

[58] This is clear, for example, from letters (Cunin-Gridaine to Intendants, May 21, 1841, May 24, 1841, November 11, 1842) surrounding the issue of the British government's demand that quarantine be dropped on the Ionian Islands since Algeria had been admitted to free pratique at Marseille. Marseille's Intendants appear not to have issued any response to the request. ADBR 200 E 208.

[59] See Gouin to the Intendants, May 25, 1840, ADBR 200 E 208.

informed Cunin-Gridaine. The incensed Minister of Commerce immediately wrote to the *Intendants*, upbraiding their "retrograde" intervention and demanding they recant. Both Britain and Austria had begun to reduce their clean bill quarantines (especially for steamship passengers). If enacted, Cunin-Gridaine noted, this change would allow travelers from the Middle East to reach Paris faster going via Trieste or Southampton than they would going by way of Marseille.[60]

Because of all of these factors, by the middle of the decade, Cunin-Gridaine's relationship with the *Intendance* had reached such a low point that he no longer bothered to inform them as the government enacted sweeping changes to French quarantine rules. In 1845, he persuaded King Louis-Philippe to issue a Royal *Ordonnance* suppressing quarantine on all ships from Tunisia, Morocco, Greece, and the Ionian Islands with clean bills of health. Slowly but surely, the distant coasts of the Mediterranean were being forcibly integrated into the zone of free pratique, a trend that the *Intendants* found impossible to accept. At a climactic meeting in June of that year, the exasperated guardians of quarantine in France's largest Mediterranean port made a last-ditch effort to assert their independence and dramatically resigned. According to a Savoyard newspaper,

The *Intendance Sanitaire* of Marseille has just handed in its resignation *en masse* ... The members of the *Intendance* have taken this action in order to disassociate themselves from all responsibility for participating in a system tending towards the abolition of quarantines. This is, they believe, a pernicious trend, which will soon subject France to all the horrors of a pestilential invasion.[61]

The *Intendants* insisted their resignation was "definitive."[62] Yet, if they expected this dramatic action to force the minister to recant, they were unsuccessful. Without much fanfare, they allowed themselves to be reconvened in the autumn of 1845 and were rendered even more impotent after French quarantine rules were drastically reduced in 1847, in the wake of a Paris Academy of Medicine report (with quarantine on the Middle East eliminated in the overwhelming majority of cases). In 1850, the *Intendance* was finally dissolved by ministerial decree when it refused to back down over a quarantine imposed on Malta during a cholera epidemic.[63]

---

[60] Cunin-Gridaine to the Intendants, June 26, 1842, ADBR 200 E 208.

[61] *Courier des Alpes*, June 7, 1845.

[62] Intendants to Cunin-Gridaine, June 9 and June 20, 1845, ADBR 200 E 194.

[63] In 1864, Dr. Évariste Bertulus dedicated a history of the *Intendance* to what he saw as the heroic former Intendants, who had resisted Parisians who were "not wanting, in 1850, to realize that they were blinded by the allure of a false doctrine." He defiantly ended his dedication by declaring that his work was "éminemment marseillaise" (fundamentally from Marseille). See Évariste Bertulus, *Marseille et son intendance sanitaire* (Marseille: Camoin Frères, 1864), v–vi.

The development of steamships, the French colonization of Algeria, and a new consensus in favor of free trade did not directly force the *Intendants* to give way; the decisive change was the growing resolve of Paris to interest itself directly in the details of quarantine practice. This was clearly related to the increasing political sympathy between Britain and France under the July Monarchy and the concurrent efforts by both countries, from the late 1830s, to organize an international conference to reform quarantine practice (although this would not occur until 1851). Mediterranean boards of health had created a system where shared norms and a tradition of transnational communication maintained the sanitary status quo. At the ministerial level, however, the decision to charge national bodies like the Academy of Medicine with investigating quarantine, alongside high-level diplomacy with the English and Austrians, finally disrupted the power of local administrations. The move from a quarantine-centric public health regime to a more multifaceted approach to the nation's health should be understood as a process in which sanitary authority was steadily centralized in national capitals even *before* we consider the specific content of new public health legislation with its "centralizing" tendencies.

Britain represents a unique case, in which, as a division of the Customs Service and as a body subject to the authority of the Privy Council, the quarantine administration was already centralized prior to the dismemberment of the system in the 1840s and 1850s. And yet, the reaction of the staff of Britain's quarantine service demonstrates the enormous disruption resulting from the reformist atmosphere of the late 1840s. It also shows the extent to which those responsible for maintaining quarantine in British ports resented the power of new health authorities like the General Board of Health.

Much like the practice in Mediterranean Europe, the (exceptionally large) upper rungs of Britain's quarantine service included long-serving superintendents, doctors, and "lazaretto masters" (an appropriate term, given that Britain's "floating lazarettos" were decommissioned ships of the Royal Navy) whose high average salaries (all made more than £100/year) put them within the early Victorian middle class. Including those officials, guardians, mariners, and boys of all work, the quarantine establishments at Stangate Creek, Milford Haven, and the Motherbank each employed dozens of workers, with smaller stations employing anywhere from five to twenty employees. All told, by the late 1840s, the total number of employees in all of Britain's quarantine stations amounted to 161, and required an annual expenditure of £15,617.[64] This sum places Britain's quarantine expenditures on par with or higher than most Continental states.

---

[64] "A Return of the Number of Persons Employed Exclusively on Quarantine Duty in the United Kingdom and the Expenses of the Quarantine Service Therein," November 4, 1848, TNA PC 1/2659.

This maintenance of a robust staff persisted despite a general trend toward contracted durations of quarantine. A copy of reformed rules issued by the PC in the fall of 1843 shows that the mandated detention for ships from the Levant with clean bills of health was only five days (with a mere twelve days for ships with a foul bill).[65] Nevertheless, in addition to these ships, any vessels lacking certificates stating that their enumerated goods were not from Anatolia or North Africa were also subjected to quarantine. And, even in a liberalized quarantine regime, the demands on quarantine workers were extensive. Since 1827, as already mentioned, ships from European ports in the Mediterranean were excluded from quarantine. Yet, by the terms of the Order in Council granting them free pratique, a medical officer had to sign off that the crew looked healthy and the trade goods had the correct certificates. In 1847, Dr. Robert Brown, the medical officer who had served in that role for twenty years, decided to retire, and preserves a sense of what his work conditions were like in a letter to the PC:

I feel that my Health requires change of air more particularly as I have been for many years at a time without sleeping a single night on shore as the Vessels with Clean Bills arriving from Christian Ports required examination without a moments [sic] detention from an early hour to sunset throughout the year.[66]

Despite the conditions under which Brown had labored, he determined that he wished his son (who was, he said, a capable surgeon with an MD from Edinburgh) to succeed him in the same position. Apparently, sleeping onboard a hospital ship for two decades and being roused at early hours to certify the salubrity of any ships that happened to arrive, still seemed like a desirable career given the dependability of the work and the relatively high salary it commanded. Across the quarantine service, the elevated level of traffic was more than enough to keep employees busy throughout the 1840s, and it is clear from the records maintained by the PC that new staff continued to be hired as late as 1847. Indeed, the junior Dr. Brown would not have immediately been laid off, as Stangate Creek retained a skeletal staff throughout the later nineteenth century and the medical officer was an indispensable role.

Yet, the drift toward the elimination of quarantine meant that most customs officials charged with managing the system began to see the writing on the wall. By the late spring of 1847, lists of quarantine staff prepared for the PC began to feature the ominous annotation "recommend reduction" next to numerous names, thus indicating that substantial layoffs were already being considered even while the lazarettos kept hiring. In May of that year, without the declaration of new Orders in Council, ships from the Middle East with clean bills of health and healthy crews were largely exempted from quarantine (this radical

---

[65] Charles Greville to Charles Scovell, September 26, 1843, TNA PC 7/5.

[66] Robert Brown to unknown (presumably Greville, as PC Secretary), May 20, 1847, TNA PC 1/ 2659.

change in quarantine practice seems to have been enacted simply by a letter from Quarantine Superintendent William Pym to the Board of Trade).[67] Despite the evident consequences of the new policy, the employees of the Quarantine Service maintained the continued relevance of their role and hoped to avoid the massive layoffs it would seem to suggest.

In this decade when quarantine workers clearly felt under siege, we see them attempting to combat accusations that their operations were overly expensive or full of unwarranted delays. In 1841, for example, a member of the staff at Stangate Creek signing only as "Veritas" drafted a letter to the editor of the *Shipping and Mercantile Gazette* attempting to rebut allegations that ships performing quarantine at Stangate Creek were subject to ludicrous delays. Protesting the charge that quarantine workers were lazy and overpaid, "Veritas" insisted that they worked "from sunrise to after sunset."[68] As we have already seen, the orientation of the General Board of Health created by the 1848 Public Health Act was rigidly antiquarantinist, and one of the first official actions of that Board was to send inspectors to Stangate Creek, presumably to collect incriminating data for the scathing *Report on Quarantine* published a year later. George Ley, a longtime administrator of the quarantine site, immediately divined their purpose after they posed a number of leading questions about the unhealthiness of the air around the quarantine harbor and their supposition that the water, too, must be of poor quality. In a letter to the Superintendent (recording this visit with some alarm), Ley noted that he stressed the excellent quality of the water and noted that he had suffered from only one "ague" throughout his seventeen years of service.[69]

When the General Board did launch its attack in 1849, Ley wrote to William Pym that "I saw the report of the General Board of Health in the *Times* and was fearful of the result." Further darkening the mood of Ley was an editorial in the *Shipping Gazette* published around the same time calling for the abolition of quarantines. Stangate Creek, he lamented, had been called the unhealthiest spot in the country, a charge that was primarily ideological and not at all borne out in the General Board of Health's own statistical reports (Figure 9.4).[70]

Less than two months later, with grim terseness, the Superintendent of the small quarantine station at St. Margaret's Hope informed Pym of the surrender of the quarantine service to the victorious General Board of Health:

[67] See Charles Greville to "Mr. Addington," August 2, 1851, TNA PC 1/4533. Greville writes that, notwithstanding the relevant orders in council, "this regulation has continued in force ever since [Pym's letter] and is the only document that can be given as the Quarantine Regulations now in force in the United Kingdom and Ireland."
[68] "Veritas," "Letter to the Editor of the *Shipping and Mercantile Gazette*," November 25, 1841, TNA PC 1/2659.
[69] George Ley to Superintendent Luck, November 22, 1848, TNA PC 1/2659.
[70] Ley to Pym, June 6, 1849, TNA PC 1/2659.

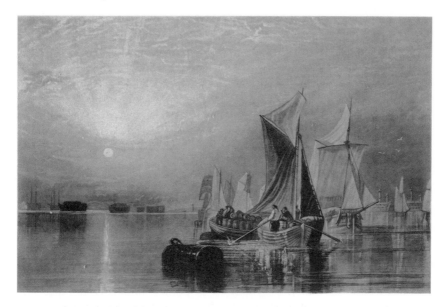

Figure 9.4 From *The Rivers of England: Stangate Creek*, 1827. Mezzotint showing the Stangate Creek Quarantine Station. After a painting by J. M. W. Turner (1775–1851), engraved by T. Lupton. Photo ©, Tate Gallery.

I beg to acknowledge the receipt of your letter of the 25th Instant, intimating to me the determination of Her Majesty's Government to discontinue all restrictions upon vessels coming from the Levant, and to abolish the quarantine stations. I shall without delay communicate this information to the officers and men in the department here, that their services will not be required after the Termination of the present year.[71]

There would be no revival of large-scale quarantine in British ports, and Pym's letter of May 1847 can serve as a final word. It bears reiterating what a blow this was to the dozens of employees who had assumed their service in Britain's floating lazarettos would be long-term; in Britain, as in the Mediterranean, a position with the quarantine service had promised to be a lifelong career. At Stangate Creek in the mid-1820s, for example, the average length of service for the twenty-three members of the quarantine office was more than twenty-one years.[72]

---

[71] B. Robertson to Pym, July 27, 1849, TNA PC 1/2659.
[72] See "An Account of the Quarantine Establishment," sent by Charles Saunders (Superintendent of Quarantine at Stangate Creek) to HM Commissioners of Customs, December 4, 1825, TNA PC 1/2659.

Quarantine formally remained on the books and, as Krista Maglen has shown, it was still deployed for select ships in the ensuing decades. Yet, the finality of the reforms of the late 1840s is impossible to miss. No further application of quarantine was without controversy, and the "English System" of mostly open barriers, port health inspectors, and medical inspections came to be a point of pride to a country holding itself open to the goods of the world.[73] When the Quarantine Act of 1825 was finally repealed under Lord Salisbury's government in 1896, few mourned its passing.

The Landscape Changes

By the time the first International Sanitary Conference convened in Paris in 1851 the British quarantine service had been transformed beyond recognition. Quarantine had been severely curtailed in French ports, and movements to reform quarantine in Italy were well under way. Part of the prevailing sense among historians that the conference accomplished little surely springs from the fact that between 1843 and 1849 so much change had already occurred. And, if negotiations to hold a similar conference had foundered after 1838, one of the reasons they were successful at the turn of the 1850s was the enormous variation that now existed between a quarantine regime that continued to be fairly rigorous in Spain and most Italian states and one that was vanishing from existence in British, French, and Austrian-controlled ports. Even so, the tenacity of tradition and the transnational patterns established by boards of health essentially made such an unprecedented conference essential if quarantine reform was to prove enduring. If the principles of mutually assured disinfection facilitated transnational sanitary control from the ground up in the decades before 1851, they also shaped the diplomatic-medical milieu of the conference that helped bring universal quarantine to a close.

Still, reformist currents were stirring even among the more traditionally "conservative" powers. Especially now that the focus of sanitary diplomacy was transferred from networks of boards of health and consuls to socially prominent doctors, high-level diplomats, and national governments, there was broad agreement on many issues. In such an atmosphere, the main concern for Britain's delegates was to ensure that other conferees would not seek to impose additional delays (such as mandatory visits by medical officers, new kinds of sanitary certificates, or new requirements for ships of war). The sanitary status quo (as achieved through unilateral action undertaken in the course of the 1840s) was satisfactory from the perspective of the British delegates. That said, the 1851 conference imposed a sense of

[73] See Maglen, *The English System.*

international legitimacy on the reform that had already begun. Although its conclusions were formally adopted by only two of the powers that attended, it was recognized throughout the long nineteenth century as the conclusive moment that replaced the previous quarantine regime. As an American doctor wrote, in a 1905 report to the US Public Health and Marine Hospital Service, the 1851–52 conference marked "a revolution in quarantine methods on the Continent" and signified "the close of the old régime of quarantine," in which it had been practiced on a "uniform basis" across the Mediterranean.[74] Indeed, the first International Sanitary Conference's significance extends far beyond the formal incorporation of its conclusions into national law.

The 1850 proposal by the government of France's Second Republic to convene an international sanitary conference precipitated a series of such conferences that lasted into the twentieth century. Again, the World Health Organization (WHO) has acknowledged this series of meetings to be an institutional precedent. While later conferences were held to respond to specific epidemic threats, the initial event, eventually convened in 1851, was devoted to an attempt to standardize European quarantines. Especially after the French and British reforms of the 1840s, practice varied substantially across the Mediterranean in 1851, and the Conference was an opportunity to ratify and generalize a new sanitary regime. As F. J. Martinez has persuasively argued, the initiative for the first International Sanitary Conference in 1851 also sprang from France's ambitions to increase its Mediterranean trade.[75] Even so, British, Austrian, Spanish, and Italian officials (among others) were happy to pursue this opportunity for regularization. Again, we can see the 1851 Conference as an attempt to impose a new sanitary order on the Mediterranean after the unilateral actions of national governments over the last decade had upset the balance achieved by long-standing interactions among local boards of health.

Invitations to the Conference were extended to all powers with a Mediterranean or Black Sea coast, to the Portuguese, and to the British as well, in recognition of Britain's colonies in the region. Spain, Portugal, Britain, France, Tuscany, the Papal States, the Kingdom of the Two Sicilies, Sardinia, Greece, Russia, and the Ottoman Empire were represented, with a medical

---

[74] John Macaulay Eager, *The Early History of Quarantine: Origin of Sanitary Measures Directed against Yellow Fever* (Washington, DC: US Government Printing Office, 1903), 24–25. The idea that the 1851–52 Conference marked a major transformation in quarantine practice was expressed roughly contemporaneously by the French advocate of Middle Eastern sanitary surveillance, Dr. Adrien Proust (father of Marcel Proust). See A. Proust, *La défense de l'Europe contre la peste et la conférence de Venise de 1897* (Paris: Masson, 1897), 348.

[75] See F. J. Martinez, "International or French?" For another account of the origin of the 1851 conference and a detailed study of many of its participants, see João Rangel de Almeida, "The 1851 International Sanitary Conference and the Construction of an International Sphere of Public Health," PhD diss., Edinburgh, 2012, esp. chapter 1.

delegate and a diplomatic representative from each government. In this way, the structure of boards of health, with their mix of politicians, diplomats, and medical members, was, to a notable extent, mapped onto the International Sanitary Conference (though there were fewer aristocrats and no mercantile representation). The principle of quarantine management as a twin matter of diplomacy and medicine thus helped lay the foundation of international health.

Britain's medical and diplomatic delegates to the first and second International Sanitary Conferences (1851 and 1859) were the anticontagionist doctor John Sutherland, a member of the General Board of Health, and Sir Anthony Perrier, the British consul at Brest. Arriving armed with a copy of the GBH Report of 1849, Sutherland and Perrier saw themselves as part of a reformist bloc that included the Austrian and French delegates. In the spirit of alliance, the British supported a proposal to give the President of the Congress a vote (in effect giving France a larger number of votes than any other power) "because France is evidently inclined to cooperate with Great Britain in 'liberalizing' Quarantine Regulations."[76]

At the conference's opening on August 5, 1851, the French Foreign Minister began with a paean to the spirit of internationalism sweeping across a Europe fully recovered from the crises of 1848. The Great Exhibition, then under way in London, he claimed, proceeded from the same international spirit that motivated the conference. Moreover, massive technological change had revolutionized transportation across the world, "but to complete this magnificent work of humanity" further rationalization of "sanitary obstacles" was imperative.[77]

Following the approach of Ségur-Dupeyron almost two decades earlier, the delegates attempted to impose order and system on a medical landscape still fraught with uncertainty. Through an untested power of consensus, of definitive votes and declarations by elite figures, they hoped to overwhelm nosological and epidemiological ambiguity. Perrier immediately found himself included on a more exclusive subcommittee of seven (four doctors and three consuls) tasked with making the consequential decisions of which diseases should be subject to quarantine and what canonical procedures ought to be deployed for those diseases. Perrier's dispatches to Lord Palmerston confirm, as we might expect, that the Committee resolved the subject of plague most crisply: on the appearance both of epidemic or even "sporadic" reports of disease, the plague should be subject to sanitary regulation in the form of quarantines. Yellow fever would be subject to possible quarantines in the case of a ship departing from a port in the midst of an epidemic, though unlike plague, "sporadic" reports would not be enough. Cholera, on the other hand, was emphatically declared by

---

[76] J. Sutherland and A. Perrier to Lord Palmerston, August 11, 1851, TNA PC 1/4533.
[77] *Moniteur*, August 6, 1851. Contained in TNA PC 1/4533.

most delegates not to be a "quarantinable" disease. Disinfection of clothes, letters, and merchandise was restricted to plague and only to plague.[78] Most of these measures passed the subcommittee by wide majorities (on 6–1 or 5–2 votes) indicating many of the delegates had come to the conference already eager to standardize the reduction of quarantine and to firmly limit it to extraordinary circumstances. In that vein, some skepticism about the different treatment accorded to cholera here is very much in order; unlike plague or yellow fever, cholera was, by now, a routine scourge of cities in Europe, and were it to have been declared "quarantinable," the quarantine system would have been brought back to life as a constant of intra-European travel. Both the British delegates and French conference organizers feared this outcome, and the latter tried to organize the crucial subcommittee in such a way as to prevent it.[79]

While it was true (as Perrier assessed) that most of the delegates were contagionists to the extent that they agreed isolation was an effective strategy against the plague (and potentially yellow fever), they were sufficiently "contingent" contagionists to accept wide-ranging reforms. In the measures discussed for the quarantine in cases of plague, an agreement was struck to let the fumigation of cotton remain up to individual countries (with a guarantee of no retaliatory quarantines). In passing this measure, delegates from more conservative states were clearly signaling that they believed there was no risk from contagion imported through cotton, but that the end of the traditional system of enumerated goods might appear a bridge too far back home. This disjunction between the reformist impulses of delegates and the ostensible caution of the publics they represented caused both Perrier and Sutherland to support a measure allowing delegates to vote in secret.[80]

All told then, the conference was off to a very promising start as far as the British delegates were concerned. By mid-October, Perrier and Sutherland enthused to Lord Palmerston about how many Britons would gain from "the advantages which commerce will derive from the changes already agreed to by the Conference."[81] Such letters were sent not only to Britain's ponderous Foreign Secretary but also submitted to the inquiring eyes at the General Board of Health (Sutherland himself was an inspector for the GBH). Chadwick and Southwood Smith clearly intended that the GBH should be involved in setting the nation's quarantine policy, and alongside Palmerston, they must have been happy with what they were reading of their colleague's activities. Again, there had been clear wins on such British priorities as fixed

---

[78] A summary of these decisions and votes is included in Anthony Perrier to Lord Palmerston, September 1, 1851, TNA PC 1/4533.
[79] See Rangel de Almeida, "1851 International Sanitary Conference," 130.
[80] Perrier and Sutherland to Palmerston, August 11, 1851, TNA PC 1/4533.
[81] Perrier and Sutherland to Palmerston, October 15, 1851, TNA MH 255/13, ff. 210–12.

limits on lengths of detention, severe limits on quarantines for ships with clean bills of health, the dispensation to land cotton in free pratique, and the limiting of yellow fever quarantine to the summer months.

While the conference retained the possible "extra and special precaution" of limited clean bill quarantines on ships from the Ottoman Empire, such quarantines were always to be inclusive of the sea voyage, rendering them essentially moot at many ports. Furthermore, clean bill quarantines were to be totally abolished after the creation of a new "sanitary organization" throughout the Ottoman state, a European surveillance network of consuls who could report on any outbreaks of epidemic disease.[82] While more reformist powers had no intention of deploying even limited clean bill quarantines, that even the conservative delegates from Naples and the Papal States were willing to accept such reforms indicated a growing confidence that the "remarkable cessation" of plague in Egypt and Anatolia would prove permanent.[83] Conferees studied the latest medical reports on plague and yellow fever – reading in detail, for example, a study by a French doctor, which emphasized that Egypt had not experienced epidemic plague since 1839 or even sporadic plague since 1844.[84] The claim was ratified with testimony from none other than Ségur-Dupeyron himself, who, from his new perch as Inspector of Lazarettos, had conducted a mission to observe the new Ottoman sanitary apparatus in 1845 and found not a single case of plague across the Empire. Other medical testimony was added to the accumulating evidence that this one-time "reservoir" of the plague was now free of it. The effects of recognizing such a change, as we have already seen, were momentous. When a proposal was made to allow countries near or contiguous to the Ottoman Empire to preserve some traditional standards of quarantine, the measure was roundly defeated, though it returned to the agenda for the Second International Sanitary Conference in 1859 as a new plague epidemic broke out in Benghazi.[85]

The initial work on the length of quarantine, the abolition of "suspected" bills of health, and new rules for enumerated goods remained the most consequential results of the conference. Part of the reason, perhaps, that the conference has been treated as relatively inconsequential is that its long duration saw an early flurry of important agreement followed by unresolved discussion and discord. The participants were still sitting, it should be noted, during Louis Bonaparte's brazen coup of December 2. In this way, the delegates had the dubious honor of contributing to an apparent international blessing of the fall of the Second Republic to its new Prince President.

Yet, it was some of the later work of the conference on sanitary surveillance in the Middle East that laid the groundwork for future events. Indeed,

---

[82] Milroy, *International Quarantine Conference*, 5.   [83] Ibid., 6.
[84] See Report by F. Meuriey, TNA MH 255/13, ff. 249–80.   [85] See TNA PC 1/2670.

Sylvia Chiffoleau has argued that the long-term internationalization of public health into the twentieth century derived from an enduring attention to what she calls "the sanitary question of the Orient."[86] This "Orient" was much larger than the one feared as a source of plague a generation earlier. If plague epidemics in port cities and along coasts constituted the central dilemmas of the quarantine system explored in the preceding pages, from the 1860s on, large movements of people such as occurred during the *Hajj* were now the center of attention as the fear shifted to the global pathways of cholera.[87] The failure of Mediterranean quarantine to stop cholera in the 1830s and 1840s meant the resurgence of the disease in the fourth pandemic of the 1860s did not generate momentum for reviving the regular, universal quarantine that is the chief focus of this book. And yet, the new centrality of cholera in public health discourse and the manner in which its transmission was focused primarily on the movement of colonized peoples help us understand how quarantine became significantly more racialized in the latter part of the nineteenth century. European navies, traders, and travelers were unlikely to be caught up in a new system designed to regulate the travel of pilgrims on the *Hajj* and centered on stopping cholera before it could reach the Mediterranean Basin. Among the only Europeans to be subjected to a regular quarantine of this new, seasonal, and particularized style were Bosnian Muslims returning from the *Hajj* each year.[88]

In some cases, the removal of the possibility that quarantine could ensnare most white Europeans appears to have made old opponents of the system more open to its appeal. Perhaps this lay behind the new willingness of Gavin Milroy, longtime opponent of quarantine, to convene a commission to decide whether it was necessary in the late 1850s, during the plague epidemic of Benghazi.[89] Both the British and French governments used the position their diplomats had on new Ottoman health boards after the 1838–39 quarantine reforms to keep tabs on any outbreaks of disease along Red Sea routes of pilgrimage and migration. Given that most Southern European lazarettos remained in operation for occasional ships with foul bills of health and that the Mediterranean and Aegean Seas remained the primary frontiers across which cholera reached the Continent

---

[86] Chiffoleau, *Genèse de la Santé Publique*, chapter 2.
[87] On the way fears about cholera transmission during the *Hajj* came to be central to debates about quarantine in the 1860s, see Chiffoleau, *Genèse de la Santé Publique*, 90–93.
[88] On this phenomenon, see Christian Promitzer, "Prevention and Stigma: The Sanitary Control of Muslim Pilgrims from the Balkans 1830–1914," in Chircop and Martínez, *Mediterranean Quarantines*, 145–65.
[89] On Milroy's commission, see McDonald, "History of Quarantine," 35–36. Again, though, there was no real push to bring back a quarantine system on the permanent footing that had existed before.

during the fourth pandemic, it is right to say the broader Mediterranean region had expanded to include the Red Sea.

Sylvia Chiffoleau aptly sums up the period in the wake of the 1847 French Academy of Medicine Report (discussed above) and the broader moves in Britain and Austria to reform quarantine rules as fundamentally about "externalization."[90] Across Western and Central Europe, the demolition of quarantine barriers was directly associated with increasing sanitary surveillance of the Ottoman Empire and North Africa. The 1847 Report explicitly adopted this policy, calling for the "transfer onto the coasts of the Orient, that is to say the point of departure, the precautions, which, in the past, have been taken on arrival."[91] This was precisely the same logic that had enabled Metternich, in 1838, to cast his newfound eagerness for an international conference to reduce quarantine lengths as the direct consequence of the signing of a treaty laying out Austrian assistance to the Ottomans in setting up a quarantine system in Anatolia.

In the event, numerous French, Italian, Austrian, and British doctors and diplomats cooperated with Ottoman officials to set up a complex network of sanitary barriers surrounding the Arabian peninsula, much as regions across the Mediterranean Basin and Balkan Peninsula constructed procedures to detain returning *Hajjis*. Intense transnational planning went into a quarantine site on the island of Mogador off the coast of Morocco.[92] Meanwhile, Indians were subjected to decades of detention at the Ottoman-run quarantine island of Kamaran (off the coast of what is now Yemen). Though some pilgrims from India managed to skirt this quarantine site by traveling first to Muscat and then onward to Jeddah, during the 1890s, it ensnared between 20 and 30,000 pilgrims each year, and even greater numbers in the run-up to the First World War.[93] This detention site actually reached its period of peak use in the early twentieth century when more than 56,000 Indian pilgrims were detained in 1912. The Tor quarantine site adjacent to the Suez Canal was staffed by Christian Greek doctors and was constructed as a pre-*Hajj* point of sanitary control and detention for would-be pilgrims from across North Africa. As Saurabh Mishra has

---

[90] Chiffoleau, *Genèse de la Santé Publique*, 65. João Rangel de Almeida makes a similar argument about the 1851 Conference and the way it fostered a rationale that the presence of cholera justified Western intervention in Ottoman public health, even as it facilitated a freer circulation of trade goods to European ports. See Rangel de Almeida, "Epidemic Opportunities: Panic, Quarantines, and the 1851 International Sanitary Conferences," in Peckham, *Empires of Panic*, 57–86.

[91] Bulletin of *Académie de médicine*. Quoted in Chiffoleau, *Genèse de la Santé Publique*, 67.

[92] See Francisco Javier Martínez, "Mending 'Moors' in Mogador: *Hajj*, Cholera, and Spanish-Moroccan Regeneration," in Chircop and Martínez, *Mediterranean Quarantines*, 66–106.

[93] Gülden Sarıyıldız and Oya Dağlar Macar, "Cholera, Pilgrimage, and International Politics of Sanitation: The Quarantine Station on the Island of Kamaran," in Varlık, *Plague and Contagion in the Islamic Mediterranean*, 252 and 262.

shown, both of these quarantine sites were flashpoints for violence and resistance – by the late nineteenth century, it is clear that those who continued to experience quarantine (entering and moving through the Ottoman state) were no longer the primarily Western travelers of yore, but colonial subjects, many of them indigent and unable to pay quarantine fees.[94] To defend quarantine from the 1870s onward was largely to endorse a deep global inequality that showed no signs of abating.

One of this book's central contentions is that Britain should not be seen as monolithically opposed to quarantine in favor of sanitarianism. To an extent, that remained true later in the nineteenth century and into the twentieth. At the same time, it is clearly the case that from the 1840s on, Britain's diplomatic orientation at International Sanitary Conferences and as a member of health boards in Egyptian and Ottoman port cities was to oppose the broader application of quarantine in favor of more open trade. This sometimes led to derisive comments from other European consuls and doctors that Britain was content to rely on its more remote geographical position and leave the rest of Europe open to epidemic contagion. Indeed, some British officials were proud of what they saw as a legacy of opposing more rigorous quarantines. Walter Miéville, British representative on the Alexandria Board of Health, referred to his career there as "my struggles, single-handed against twenty colleagues, on behalf of navigation."[95] Miéville noted, with apparent unconcern, that a French newspaper had considered his nomination to the health board to be "the triumph of cholera."[96]

That said, the disagreement Miéville was fixated on was one of degree more than kind. He was by no means opposed to all quarantines while on the health board, and while in many venues, Britain was pushing the most consistently antiquarantinist line of the European powers, in other areas, Britons were keen to institute quarantines. In Chapter 8, we saw that throughout the later nineteenth century, numerous Britons considered massive sanitary cordons to be essential responses to endemic plague in northern India. British officials were largely responsible for running the *Hajj* quarantine site at Kamaran from the middle of the First World War on, and rather than beginning to deconstruct the facility, they invested significant funds in upgrading it. The picture of British behavior during the third plague pandemic at the end of the century is mixed, however quarantines and isolation were certainly (and controversially) used to contain the plague in India, Cape Town, and Hong Kong. British politicians and administrators may have been proud of the "English System" of port health sanitation, but depending on place and context (and, above all, the extent to

---

[94] Saurabh Mishra, "Incarceration and Resistance in a Red Sea Lazaretto, 1880–1930," in *Quarantine: Local and Global Histories*, ed. Alison Bashford (New York: Palgrave, 2016), 54–65. See also Mark Harrison, "Quarantine, Pilgrimage, and Colonial Trade: India 1866–1900," *The Indian Economic and Social History Review* 29, no. 2 (1992): 117–44.
[95] Miéville, *Under Queen and Khedive*, 139.   [96] Ibid., 146.

which the subjects of their proposed quarantines were not white), they remained open to quarantine when it came to plague.

The 1866 International Sanitary Conference in Constantinople marked a growing international consensus in favor of contagionism,[97] which included a number of Britons. This was motivated primarily by fears of cholera importation during the *Hajj*. But the new momentum toward contagionism was also linked to a resurgence of plague in the Ottoman hinterland that occurred at the same time. In 1866 and 1867, a major outbreak occurred around Baghdad in Mesopotamia, prompting, at least temporarily, a fear that the absence of the plague enjoyed by the center of the Ottoman state since 1839 might well be illusory.[98] On observing the apparent resurrection of enthusiasm for quarantine, an aging Clot Bey, acolyte of anticontagion that he was, took the opportunity to lament that the 1851 Conference, in retrospect, represented the high-water mark of progressive public health. Now, he lamented, delegates to the 1866 Conference were endorsing "the renewal of the laws of the Middle Ages," something Clot found "deplorable."[99] Yet the weight of the future was not with him. As bacteriology made its halting way toward consensus in the 1870s and 1880s, later conferences were more likely to propose isolated, particular quarantines and to include cholera as a disease subject to isolation and detention (a trend that conveniently occurred after most European cities had experienced their final cholera epidemics).

On their winding path from poorly veiled anticontagionism in 1851 to contagionist principles as early as the 1860s, the International Sanitary Conferences transformed quarantine from a continuous system to an occasional instrument. Gone was even a tattered *cordon sanitaire*. Yet quarantine itself lingered. And as a situational tool, rather than an implacable barrier, it was more capable of making distinctions among the people singled out for isolation. This change explains why so many twentieth-century scholars of quarantine focus their studies on the race-based distinctions that such later iterations of the practice foregrounded. As a tool, quarantine could be applied to all manner of supposed threats. From "contagious Arabs" seeking entry to Europe,[100] to numerous immigrants to Australia and Canada, to Chinese immigrants in the western US (particularly in the era of the third plague pandemic), medical proscriptions were a convenient way to cloak racial anxiety.

---

[97] See Patrick Zylberman, "Civilizing the State: Borders, Weak States, and International Health in Modern Europe," in *Medicine at the Border*, ed. Alison Bashford (New York: Palgrave Macmillan, 2006), 25.
[98] The Ottoman Board of Health in Constantinople dispatched its chief medical advisor to observe the plague in Baghdad. On this epidemic, see J. B. Tholozan, *Une épidémie de Peste en Mesopotamie en 1867* (Paris: Victor Massin et Fils, 1869).
[99] Bey, *Deniers mots*, iv.   [100] See Chircop, "Quarantine, Sanitization," esp. 217.

In describing the later phases of quarantine this way, I am not attempting to exonerate the earlier practices that are the focus of this book. While the majority of those ensnared by the Mediterranean lazarettos were Europeans traveling between European ports or those returning from trade, travel, military service, or diplomacy in the Middle East, early nineteenth-century quarantine's enduring legacy has been the concept of a healthy Europe facing a suspect East and South. As I have written this book, the world has witnessed a surge of desperate migrants and refugees from the Middle East and Africa attempting to cross the Mediterranean along the same routes plied by ships subject to quarantine in the nineteenth century. They, too, are subject to a cordon of exclusion and suspicion, and unlike those who experienced universal quarantine, their detention does not come with a predetermined expiration date. In the language of nautical symbols, the yellow flag itself has changed its meaning from a ship in quarantine to one that is free of disease. But, in many ways, the freedom of movement that opponents of quarantine claimed they sought has been elusive in our own time. The ramparts of twenty-first century "Fortress Europe" are built, in part, along the same sanitary cordon, whose fortresses we have investigated, inhabited, and seen shuttered in the pages before.

Conclusion: Plagueomania

Adieu thou damndest quarantine / That gave me fever, and the spleen

Lord Byron, "A Farewell to Malta"

Did quarantine work and was it worth it? The enforcement of rigorous sanitation laws after the Marseille plague epidemic of the early eighteenth century did coincide with an epidemiological shift that left Western Europe (for the most part) free of the plague. While most quarantine procedures were irrelevant or gratuitous, the basic delays the system imposed clearly kept plague within lazarettos on several occasions when it otherwise could have spread further.[1] As we have seen in the final chapter, the end of universal quarantine did not depend on anticontagionist persuasiveness or ideological change so much as it responded to the medical state of affairs in the Middle East. Plague retains its status as a preeminent dread disease even today.

Mediterranean quarantine may literally have been "border medicine," but quarantined borders shifted constantly – imperialism, epidemiological change, and diplomacy made the boundaries between the medically secure and the suspiciously contagious ever subject to negotiation. The border with the longest staying power, of course, was that between "the Levant and Barbary" and the West. The consequences of the epidemiological imbalance between those parts of the world and Western Europe fed directly into long-standing tropes of Orientalist exoticism and decline, as I have shown. In a way, this geography has proved the most intractable, as the hardest Mediterranean borders today mimic the geography of quarantine.

Like all border regimes, quarantine reverberated far from the frontier. Whether or not it was an essential guarantor of national health, we have seen how it transformed debates about public health, how it helped shape diplomacy, and how it constituted a painful reality for hundreds of thousands of mobile Europeans, North Africans, and Ottomans who were ensnared in lazarettos for weeks and months. Quarantine renders visible the patterns and concerns of

---

[1] Other factors were undoubtedly also involved, including the evolution of the *Y. Pestis* bacteria, the displacement of the black rat by the brown rat in many parts of Europe, and a broad trend toward building in materials other than wood, rendering cities less congenial for fleas.

278

Mediterranean mobility during the great wave of globalization in the nineteenth century. Above all, this book has made a clear case that plague was experienced in the nineteenth century as a modern phenomenon. Mediterranean quarantine functioned as a transnational system, which influenced practice in metropolitan centers like London and also in colonial spaces from Cape Town to the Himalayas. A system defined by isolation and separation could also be a force toward coordination and connection – we have seen how the rhythms and precedents set by quarantine reveal the functioning of the Mediterranean as a multipolar world, even from the perspective of the dominant British Empire at the onset of the period of high imperialism.

Quarantine became a moral and philosophical touchstone. It was a common tactic of anticontagionists, as we have seen, to cast it as fundamentally opposed to liberalism. Many travelers who experienced the system agreed that it represented the surrender of personal freedom for an abstract idea of sanitary security. Yet, for the far greater portion of the public that did not experience quarantine at the border, exclusion seems to have sated public anxiety; universal quarantine was popular. Aside from additional costs on Levantine merchandise (which rarely commanded a mass market), there were few downsides to the system as far as the majority was concerned. This popularity is apparent from the text of the *1824 Select Committee Report*, in which MPs and doctors return again and again to the question of whether reform of the Quarantine Laws would stoke public "fears." This evidently did come to pass by the onset of the reforms of the 1840s – the first time quarantine was substantially reduced. When, in the 1840s, the British government first mooted plans to allow P&O steamers proceeding directly from Alexandria to land without quarantine at Southampton, a local outcry occurred. As the *Hampshire Advertiser* put it, "the plagueomania exploded the day steam-voyaging to Alexandria commenced."[2]

Quarantine had been designed to protect the entire populace, and apparently (at least in Southampton), most of that populace supported its continuation. Both the Tory *Advertiser* and the more liberal *Hampshire Independent* cohered around an opinion that the quarantine laws were useless: "unnecessary, and (for any practical purpose) ineffective," as the *Advertiser* put it,[3] while the *Independent* considered all lazarettos to be "absurd establishments."[4] Crucially, both newspapers place the blame for the continuing necessity of quarantine not on diplomatic imperatives but rather on popular fears within Britain. Not only did the *Advertiser* lament the "plagueomania" that had broken out in Southampton over the idea that the new steamers would be admitted without quarantine but the *Independent* also disdainfully ascribed the need to

---

[2] "Proposed Lazarette on the Southampton Water," *Hampshire Advertiser*, February 24, 1844.
[3] Ibid.   [4] "Southampton," *Hampshire Independent*, February 24, 1844.

continue quarantine to "the old-womanish fears of the timid portion of the community."[5]

It is not surprising that quarantine was most popular among the proportion of the population who did not have to experience it, but it is useful to remember the strong support it garnered, given the recurrent emphases in anticontagionist rhetoric (or in the historiography on quarantine reform) that a widespread consensus existed by the 1840s in favor of repealing the quarantine laws. A *limited* elite consensus is visible in the convergence of opinion between the Tory and Whig-Liberal press, but there is no reason to believe that, outside the halls of Parliament, the Foreign Office, or elite institutions of commerce and medicine, a mass public was on board with such a repeal.

Political debates about quarantine (in the present as in the past) often feature an uneasy populism. Yet, this book has shown that the impulses behind the Mediterranean system of universal quarantine were complex. A nuanced view becomes possible when we carefully consider the different registers on which quarantine politics can apply (abstract vs. particular; local vs. national). Rather than attempt to categorize nations as monolithically "quarantinist" or "sanitationist," we should accept that opinions about quarantine were shaped by much more than one's national origin. Around the Mediterranean, local boards of health were responsive to the concerns of their cities and imbued with the responsibility of being the final line of defense against epidemic disease (unlike national ministers, who had competing priorities). It should not surprise us, then, that these boards were responsible for the construction of quarantine as a transnational system. If epidemics did not respect borders, as board members knew they did not, it was all the more incumbent on local authorities to seek to forge links with colleagues across the Mediterranean, to cast their ambitions in favor of a universal system along a seamless frontier.

It is essential to approach the study of the early nineteenth-century system of universal quarantine in a way that crosses the frames of the local, national, and transnational. Such a multilevel lens is important not least because those who governed and experienced quarantine also traversed these frames of reference: health board members, diplomats, colonial officials, and travelers of all kinds. By situating this work in the interstices between transnational Mediterranean history and British history, we can see the wide reach of quarantine from the Middle Sea into domestic politics, and then around a global empire. British epidemic administrators on the Himalayan frontiers of their empire responded to plague similarly to the members of Mediterranean boards of health and were earnestly interested in their example.

Quarantine applies a blunt vision to the sensitive process of demarcating zones of health and disease. Over the centuries, it has severely impinged on the

---

[5] Ibid.

lives of many (and many others have passed their last days in a lazaretto or onboard a quarantined ship, far from their friends and family). Yet as a historical lens, quarantine has a salutary effect. This book has used it as a vehicle for understanding movement, diplomacy, and imaginative geography. Similarly, the study of quarantine should not be cordoned off from broader questions about the growth of the state, Orientalism, European integration, public health reform, and the history of borderlands. As a system located on the frontier of countries and continents, its study draws different fields of inquiry together. Pursuing the history of quarantine's administration in tandem with the controversies it generated and the testimony of those it ensnared lets us look inward to national histories and outward to global stories simultaneously.

Bibliography

Primary Sources

Adam, Joseph. *An Inquiry into the Laws of Different Epidemic Diseases, with the View to Determine the Means of Preserving Individuals and Communities from Each.* London: Printed for J. Johnson et al. by W. Thorne, 1809.

Adams, Francis. *The Medical Works of Paulus Aegineta.* London: J. Welsh, 1834.

Administration Sanitaire de Marseille. *Conservation de la santé publique.* Marseille: Bertrand, 1799.

Alison, William Pulteney. *Observations on the Management of the Poor in Scotland and Its Effects on the Health of the Great Towns.* Edinburgh: William Blackwood, 1840.

Anonymous. *Considerations on the Nurseries for British Seamen; the Present State of the Levant and Carriage-Trade in the Mediterranean; and the Comparative, Military, Naval, and Commercial Powers of the Barbary States.* [London], 1766.

Anonymous [An Untainted Englishman]. *The Nature of a Quarantine, as It Is Performed in Italy; to Guard against That Very Alarming and Dreadful Contagious Distemper, Commonly Called the Plague. With Important Remarks on the Necessity of Laying Open the Trade to the East Indies.* London: J. Williams, 1767.

Anonymous. *A Letter on Spasmodic Cholera.* London: Highley, 1832.

Anonymous [A Merchant in Turkey]. *A Letter to Mr. Eton from a Merchant in Turkey, in Answer to a Chapter in His Survey of the Turkish Empire, to Prove the Necessity of Abolishing the Levant Company; and Also, On Quarantine Regulations.* London: J. Mathews, 1799.

Anonymous. *Rapport sur la transmission de la peste et de la fièvre jaune.* Marseille: Barlatier-Feissat et Demoncy, 1845.

Anonymous. *A Comparative Estimate of the Advantages Great Britain Would Derive from a Commercial Alliance with the Ottoman, in Preference to the Russian Empire.* London: J. Debrett and J. Johnson, 1791.

Anonymous. *Procès-verbaux de la Conférence sanitaire internationale ouvert à Paris, le 27 Juillet 1851.* Paris: Imprimerie Nationale, 1852.

Anonymous [An Officer of His Highness the Nizam's Army]. *Narrative of a Journey from Southampton to Bombay via Paris, Brussels, the Rhine, Part of Switzerland and Savoy, South of France, Malta, Upper Egypt, and Aden Performed between the 12th October and 13th December, 1842.* Madras: B. Lacey, 1842.

Antes, John. *Observations on the Manners and Customs of the Egyptians, the Overflowing of the Nile and Its Effects; with Remarks on the Plague and Other Subjects*. London: John Stockdale, 1800.

Aubert-Roche. *De la reforme des quarantaines et des lois sanitaires de la peste*. Paris: Just-Rouvier, 1843.

Baillie, Mrs. *A Sail to Smyrna; or, An Englishwoman's Journal*. London: Longmans, Green, 1873.

Barral, M. *Fièvre Jaune de Marseille, Observée au Lazaret*. Montpellier: Jean Martel, 1827.

Bartlett, W. H. *Gleanings, Pictorial and Antiquarian on the Overland Route*. London: Hall, Virtue, 1851.

Beggs, Thomas. *The Cholera: The Claims of the Poor upon the Rich*. London: Charles Gilpin, [1849].

Beldam, Joseph. *Recollections of Scenes and Institutions in Italy and the East*. London: James Madden, 1851.

Bertrand, J. B. *A Historical Relation of the Plague at Marseilles in the Year 1720*. Translated by Anne Plumptre. London: Joseph Mawman, 1805.

Bertulus, Évariste. *Marseille et son Intendance Sanitaire*. Marseille: Camoin Frères, 1864.

Beswick, Mary, and Tom Beswick. *Chronicles of a Journey 1839–1840*. Scarborough: AWU, 2005.

Blane, Gilbert, Henry Halford et. al. *Cholera Morbus*. Glasgow: W. R. McPhun, 1831.

Blaquiere, Edward. *Letters from the Mediterranean; Containing a Civil and Political Account of Sicily, Tripoly, Tunis, and Malta*. London: Henry Colburn, 1813.

Board of Health. *The First Report of the Board of Health Containing an Outline of a Plan to Prevent the Spreading of the Plague, or Other Contagious Diseases*. London: William Bulmer, 1805.

  Second Report of the Board of Health on the Purification of Goods and Houses. London: William Bulmer, 1805.

Bourrienne, Louis. *Memoirs of Napoleon Bonaparte*. Vol. I. Translator unknown. Glasgow: Blackie and Son, 1830.

Bowring, John. *Observations on the Oriental Plague and on Quarantines as a Means of Arresting Its Progress. An Address Given to the British Association of Science, August 15, 1838, at Newcastle*. Edinburgh: William Tait, 1838.

  Speech Given to Parliament on Submitting His Resolution Relating to Quarantine Laws and Regulations. 23rd July, 1844. London: Hansard, 1844.

  Autobiographical Reflections. London: Henry King, 1877.

Brayer, A. *Neuf années a Constantinople*. Paris: Bellizard, Barthès, Dufour, et Lowell, 1831.

Bulard, A. F. *De la peste orientale*. Paris: Béchet Jeune et Labé, 1839.

Bull, Thomas. *The Maternal Management of Children in Health and Disease*. London: Longman, Orme, Browne, Green, and Longmans, 1840.

Bulwer, H. L. *Palmerston: His Life and Times*. Philadelphia: Lippincott, 1871.

Bussolin, Giovanni. *Delle istituzioni di sanità marittima nel bacino del Mediterraneo*. Trieste: Lod. Herrmanstorfer, 1881.

Byron, Lord. "Farewell to Malta." 1811.

Carlyle, Thomas. *Chartism*. Boston: Charles Little and James Brown, 1840.

Chadwick, Edwin. *Inquiry into the Sanitary Condition of the Labouring Population of Great Britain*. London: W. Clowes, 1842.

Chervin, Nicolas. *Observations critiques sur les expériences proposées par M. le docteur Bulard dans le but de connaitre le mode de propagation de la peste*. Paris: J. B. Ballière, 1838.

Clarke, E. D. *Travels in Various Countries of Europe, Asia, and Africa*. London: T. Cadell and W. Davies, 1818.

Clot, Antoine. *De la peste observée en Égypte*. Paris: Fortin, Masson, et CIE, 1840.

    Leçon sur la peste d'Égypte et spécialement sur ce qui concerne la contagion ou la non-contagion de cette maladie. Marseille: Imprimerie Vial, 1862.

    Deniers mots sur la non-contagion de la peste. Paris: Victor Masson & Fils, 1866.

    Mémoires de A.-B. Clot Bey. Paris: IIFAO, 1949.

Cockburn, George. *A Voyage to Cadiz and Gibraltar, up the Mediterranean to Sicily and Malta, in 1810 & 11*. London: J. Harding, 1815.

Connolly, John, John Forbes, and Alexander Tweedie, eds. *Cyclopedia of Practical Medicine* . London: Sherwood, Gilbert, and Piper, 1835.

Customs Service. *Quarantine: Return to an Order of the Honorable House of Commons, dated 5 August 1831*. London: House of Commons, 1831.

Damer, the Hon. Mrs. G. L. Dawson. *Diary of a Tour in Greece, Turkey, Egypt, and the Holy Land*. 2 vols. 2nd ed. London: Henry Colburn, 1842.

Davy, John. *Notes and Observations on the Ionian Islands and Malta with Some Remarks on Constantinople and Turkey and on the System of Quarantine as at Present Conducted*. Vols. 1 and 2. London: Smith, Elder, 1842.

Delagrange, A. *Abolition des lazarets, ou, l'anticontagionisme absolu*. Paris: Duboucher, Lechevalier, et CIE, 1846.

Desgenettes, René, ed. *Histoire médicale de l'Armée d'Orient*. Paris: Croullebois, 1802.

Dew, Dyer. *A Digest of the Duties of Customs and Excise*. London: Richards and Co., 1818.

Dickens, Charles. *Little Dorrit*. Oxford: Oxford University Press, 1982.

D'Ohsson, Baron. *Tableau général de l'empire Othoman*. Paris: L'Imprimerie de Monsieur, 1787.

Doughty, Edward. *Observations and Inquiries into the Nature and Treatment of the Yellow, or Bulam Fever, in Jamaica and at Cadiz*. London: Highley and Son, 1816.

Duncan, Andrew. *Heads of Lectures on Medical Police*. Edinburgh: Adam Neill and Co., 1801.

Eager, John. *The Early History of Quarantine: Origin of Sanitary Measures Directed against Yellow Fever*. Washington, DC: US Government Printing Office, 1903.

Eton, William. *A Survey of the Turkish Empire*. 2nd ed. London: T. Caddell, 1799.

Fonblanque, J. S. M., and J. A. Paris. *Medical Jurisprudence*. London: W. Philips, 1823.

Faulkner, Arthur Brooke. *A Treatise on the Plague, Designed to Prove It Contagious, from Facts Collected during the Author's Residence in Malta, When Visited by That Malady in 1813*. London: Longman, Hurst, Rees, Orme, and Brown, 1820.

Favell, Charles. *A Treatise on the Nature, Causes, and Treatment of Spasmodic Cholera*. London: R. Groombridge, 1832.

Finlay, David Luke. *Observations on the Remittent (So-Called) and Yellow Fevers of the West Indies*. Dublin: Fannin and Co., 1853.

Forbes, Frederick. *Thesis on the Nature and History of the Plague as Observed in the North Western Provinces of India*. Edinburgh: Maclachlan, Stewart, and Co., 1840.

Forster, T. *Essay on the Origin, Symptoms, and Treatment of Cholera Morbus, and of Other Epidemic Disorders, with a View to the Improvement of Sanitary Regulations*. London: Keating and Brown, 1831.

Francis, C. R. "Endemic Plague in India." *Transactions of the Epidemiological Society of London* 4 (1881): 391–414.

Frank, Johann Peter. *A Complete System of Medical Police*. Translated by E. Vilim. Baltimore, MD: Johns Hopkins University Press, 1976.

Frankland, Charles Colville. *Travels to and from Constantinople, in the Years 1827 and 1828*. London: Henry Colburn, 1829.

Galt, John. *Voyages and Travels, in the Years 1809, 1810, and 1811; Containing Statistical, Commercial, and Miscellaneous Observations on Gibraltar, Sardinia, Sicily, Malta, Serigo, and Turkey*. London: T. Cadell and W. Davies, 1812.

General Board of Health. *Report of the General Board of Health on the Measures Adopted for the Nuisance Removal and Disease Prevention Act and the Public Health Act*. London: W. Clowes, 1849.

Report on Quarantine. London: W. Clowes, 1849.

Report of the General Board of Health on the Epidemic Cholera of 1848 and 1849. London: W. Clowes, 1850.

Gooch, Robert. "Plague, a Contagious Disease." *Quarterly Review* 33 (1825): 218–57.

Granville, Augustus Bozzi. *A Letter to the Right Honorable F. Robinson, M.P. on the Plague and Contagion, with Reference to the Quarantine Laws*. London: Richard and Arthur Taylor, 1819.

A Letter to the Right Honble. W. Huskisson. M.P., President of the Board of Trade, on the Quarantine Bill. London: J. Davy, 1825.

The Autobiography of A.B. Granville. London: Henry King, 1874.

Greville, Charles. *The Greville Diaries*. Edited by Roger Fulford. New York: Macmillan, 1963.

Griffith, Major, and Mrs. George Darby. *A Journey across the Desert from Ceylon to Marseilles: Comprising Sketches of Aden, the Red Sea, Lower Egypt, Malta, Sicily, and Italy*. London: Henry Colburn, 1845.

Haight, Sarah. *Over the Ocean, or, Glimpses of Travel in Many Lands*. London: Paine and Burgess, 1846.

Hancock, Thomas. *Researches into the Laws and Phenomena of Pestilence*. London: William Phillips, 1821.

Hanway, Jonas. *An Answer to the Appendix of a Pamphlet Entitled Reflexions upon Naturalization, Corporations, and Companies, &c. Relating to the Levant Trade and Turkey Company*. London: R. Dodsley, 1753.

Heberden, William. *Observations on the Increase and Decrease of Different Diseases, and Particularly of the Plague*. London: T. Payne, 1801.

Hennen, John. *Sketches of the Medical Topography of the Mediterranean: Comprising an Account of Gibraltar, the Ionian Islands, and Malta*. London: Thomas and George Underwood, 1830.

Hervé, Francis. *A Residence in Greece and Turkey*. [London]: Whittaker and Co., 1837.

Hirsch, August. *Handbook of Geographical and Historical Pathology*. Translated by Charles Creighton. London: New Sydenham Society, 1883.

Hofland, Mrs. *Alfred Campbell: or, Travels of a Young Pilgrim in Egypt and the Holy Land*. London: John Harris, 1826.

Holroyd, Arthur T. *The Quarantine Laws, Their Abuses and Inconsistencies: A Letter Addressed to the Rt. Hon. Sir John Cam Hobhouse, Bart. M.P.* London: Simpkin, Marshall & Co., 1839.

House of Commons. *Correspondence Relative to the Contagion of the Plague and the Quarantine Regulations of Foreign Countries, 1836–1843*. London: T. H. Harrison, 1843.

House of Commons, Select Committee Appointed to Consider the Validity of the Doctrine of Contagion in the Plague. *Report*. London: House of Commons, 1819.

House of Commons, Select Committee Appointed to Consider the Means of Improving and Maintaining the Foreign Trade of the Country. *Report*. London: House of Commons, 1824.

Howard, John. *An Account of the Principal Lazarettos in Europe with Various Papers Relative to the Plague Together with Further Observations on Some Foreign Prisons and Hospitals and Additional Remarks on the Present State of Those in Great Britain and Ireland*. Warrington: William Eyres, 1789.

Howitt, Mary, and William Howitt. *The Desolation of Eyam: The Emigrant: a Tale of the American Woods, and Other Poems*. London: Wightman and Cramp, 1827.

Kendrick, James. *Cursory Remarks on the Present Epidemic*. London: C. J. G. and F. Rivington, 1832.

Kinglake, Alexander. *Eothen; or Traces of Travel Brought Home from the East*. New York: Wiley and Putnam, 1845.

Knight, Charles, ed. *The English Cyclopaedia*. London: Charles Knight, 1854.

Lamartine, Alphonse de. *A Pilgrimage to the Holy Land; Comprising Recollections, Sketches, and Reflections Made during a Tour in the East*. New York: D. Appleton, 1847.

Larpent, George, and Sir James Porter. *Turkey; Its History and Progress*. Vol. I. London: Hurst and Blackett, 1854.

Lefevre, George William. *Observations on the Nature and Treatment of the Cholera Morbus, Now Prevailing Epidemically in St. Petersburg*. London: Longman, Rees, Orme, Brown, and Green, 1831.

Levant Company. *Proceedings of the Levant Company, Respecting the Surrender of Their Charter, 1825*. London: J. Darling, 1825.

Lind, James. *An Essay on Diseases Incidental to Europeans in Hot Climates*. London: T. Becket, 1771.

Maclean, Charles, and William Yates. *A View of the Science of Life*. Philadelphia: William Young, 1797.

A Dissertation on the Source of Epidemic and Pestilential Diseases. Philadelphia: William Young, 1797.

An Excursion in France, and Other Parts of the Continent of Europe; From the Cessation of Hostilities in 1801, to the 13th of December 1803. Including a Narrative of the Unprecedented Detention of the English Travelers in That Country as Prisoners of War. London: T. N. Longman and C. Rees, 1804.

The Affairs of Asia Considered in Their Effects on the Liberties of Britain, in a Series of Letters, Addressed to the Marquis Wellesley, Late Governor-General of India. 2nd ed. London: C. Maclean, 1806.

Suggestions for the Prevention and Mitigation of Epidemic and Pestilential Diseases. London: T. and G. Underwood, 1817.

Results of an Investigation Respecting Epidemic and Pestilential Diseases; Including Researches in the Levant. London: T. and G. Underwood, 1817.

Practical Illustrations of the Progress of Medical Improvement, for the Last Thirty Years. London: Printed for the Author, 1818.

Specimens of Systematic Misrule; or, Immense Sums Annually Expended in Upholding a Single Imposture, Discoveries of the Highest Importance to All Mankind Smothered: And Injustice Perpetrated, for Reasons of State. London: H. Hay, 1820.

Remarks on the British Quarantine Laws, and the So-Called Sanitary Laws of the Continental Nations of Europe, Especially Those of Spain. London: Published by the Author, 1823.

Evils of Quarantine Laws, and Non-existence of Pestilential Contagion; Deduced from the Phænomena of the Plague of the Levant, the Yellow Fever of Spain, and the Cholera Morbus of Asia. London: T. and G. Underwood, 1824.

Macdonald, John. *Outlines of Naval Hygiene.* London: Smith, Elder, & co., 1881.

Madden, R. R. *Travels in Turkey, Egypt, Nubia, and Palestine, in 1824, 1825, 1826, and 1827.* Vol. I. London: Henry Colburn, 1829.

Mavor, William. *The Catechism of Health; Containing Simple and Easy Rules and Directions for the Management of Children and Observations on the Conduct of Health in General. For the Use of Schools and Families.* London: Lackington, Allen, and Co., 1809.

Meryon, Charles. *Travels of Lady Hester Stanhope.* Vol. I. London: Henry Colburn, 1845.

Michelet, Jules. *Bible de l'humanité.* Paris: F. Chamerot, 1864.

Miéville, Walter. *Under Queen and Khedive: The Autobiography of an Anglo-Egyptian Official.* London: William Heinemann, 1899.

Milroy, Gavin. *Quarantine and the Plague: Being a Summary of the Report on These Subjects Recently Addressed to the Royal Academy of Medicine in France.* London: Samuel Highley, 1846.

The International Quarantine Conference of Paris in 1851–2: with Remarks. London: Savile and Edwards, 1859.

Moncrieff, W. T. *The Pestilence of Marseilles; or, the Four Thieves: A Melo-Drama, in Three Acts.* London: Thomas Richardson, 1829.

Montague, Edward P. *Narrative of the Late Expedition to the Dead Sea, from a Diary by One of the Party.* Philadelphia: Carey and Hart, 1849.

Montague, Lady Mary Wortley. *The Turkish Embassy Letters.* Edited by Malcolm Jack. London: Virago, 1994.

Montefiore, Sir Moses and Lady. *Diaries of Sir Moses and Lady Montefiore.* Edited by Louis Loewe. London: Jewish Historical Society of England, 1983.

Moulon, Amedée Mathieu. *De la Peste Orientale et de la Nécessité d'une Réforme dans les Quarantaines.* Trieste: Jean Maldini, 1845.

Morris, Edward J. *Notes of a Tour through Turkey, Greece, Egypt, Etc.* Aberdeen: George Clark, 1847.

Mortimer, Thomas. *General Dictionary of Commerce, Trade, and Manufactures.* London: Richard Philips, 1810.

Murray, John. *The Plague and Quarantine: Remarks on Some Epidemic and Endemic Disease; (Including the Plague of the Levant,) and the Means of Disinfection with a Description of the Preservative Phial*. London: Rolfe and Fletcher, 1839.

Murray, John (firm). *A Handbook for Travellers in Turkey*. London: John Murray, 1854.

Nair, Aparna. "An Egyptian Infection: War, Plague, and the Quarantines of the English East India Company at Madras and Bombay, 1802." *Hygiea Internationalis* 8, no. 1 (2009): 7–29.

Newman, Cardinal John Henry. *Letters and Correspondence of Cardinal John Henry Newman*. Edited by Anne Mozley. London: Longmans, Green, 1891.

Papon, Jean-Pierre. *De la peste, ou époques mémorables de ce fléau et les moyens de s'en préserver*. Paris: Lavillete et Compagnie, 1800.

Pariset, Étienne. *Mémoire sur les causes de la peste et sur les moyens de la détruire*. Paris: J.-B. Baillière, 1837.

Penneck, Henry. *An Essay on the Nature and Treatment of the Indian Pestilence, Commonly Called Cholera*. London: S. Highley, 1831.

Penn, Granville. *The Policy and Interest of Great Britain with Respect to Malta, Summarily Considered*. London: J. Hatchard, 1805.

Pettigrew, T. J. *Observations on Cholera; Comprising a Description of the Epidemic Cholera of India, the Mode of Treatment, and the Means of Prevention*. London: S. Highley, 1831.

Pouqueville, F. C. *Travels in the Morea, Albania, and Other Parts of the Ottoman Empire*. Translated by Anne Plumptre. London: Henry Colburn, 1813.

Privy Council. *Official Reports Made to Government by Drs. Russell and Barry on the Disease Called Cholera Spasmodica*. London: Privy Council, 1832.

Proust, Achille. *La défense de l'Europe contre la peste et la Conférence de Venise de 1897*. Paris: Masson, 1897.

Ranken, James. *Report on the Malignant Fever Called the Pali Plague*. Calcutta: Bengal Military Orphan Press, 1838.

Redcliffe, Viscount Stratford de. *The Eastern Question*. London: John Murray, 1881.

Registrar General. *Tenth Annual Report of the Registrar General*. London: Longman, Green, Brown, and Longmans, 1852.

Renny, Charles. *Medical Report on the Mahamurree in Gurhwal, in 1849–50*. Agra: Secundra Orphan Press, 1851.

Richardson, David Lester. *The Anglo-Indian Passage; Homeward and Outward; or, A Card for the Overland Traveler*. London: Madden and Malcolm, 1845.

Rowed, Richard. *Cholera, Plague, Pestilence, and Fevers Mitigated by Adopting Rowed's Comprehensive Plans for the Improvement of the Health of the Metropolis and Large Towns*. London: James Watson, [1849].

Russell, Alexander. *The Natural History of Aleppo, and Parts Adjacent*. London: A. Millar, 1756.

Russell, Patrick. *A Treatise of the Plague*. London: G. G. J. and J. Robinson, 1791.

Sandwith, F. M. *Egypt as a Winter Resort*. London: Kegan, Paul, Trench, 1889.

Schembri, G. B. *Ragionamento pratico-sanitario sopra varie osservazioni riguardanti la Peste-Bubonica, e metodo con cui s'arresta, s'attacca, e si estingue in questo Lazzaretto di Malta*. Malta, 1842.

Scott, C. Rochfort. *Rambles in Egypt and Candia*. Vol. I. London: Henry Colburn, 1837.

Ségur-Dupeyron, Pierre. *Des quarantaines et des pertes qu'elles occasionnent au commerce*. Paris: Madame Huzard, 1833.

Rapport adressé a son Exc. Le Ministre du Commerce, chargé de procéder a une enquête sur les divers régimes sanitaires de la Méditerranée, et sur les modifications qui pourraient être apportées aux tableaux qui fixent la durée de quarantaine en France. Paris: Imprimerie Royale, 1834.

Rapport adressé à S. Exc. le Ministère du Commerce et l'Agriculture sur des modifications à apporter aux règlements sanitaires. Paris: Imprimerie Nationale, 1839.

Semple, Robert. *Observations on a Journey through Spain and Italy to Naples; and Thence to Smyrna and Constantinople*. London: C. and R. Baldwin, 1808.

Shaw, Thomas. *Travels and Observations*. London: J. Ritchie, 1808.

Shelley, Mary. *The Last Man*. London: University of Nebraska Press, 1965.

Simpson, W. J. *A Treatise on the Plague*. Cambridge: Cambridge University Press, 1905.

Slade, Adolphus. *Turkey, Greece, and Malta*. London: Saunders and Otley, 1837.

Smith, Albert. *A Hand-book to Mr. Albert Smith's Entertainment*. London, 1850.

Smith, Thomas Southwood. *The Philosophy of Health*. Vol. I. London: Charles Knight, 1835.

The Common Nature of Epidemics, and Their Relation to Climate and Civilization; Also, Remarks on Contagion and Quarantine. Philadelphia: Lippincott, 1866.

Snow, Robert. *Journal of a Steam Voyage Down the Danube to Constantinople, and Thence by Way of Malta and Marseilles to England*. London: Moyes and Barclay, 1842.

Souvestre, Émile. *The Isle of the Dead, or The Keeper of the Lazaretto*. Translated by Emily Bowles. London: Burns & Oates, 1907.

Stiven, W. S. *Report on the Epidemic in the Moradabad District in 1854*. Agra: Secundra Orphan Press, 1854.

Terry, Charles. *Scenes and Thoughts in Foreign Lands*. London: William Pickering, 1848.

Theal, George. *Records of the Cape Colony*. Vol. 13. Cape Town: Government of the Cape Colony, 1902.

Tholozan, J. B. *Une épidémie de peste en Mesopotamie en 1867*. Paris: Victor Massin et Fils, 1869.

Thornton, Thomas. *The Present State of Turkey*. 2 vols. London: Joseph Mawman, 1809.

Tott, Baron de. *Memoirs of the Baron de Tott*. London: G. G. J. and J. Robinson, 1786.

Tulloch, Alexander. *Statistical Report on the Sickness, Mortality, and Invaliding among the Troops in the West Indies*. London: W. Clowes, 1838.

Tully, J. D. *History of the Plague as It Has Lately Appeared in the Islands of Malta, Gozo, Corfu, Cephalonia, &c*. London: Longman, Hurst, Rees, Orme, and Brown. 1821.

Urquhart, David. *Turkey and Its Resources*. London: Saunders and Otley, 1833.

Walsh, Robert. *Account of the Levant Company with Some Notices of the Benefits Conferred Upon Society by Its Officers in Promoting the Cause of Humanity, Literature, and the Fine Arts*. London: J. and A. Arch, 1825.

Narrative of a Journey from Constantinople to England. 4th ed. London: Frederick Wesley and A. H. Davis, 1831.

A Residence at Constantinople. London: Frederick Wesley and A. H. Davis, 1836.

Warburton, Eliot. *The Crescent and the Cross*. London: Henry Colburn, 1845.

Watkins, Thomas. *Travels through Switzerland, Italy, Sicily, the Greek Islands, to Constantinople; through Part of Greece, Ragusa, and the Dalmatian Isles; in a Series of Letters to Pennoyre Watkins*. London: T. Cadell, 1792.

Wells, T. S. "On the Practical Results of Quarantine." *Association Medical Journal* 2, no. 89 (1854): 831–34.

White, Andrew. *A Treatise on the Plague: More Especially on the Police Management of that Disease*. London: John Churchill, 1846.

White, Charles. *Three Years in Constantinople: or, Domestic Manners of the Turks in 1844*. London: Henry Colburn, 1845.

Wilkinson, John Gardner. *A Handbook for Travelers in Egypt*. London: John Murray, 1847.

Wilson, Erasmus. *The Eastern, or Turkish Bath: Its History, Revival in Britain, and Application to the Purposes of Health*. London: John Churchill, 1861.

Wilson, James C. "Plague." In *A System of Practical Medicine*, Vol. I, edited by William Pepper and Louis Starr, 771–84. Philadelphia: Lea Brothers, 1885.

Wittman, William. *Travels in Turkey, Asia-Minor, Syria, and across the Desert into Egypt during the Years 1799, 1800, and 1801, in Company with the Turkish Army, and the British Military Mission*. London: Richard Phillips, 1803.

Wood, Mark. *The Importance of Malta Considered, in the Years 1796 and 1798*. London: John Stockdale, 1803.

Yates, William. *The Modern History and Condition of Egypt, Its Climate, Diseases, and Capabilities*. London: Smith, Elder, and Co., 1843.

Secondary Material

Ackerknecht, Erwin. "Anticontagionism between 1821 and 1867." *Bulletin of the History of Medicine* 22 (1948): 562–93.

Agamben, Giorgio. *State of Exception*. Translated by Kevin Attell. Chicago: University of Chicago Press, 2005.

Aisenberg, Andrew. *Contagion: Disease, Government, and the "Social Question" in Nineteenth-Century France*. Stanford, CA: Stanford University Press, 1999.

AOM Architects. *Sourcebook for the Reconstruction of the Malta Lazaretto*. 2005. (Unpublished).

Apel, Thomas. *Feverish Bodies, Enlightened Minds: Science and the Yellow Fever Controversy in the Early American Republic*. Stanford, CA: Stanford University Press, 2016.

Arner, Katherine. "The Malady of Revolutions: Yellow Fever in the Atlantic World, 1793–1828." PhD diss., Johns Hopkins University, 2014.

Arnold, David. *Colonizing the Body: State, Medicine, and Epidemic Disease in Nineteenth-Century India*. Berkeley: University of California Press, 1993.

  The Tropics and the Traveling Gaze: India, Landscape, and Science, 1800–1856. Seattle: University of Washington Press, 2006.

Baldwin, Peter. *Contagion and the State in Europe: 1830–1930*. Cambridge: Cambridge University Press, 1999.

  "The Victorian State in Comparative Perspective." In *Liberty and Authority in Victorian Britain*, edited by Peter Mandler, 51–70. Oxford: Oxford University Press, 2006.

Barnes, David S. *The Great Stink of Paris and the Nineteenth-Century Struggle against Filth and Germs*. Baltimore, MD: Johns Hopkins University Press, 2006.

"Cargo, 'Infection,' and the Logic of Quarantine in the Nineteenth Century." *Bulletin of the History of Medicine* 88, no. 1 (2014): 75–101.

"'Until Cleansed and Purified': Landscapes of Health in the Interpermeable World." *Change over Time* 6, no. 2 (2016): 138–52.

Bartle, George. "Bowring and the Near Eastern Crisis of 1838–1840." *English Historical Review* 79, no. 313 (1964): 761–74.

Bashford, Alison. *Purity and Pollution: Gender, Embodiment, and Victorian Medicine*. New York: St. Martin's, 1998.

"At the Border: Contagion, Immigration, Nation." *Australian Historical Studies* 33, no. 120 (2002): 344–58.

ed. *Medicine at the Border: Disease, Globalization, and Security, 1850 to the Present*. New York: Palgrave Macmillan, 2006.

Bashford, Alison, and Clare Hooker, eds. *Contagion: Cultural and Historical Studies*. New York: Taylor and Francis, 2002.

Bayly, C. A. *Imperial Meridian: The British Empire and the World, 1780–1830*. New York: Longman, 1989.

Bell, David A. *The First Total War*. Boston: Houghton Mifflin, 2007.

Ben-Arieh, Yehoshua. "Jerusalem Travel Literature as Historical Source and Cultural Phenomenon." In *Jerusalem in the Mind of the Western World: 1800–1948*, edited by Yehoshua Ben-Arieh, 25–46. Westport, CT: Praeger, 1997.

Ben-Yahoyada, Naor. "Mediterranean Modernity." In *A Companion to Mediterranean History*, edited by P. Horden and S. Kinoshita, 107–21. Hoboken, NJ: Wiley-Blackwell, 2014.

Benedict, Carol. *Bubonic Plague in Nineteenth-Century China*. Stanford, CA: Stanford University Press, 1996.

Biraben, Jean-Noël. *Les hommes et la peste en France et dans les pays Européens et Méditerranéens*. Mouton: Mouton/EHESS, 1975.

Bonastra, Quim. "Recintos sanitarios y espacios de control. Un estudio morfológico de la arquitectura cuarentenaria." *Dynamis* 30 (2010): 17–40.

Booker, John. *Maritime Quarantine: The British Experience, c.1650–1900*. Aldershot, UK: Ashgate, 2007.

Braudel, Fernand. *The Mediterranean in the Age of Philip II*. Translated by Sian Reynolds. New York: Harper and Row, 1972.

Briggs, Asa. "Cholera and Society." In *European Political History, 1815–1870: Aspects of Liberalism*, edited by Eugene C. Black, 37–61. New York: Harper and Row, 1967.

Brockington, Fraser. "Public Health at the Privy Council, 1805–6." *Medical History* 7, no. 1 (1963): 13–31.

"Public Health at the Privy Council, 1831–34." *Journal of the History of Medicine and Allied Sciences* 16, no. 2 (1961): 161–85.

Brown, Michael. "From Foetid Air to Filth: The Cultural Transformation of British Epidemiological Thought, ca. 1780–1848." *Bulletin of the History of Medicine* 82, no. 3 (2008): 515–44.

Bulmuş, Birsen. *Plague, Quarantines, and Geopolitics in the Ottoman Empire*. Edinburgh: Edinburgh University Press, 2012.

Caquet, P. E. "The Napoleonic Legend and the War Scare of 1840." *International History Review* 35, no. 4 (2013): 702–22.

Carminati, Lucia. "Alexandria, 1898: Nodes, Networks, and Scales in Nineteenth-Century Egypt and the Mediterranean." *Comparative Studies in History and Society* 59, no. 1 (2017): 127–53.

Cassar, Paul. *A Medical History of Malta*. London: Wellcome, 1964.

Chahrour, Marcel. "A Civilizing Mission? Austrian Medicine and the Reform of Medical Structures in the Ottoman Empire, 1838–1850." *Studies in History and Philosophy of Biological and Biomedical Sciences* 38 (2007): 687–705.

Chandavarkar, Rajnarayan, "Plague Panic and Epidemic Politics in India, 1896–1916." In *Epidemics and Ideas*, edited by Terence Ranger and Paul Slack, 203–40. Cambridge: Cambridge University Press, 1992.

Chevalier, Louis. *Le Choléra: Première Épidemie de XIXe Siècle*. La Roche sur Yon: Imprimerie de l'Ouest, 1958.

Chiffoleau, Sylvia. *Genèse de la santé publique internationale. De la peste d'Orient à l'OMS*. Beirut: Institut Français du Proche-Orient, 2013.

Chircop, John, and Francisco Javier Martínez, eds. *Mediterranean Quarantines, 1750–1914*, 199–231. Manchester, UK: Manchester University Press, 2018.

Choay, Françoise. *The Invention of the Historic Monument*. Translated by Lauren O'Connell. Cambridge: Cambridge University Press, 2001.

Christensen, Allan Conrad. *"Our Feverish Contact": Nineteenth-Century Narratives of Contagion*. New York: Routledge, 2005.

Cipolla, Carlo. *Fighting the Plague in Seventeenth-Century Italy*. Madison: University of Wisconsin Press, 1981.

Clancy-Smith, Julia. *Mediterraneans: Europe and North Africa in an Age of Migration, c. 1800–1900*. Berkeley: University of California Press, 2010.

Cohn, Samuel. *Cultures of Plague*. Oxford: Oxford University Press, 2010.

Colley, Linda. *Britons: Forging the Nation, 1707–1832*. New Haven, CT: Yale University Press, 1992.

Collins, Bruce. "The Limits of British Power: Intervention in Portugal, 1820–30." *International History Review* 35, no. 4 (2013): 744–65.

Cranshaw, Jane. "The Renaissance Invention of Quarantine." In *The Fifteenth Century XII: Society in an Age of Plague*, edited by Linda Clark and Carole Rawcliffe, 161–74. Rochester, NY: Boydell Press, 2013.

Crook, Tim. *Governing Systems: Modernity and the Making of Public Health in England, 1830–1910*. Oakland: University of California Press, 2016.

Cunningham, Allan. "The Sick Man and the British Physician." *Middle Eastern Studies* 17, no. 2 (1981): 147–73.

Curtin, Philip D. "Epidemiology and the Slave Trade." *Political Science Quarterly* 83, no. 2 (1968): 190–216.

Daunton, Martin. *Trusting Leviathan: The Politics of Taxation in Britain, 1799–1914*. Cambridge: Cambridge University Press, 2001.

Davis, Ralph. *Aleppo and Devonshire Square*. London: Macmillan, 1967.

Davison, R. H. "Ottoman Public Relations in the Nineteenth Century: How the Sublime Porte Tried to Influence European Public Opinion." In *Histoire economique et sociale de l'Empire Ottoman et de la Turquie, 1326–1960*, Edited by Daniel Panzac, 593–603. Paris: Peeters, 1995.

DeLacy, Margaret. *The Germ of an Idea: Contagionism, Religion, and Society in Britain, 1660–1730*. New York: Palgrave, 2016.

Contagionism Catches On: Medical Ideology in Britain, 1730–1800. New York: Palgrave, 2017.

Delaporte, François. *The Cholera in Paris, 1832*. Cambridge, MA: Harvard University Press, 1986.

Dodero, Giuseppe. *I Lazzaretti: Epidemie e Quarantene in Sardegna*. Cagliari: Aipsa Edizione, 2001.

Dols, Michael. "The Second Plague Pandemic and Its Recurrences in the Middle East, 1347–1894." *Journal of the Economic and Social History of the Orient* 22 (1979): 162–89.

Durey, Michael. *The Return of the Plague: British Society and the Cholera, 1831–2*. Dublin: Gill and Macmillan, 1979.

Evans, Richard J. *Death in Hamburg: Society and Politics in the Cholera Years, 1830–1910*. London: Penguin Books, 1987.

Faroqhi, Suraiya. *Approaching Ottoman History: An Introduction to the Sources*. Cambridge: Cambridge University Press, 1999.

Flinn, Michael. *The European Demographic System, 1500–1820*. Baltimore, MD: Johns Hopkins University Press, 1981.

Foxhall, Katherine. "Fever, Immigration and Quarantine in New South Wales, 1837–1840." *Social History of Medicine* 24, no. 3 (2011): 624–42.

Foucault, Michel. *Discipline and Punish: The Birth of the Prison*. Translated by Alan Sheridan. New York: Random House, 1977.

Galani, Katerina. *British Shipping in the Mediterranean during the Napoleonic Wars: The Untold Story of a Successful Adaptation*. Leiden: Brill, 2017.

Gallagher, Nancy. *Medicine and Power in Tunisia, 1780–1900*. New York: Cambridge University Press, 1983.

Egypt's Other Wars. Syracuse, NY: Syracuse University Press, 1990.

Gallant, Thomas. *Experiencing Dominion: Culture, Identity, and Power in the British Mediterranean*. Notre Dame, IN: University of Notre Dame Press, 2002.

Gazel, Louis. *Le Baron des Genettes, 1762–1837: Notes Biographiques*. Paris: Henry Paulin, 1912.

Gilbert, Pamela. *Cholera and Nation: Doctoring the Social Body in Victorian England*. Albany: SUNY Press, 2008.

Gordon, Daniel. "Confrontations with the Plague in Eighteenth-Century France." In *Dreadful Visitations: Confronting Natural Catastrophe in the Age of Enlightenment*, edited by Alessa Johns, 3–30. New York: Routledge, 1999.

Gregory, Desmond. *Malta, Britain, and the European Powers*. Madison, NJ: Fairleigh Dickinson University Press, 1996.

Grigsby, Darcy. "Out of the Earth." In *Edges of Empire: Orientalism and Visual Culture*, edited by Jocelyn Hackforth-Jones and Mary Roberts, 38–69. London: Blackwell, 2005.

Haley, Bruce. *The Healthy Body and Victorian Culture*. Cambridge, MA: Harvard University Press, 1978.

Hamlin, Christopher. *Public Health and Social Justice in the Age of Chadwick*. Cambridge: Cambridge University Press, 1998.

"Ackerknecht and Anticontagionism: A Tale of Two Dichotomies." *International Journal of Epidemiology* 38, no. 1 (2009): 22–27.

Hanley, James. *Healthy Boundaries: Property, Law, and Public Health in England and Wales, 1815–1872*. Rochester, NY: University of Rochester Press, 2016.

Hardy, Anne. "Cholera, Quarantine, and the English Preventive System, 1850–1895." *Medical History* 37 (1993): 250–69.

Harrison, Mark. "Quarantine, Pilgrimage, and Colonial Trade: India 1866–1900." *Indian Economic and Social History Review* 29, no. 2 (1992): 117–44.

"Disease, Diplomacy, and International Commerce." *Journal of Global History* 1, no. 2 (2006): 197–217.

Contagion: How Commerce Has Spread Disease. New Haven, CT: Yale University Press, 2012.

Harrison, Robert. *Gladstone's Imperialism in Egypt*. Westport, CT: Greenwood Press, 1995.

Henriques, Ursula R. Q. *Before the Welfare State*. London: Longman, 1979.

Hildesheimer, Françoise. *Le Bureau de la Santé de Marseille sous l'Ancien Régime: Le renfermement de la contagion*. Marseille: Fédération Historique de Provence, 1980.

Hilton, Boyd. *A Mad, Bad, and Dangerous People? England 1783–1846*. Oxford: Oxford University Press, 2006.

Hodgkinson, Ruth. *The Origins of the National Health Service*. London: Wellcome, 1967.

Holland, Robert. *Blue-Water Empire: The British in the Mediterranean Since 1800*. New York: Penguin, 2012.

Hoock, Holger. *Empires of the Imagination*. London: Profile Books, 2010.

Horden, Peregrine, and Nicholas Purcell. *The Corrupting Sea*. Oxford: Blackwell, 2000.

Howard-Jones, Norman. *The Scientific Background of the International Sanitary Conferences, 1851–1938*. Geneva: WHO, 1975.

Huber, Valeska. "The Unification of the Globe by Disease? The International Sanitary Conferences on Cholera, 1851–1894." *Historical Journal* 49 (2006): 453–76.

Huet, Marie-Hélène. *The Culture of Disaster*. Chicago: University of Chicago Press, 2012.

Inalcik, Halil, and Donald Quataert, eds. *An Economic and Social History of the Ottoman Empire (1300–1914)*. Cambridge: Cambridge University Press, 1994.

Jasanoff, Maya. *The Edge of Empire: Lives, Culture, and Conquest in the East 1750–1850*. New York: Knopf, 2005.

Jones, Colin. "Plague and Its Metaphors in Early Modern France." *Representations* 53 (1996): 97–127.

Jones, Raymond A. *The British Diplomatic Service, 1815–1914*. Gerrards Cross, UK: Colin Smythe, 1983.

Kasaba, Resat. *The Ottoman Empire and the World Economy: The Nineteenth Century*. Albany: SUNY Press, 1988.

Kashani-Sabet, Firoozeh. "'City of the Dead': The Frontier Polemics of Quarantines in the Ottoman Empire and Iran." *Comparative Studies of South Asia, Africa and the Middle East* 18, no. 2 (1998): 51–58.

Kelly, Catherine. "'Not from the College, but through the Public and the Legislature': Charles Maclean and the Relocation of Medical Debate in the Early Nineteenth Century." *Bulletin of the History of Medicine* 82 (2008): 545–69.

War and the Militarization of British Army Medicine, 1793–1830. London: Pickering and Chatto, 2011.

Kerr, Matthew Newsom. *Contagion, Isolation, and Biopolitics in Victorian London*. New York: Palgrave Macmillan, 2017.

Koch, Tom. *Cartographies of Disease: Maps, Mapping, and Medicine*. Redlands, CA: Esri Press, 2005.

Kohn, George C. *Encyclopedia of Plague and Pestilence*. New York: Facts on File, 1995.

Kuhnke, LaVerne. *Lives at Risk: Public Health in Nineteenth-Century Egypt*. Berkeley: University of California Press, 1990.

Laget, Pierre-Louis. "Les lazarets et l'émergence de nouvelles maladies pestilentielles au XIXe et au début du XXe siècle." *In Situ* 2 (2002): 1–12.

Laidlaw, Christine. *Trade and Perceptions of the Ottoman Empire*. New York: Tauris, 2010.

Leask, Nigel. *Curiosity and the Aesthetics of Travel Writing: 1770–1840*. Oxford: Oxford University Press, 2002.

British Romantic Writers and the East: Anxieties of Empire. Cambridge: Cambridge University Press, 1992.

Longmate, Norman. *King Cholera: The Biography of a Disease*. London: Hamish Hamilton, 1966.

Lubenow, William. *The Politics of Government Growth*. Hamden, CT: Archon, 1971.

Maglen, Krista. *The English System: Quarantine, Immigration, and the Making of a Port Sanitary Zone*. Manchester, UK: Manchester University Press, 2014.

Mandler, Peter. *Aristocratic Government in the Age of Reform*. Oxford: Oxford University Press, 1990.

ed. *Liberty and Authority in Victorian Britain*. Oxford: Oxford University Press, 2006.

Mansfield, Julia. "The Disease of Commerce: Yellow Fever in the Atlantic World, 1793–1805." PhD diss., Stanford University, 2017.

Markel, Howard. *Quarantine! East European Jewish Immigrants and the New York City Epidemics of 1892*. Baltimore, MD: Johns Hopkins University Press, 1999.

Marks, Shula. "What Is Colonial about Colonial Medicine? And What Has Happened to Imperialism and Health?" *Social History of Medicine* 10, no. 2 (1997): 205–19.

Marlowe, John. *Perfidious Albion: The Origins of Anglo-French Rivalry in the Levant*. London: Elek Books, 1971.

Martínez, F. J. "International or French? The Early International Sanitary Conferences and France's Struggle for Hegemony in the Mid-Nineteenth Century Mediterranean." *French History* 30, no. 1 (2016): 77–98.

Masters, Bruce. *The Origins of Western Economic Dominance in the Middle East*. New York: NYU Press, 1988.

Mather, James. *Pashas: Traders and Travelers in the Levantine World*. New Haven, CT: Yale University Press, 2009.

McDonald, J. C. "The History of Quarantine in Britain during the Nineteenth Century." *Bulletin of the History of Medicine* 25 (1951): 22–44.

McGrew, Roderick. *Russia and the Cholera: 1823–32*. Madison: University of Wisconsin Press, 1965.

McLean, David. *Public Health and Politics in the Age of Reform: Cholera, the State, and the Royal Navy in Victorian Britain*. New York: Tauris, 2006.

Meyer, Karl. *Disinfected Mail*. Holton, KS: Gossip Printery, 1962.
Mikhail, Alan. "The Nature of Plague in Late Eighteenth Century Egypt." *Bulletin of the History of Medicine* 82, no. 2 (2008): 249–75.
Mishra, Saurabh. "Incarceration and Resistance in a Red Sea Lazaretto, 1880–1930." In *Quarantine: Local and Global Histories*, edited by Alison Bashford, 54–65. New York: Palgrave, 2016.
Mitchell, Peta. *Contagious Metaphor*. London: Bloomsbury, 2012.
Mooney, Graham. *Intrusive Interventions: Public Health, Domestic Space, and Infectious Disease Surveillance in England, 1840–1914*. Rochester, NY: University of Rochester Press, 2015.
Morris, R. J. *Cholera, 1832: The Social Response to an Epidemic*. New York: Holmes and Meier, 1976.
Mukharji, Projit Bihari. "The 'Cholera Cloud' in the Nineteenth-Century 'British World': History of an Object-without-an-Essence." *Bulletin of the History of Medicine* 86, no. 3 (2012): 303–32.
Mullett, Charles F. "A Century of English Quarantine, 1709–1825." *Bulletin of the History of Medicine* 23 (1949): 527–45.
"Politics, Economics, and Medicine: Charles Maclean and Anticontagion in England." *Osiris* 10, no. 1 (1952): 224–51.
Nair, Aparna. "An Egyptian Infection: War, Plague, and the Quarantines of the English East India Company at Madras and Bombay, 1802." *Hygiea Internationalis* 8, no. 1 (2009): 7–29.
O'Connor, Erin. *Raw Material: Producing Pathology in Victorian Culture*. Durham, NC: Duke University Press, 2000.
Otis, Laura. *Membranes: Metaphors of Invasion in Nineteenth-Century Literature, Science, and Politics*. Baltimore, MD: Johns Hopkins University Press, 1999.
Owen, Roger. *The Middle East in the World Economy, 1800–1914*. New York: Methuen, 1981.
Pamuk, Şevket. *The Ottoman Empire and European Capitalism, 1820–1913*. Cambridge: Cambridge University Press, 1987.
Panzac, Daniel. *La peste dans l'empire Ottoman*. Leuven: Editions Peeters, 1985.
Quarantaines et lazarets: l'Europe et de la peste d'Orient. Aix-en-Provence, France: Édisud, 1986.
Population et santé dans l'empire Ottoman (XVIII à XXè siècles). Istanbul: Isis, 1996.
Les corsaires Barbaresques. La fin d'une épopée. Paris: CNRS Editions, 1999.
Pati, Biswamoy, and Mark Harrison, eds. *Health, Medicine and Empire: Perspectives on Colonial India*. London: Sangam Books, 2001.
Peckham, Robert, ed. *Empires of Panic: Epidemics and Colonial Anxieties*. Hong Kong: Hong Kong University, 2015.
Pelling, Margaret. *Cholera, Fever, and English Medicine: 1825–1865*. Oxford: Oxford University Press, 1978.
"The Meaning of Contagion: Reproduction, Medicine, and Metaphor." In *Contagion: Historical and Cultural Studies*, edited by Alison Bashford and Claire Hooker, 15–38. London: Routledge, 2001.
Pemble, John. *The Mediterranean Passion: Victorians and Edwardians in the South*. Oxford: Clarendon Press, 1987.

Penson, Lillian, and Harold Temperley. *British Foreign Policy from Pitt to Salisbury.* Cambridge: Cambridge University Press, 1938.

Pesalj, Jovan. "Some Observations on the Habsburg-Ottoman Border and Mobility Control Policies." In *Transgressing Boundaries*, edited by Marija Wakounig and Markus Beham, 245–56. Zurich: GmbH & Co., 2013.

Platt, D. C. M. *The Cinderella Service: British Consuls since 1825.* London: Longman, 1971.

Poovey, Mary. *Making a Social Body: British Cultural Formation, 1830–1864.* Chicago: University of Chicago Press, 1995.

Porter, Bernard. "'Bureau and Barrack': Early Victorian Attitudes toward the Continent." *Victorian Studies* 27, no. 4 (1984): 407–33.

Porter, Dorothy. *Health, Civilization, and the State: A History of Public Health from Ancient to Modern Times.* London: Routledge, 1999.

Pratt, Mary Louise. *Imperial Eyes.* New York: Routledge, 1992.

Ragsdale, Hugh. *Tsar Paul and the Question of Madness.* New York: Greenwood, 1988.

Reid, Donald. *Whose Pharaohs?* Berkeley: University of California Press, 2002.

Restifo, Giuseppe. *Le ultime piaghe: le pesti nel Mediterraneo (1720–1820).* Milan: Selene Edizioni, 1994.

 I porti della peste: epidemie Mediterranee fra sette e ottocento. Messina, Italy: Mesogea, 2005.

Riall, Lucy. *Under the Volcano: Revolution in a Sicilian Town.* Oxford: Oxford University Press, 2013.

Robarts, Andrew. *Migration and Disease in the Black Sea Region.* London: Bloomsbury, 2017.

Roberts, David. "Tory Paternalism and Social Reform." *AHR* 63, no. 2 (1958): 323–37.

Rodogno, Davide. *Against Massacre: Humanitarian Interventions in the Ottoman Empire, 1815–1914.* Princeton, NJ: Princeton University Press, 2012.

Rosenberg, Charles. *The Cholera Years.* Chicago: University of Chicago Press, 1987.

 Explaining Epidemics and Other Studies in the History of Medicine. Cambridge: Cambridge University Press, 1992.

Rothenburg, Gunther. "The Austrian Sanitary Cordon and the Control of the Bubonic Plague, 1710–1871." *Journal of the History of Medicine* 28, no. 1 (1973): 15–23.

Russell, Ina. "The Later History of the Levant Company." PhD diss., University of Manchester, 1935.

Sakula, A. "Augustus Bozzi Granville (1783–1872): London Physician-Accoucheur and Italian Patriot." *Journal of the Royal Society of Medicine* 76 (1998): 876–82.

Said, Edward. *Orientalism.* New York: Vintage Books, 1978.

Sattin, Anthony. *Lifting the Veil: British Society in Egypt 1768–1956.* London: J. M. Dent, 1988.

Schepin, Oleg P., and Waldemar V. Yermakov. *International Quarantine.* Translated by Boris Meerovich and Vladimir Bobrov. Madison, CT: International Universities Press, 1991.

Schiffer, Reinhold. *Oriental Panorama: British Travelers in 19th Century Turkey.* Atlanta, GA: Rodopi, 1999.

Searight, Sarah, and Malcolm Wagstaff, eds. *Travelers in the Levant: Voyagers and Visionaries.* Durham, NC: Astene, 2001.

Sechel, Teodora D., ed. *Medicine within and between the Habsburg and Ottoman Empires, 18th–19th Centuries.* Bochum, Germany: Winkler, 2011.

Shah, Nayan. *Contagious Divides: Epidemics and Race in San Francisco*. Berkeley: University of California Press, 2001.

Shefer-Mossensohn, Miri. *Ottoman Medicine, 1500–1700*. Albany: SUNY Press, 2009.

Sheridan, Richard. *Doctors and Slaves: A Medical and Demographic History of Slavery in the British West Indies, 1680–1834*. Cambridge: Cambridge University Press, 1985.

Siena, Kevin. *Rotten Bodies: Class and Contagion in 18th-Century Britain*. New Haven, CT: Yale University Press, 2019.

Snowden, Frank. *Naples in the Time of Cholera: 1884–1911*. Cambridge: Cambridge University Press, 1995.

Speziale, Salvatore. "Epidemics and Quarantine in Mediterranean Africa from the Eighteenth to the Mid-Nineteenth Century." *Journal of Mediterranean Studies* 16 (2006): 249–58.

Stafford, Barbara. *Voyage into Substance*. Cambridge, MA: MIT Press, 1984.

Starkey, Janet C. M. "No Myopic Mirage: Alexander and Patrick Russell at Aleppo." *History and Anthropology* 13, no. 4 (2002): 257–73.

Sultana, Donald. *Benjamin Disraeli in Spain, Malta, and Albania: 1830–32*. London: Tamesis, 1976.

Takeda, Junko. *Between Crown and Commerce: Marseille and the Early Modern Mediterranean*. Baltimore, MD: Johns Hopkins University Press, 2011.

Tenenti, Alberto. *Piracy and the Decline of Venice, 1580–1615*. Translated by Janet and Brian Pullan. Berkeley: University of California Press, 1967.

Thomson, Ann. *Barbary and Enlightenment: European Attitudes to the Maghreb in the 18th Century*. Leiden, Netherlands: Brill, 1987.

Thompson, Carl. *The Suffering Traveler in the English Romantic Imagination*. Oxford: Oxford University Press, 2007.

Todd, David. "John Bowring and the Global Dissemination of Free Trade." *Historical Journal* 51, no. 2 (2008): 373–97.

Todorova, Maria. *Imagining the Balkans*. Oxford: Oxford University Press, 1997.

Tomić, Zlata Blažina, and Vesna Blažina. *Expelling the Plague*. Montreal: McGill-Queen's University Press, 2015.

Tusan, Michelle. *Smyrna's Ashes: Humanitarianism, Genocide, and the Birth of the Middle East*. Berkeley: University of California Press, 2012.

Valensi, Lucette. *The Birth of the Despot: Venice and the Sublime Porte*. Translated by Arthur Denner. Ithaca, NY: Cornell University Press, 1993.

Vandervelde, V. Denis. "The River Danube Quarantine Stations." *Pratique: The Journal of the Disinfected Mail Study Circle* 21, no. 2 (1996): 44–50.

"Moslem Attitudes to Disinfection in the Nineteenth Century." *Pratique* 22, no. 3 (1997): 100–103.

"Quarantine at the Motherbank, 1845–53." *Pratique* 35, no. 1 (2011): 5.

"Quarantine and Disinfection in Egypt, 1747–1881." *Pratique* 35, no. 1 (2011): 5–25.

Varlık, Nükhet. *Plague and Empire in the Early Modern Mediterranean World: The Ottoman Experience, 1367–1600*. Cambridge: Cambridge University Press, 2016.

ed., *Plague and Contagion in the Islamic Mediterranean*. Kalamazoo, MI: ARC Humanities Press, 2017.

Vlami, Despina. *Trading with the Ottomans: The Levant Company in the Middle East*. New York: I. B. Tauris, 2014.

Wallis, Patrick. "A Dreadful Heritage: Interpreting Epidemic Disease at Eyam, 1666–2000." *History Workshop Journal* 61, no.1 (2006): 31–56.

Wohl, A. S. *Endangered Lives: Public Health in Victorian Britain*. Cambridge, MA: Harvard University Press, 1983.

Wood, A. C. *A History of the Levant Company*. Oxford: Frank Cass, 1935.

Worboys, Michael. *Spreading Germs: Disease Theories and Medical Practice in Britain, 1865–1900*. Cambridge: Cambridge University Press, 2000.

Archives Consulted

Archives Nationales, Paris
Archives Nationales, Pierrefitte-sur-Seine
Archives Départementales du Bouches-du-Rhône, Marseille
Archivio di Stato di Genova, Genoa
Archivio di Stato di Livorno, Livorno
Archivio di Stato di Napoli, Naples
Archivio di Stato di Venezia, Venice
British Library, London
Haus-, Hof-, und Staatsarchiv, Vienna
National Archives of Malta, Rabat
National Library of Malta, Valletta
National Maritime Museum Archives, Caird Library, London
Princeton University Archives, Princeton
Royal College of Physicians Archive, London
UK National Archives, London
University of Glasgow Archives, Glasgow
Wellcome Archives, London

Newspapers and Periodicals

Annali universali di medicina
Association Medical Journal
British and Foreign Medical Review
Caledonian Mercury
Courier des Alpes
Edinburgh Medical and Social Journal
Edinburgh Review
Galignani's Messenger
Hampshire Advertiser
Hampshire Independent
Hansard
Kaleidoscope, The
Lancet, The
Literary Gazette
London Times
Medical Repository

Medico-Chirurgical Review
Morning Post
Oriental Herald
Pamphleteer, The
Quarterly Review
Revue de l'Orient
Westminster Review

Index